Immunology of Malignant Diseases

IMMUNOLOGY AND MEDICINE SERIES

IMMUNOLOGY
· SERIES · SERIES · SERIES · SERIES · **AND** · SERIES · SERIES · SERIES · SERIES ·
MEDICINE

Immunology of Malignant Diseases

Edited by

V. S. Byers   and   R. W. Baldwin

Xoma Corporation
Berkeley, California
USA

Cancer Research Campaign
Laboratories
University of Nottingham
Nottingham, UK

Series Editor: Professor W. G. Reeves

 MTP PRESS LIMITED
a member of the KLUWER ACADEMIC PUBLISHERS GROUP
LANCASTER / BOSTON / THE HAGUE / DORDRECHT

Published in the UK and Europe by
MTP Press Limited
Falcon House
Lancaster, England

British Library Cataloguing in Publication Data

Immunology of malignant diseases.—
   (Immunology and medicine series).
   1. Cancer—Immunological aspects
   I. Byers, Vera S. II. Baldwin, R. W.
   (Robert William)   III. Series
   616.99′4079   RC268.3

   ISBN 0-85200-964-X
   ISBN 0-85200-824-4 Series

Published in the USA by
MTP Press
A division of Kluwer Academic Publishers
101 Philip Drive
Norwell, MA 02061, USA

Library of Congress Cataloging-in-Publication Data

Immunology of malignant diseases.

   (Immunology and medicine series)
   Includes bibliographies and index.
   1. Cancer—Immunological aspects. I. Byers, Vera S.
II. Baldwin, R. W. (Robert William), 1927–
III. Series. [DNLM: 1. Neoplasms—immunology.
QZ 200 I34524]
RC268.2.I4627   1987   616.99′4079   87–3161
ISBN 0-85200-964-X

Typeset by Witwell Ltd, Liverpool
Printed and bound by Butler and Tanner Limited, Frome and London

Contents

Preface

Over the past 5 years, clinical immunology, as a whole, has advanced more rapidly than over the past 20 years. Many of these advances have been due to monoclonal antibody technology with its ability to identify antigens on tumour cells with a precision never before available. Monoclonal antibodies have the ability to identify subsets of human T-lymphocytes and aid in diagnosis of both immunodeficiency disorders such as AIDS, or autoimmune diseases, and they can be adapted as drug targeting agents. Additionally, however, major advances have been made in identifying immunomodulating agents, and the last year has seen two such agents, IL-2 and OKT3, made available commercially for such intervention. Furthermore, another immunomodulating technique, bone marrow transplantation, has now been established as a curative modality in leukaemia treatment.

A central issue in tumour immunology is whether human tumours express antigens which can be termed tumour-specific. This has important implications for both tumour immunity as well as drug targeting. This issue is considered in detail by R. A. Robins in the introductory chapter in which the expression of antigens in human tumours is compared with that in experimentally induced animal tumours. This controversial issue is also considered in later chapters by Bast in breast carcinoma, Rümke and de Vries in melanoma, Vánky in lung cancer, Armitage in colorectal cancer, and Paulie and Perlmann in bladder carcinoma. The current consensus is that such antigens do not exist, in that all 'neoantigens' on these tumours are shared to some extent with normal tissues.

Another theme of these chapters has been the extent to which the immune response can be manipulated to induce tumour rejection. This issue is first addressed in the initial chapter in which a description of the various types of effector cell mechanisms is given and forms a central theme in many of the clinical chapters, being described in detail in lung cancer and melanoma along with description of the graft vs. leukaemia effect seen in bone marrow transplantation in leukaemia.

Despite the limitations in generating specifically sensitized lymphocytes in human cancer, the use of activated killer cells (LAK cells) generated by

vii

lymphocyte activation with the lymphokine interleukin-2 is being explored. This approach has been actively promoted by Rosenberg and this is reflected in the reviews of LAK cells in terms of immunomodulating agents by Vose and by their use in the treatment of malignant melanoma, and colorectal cancer. This approach emphasizes the current interest in developing immuno-modulating agents for cancer treatment (Vose) and these approaches are considered with respect to malignant melanoma, breast cancer and colorectal cancer.

Some of the most exciting advances in clinical immunology have been the development of drug targeting by monoclonal antibodies, and/or bone marrow transplantation in the treatment of leukaemia. Immunoscintigraphy is developing into an established diagnostic modality in which either ^{111}In or ^{131}I is coupled to antibody and successfully targeted to tumours for imaging. To date this has been used for diagnosis with a number of tumours and at least one such product is commercially available in the UK for use in colon cancer. Therapeutic applications are still under development, but several groups are currently moving into phase I trials in drug targeting with ricin A-chain, methotrexate, or vindesine linked to antibodies. These develop-ments are discussed in the chapter on immunoscintigraphy by Pimm, and that on drug targeting by Baldwin and Byers. As exciting is the growing importance of bone marrow transplantation in leukaemia. This modality has long been established as standard therapy in aplastic anaemia and SCIDS, but the last 5 years have seen its firm establishment as curative therapy in leukaemia. This is discussed in the chapter by Byers, along with new techniques to deal with its principal complication, graft vs. host disease.

The most frightening disease of the last decade has certainly been AIDS, with its 100% mortality and the possibility of its spread to the heterosexual population. Although no therapy is yet in sight, important advances have been made as to controlling its spread by understanding its mechanism of transmission, identifying infected individuals, and developing screening techniques to make the nation's blood banks safe. These advances are discussed in the chapter by Chachoua *et al.* which provides a state-of-the-art view of this devastating disease.

V. S. Byers
R. W. Baldwin

Series Editor's Note

The modern clinician is expected to be the fount of all wisdom concerning conventional diagnosis and management relevant to his sphere of practice. In addition, he or she has the daunting task of comprehending and keeping pace with advances in basic science relevant to the pathogenesis of disease and ways in which these processes can be regulated or prevented. Immunology has grown from the era of anti-toxins and serum sickness to a state where the study of many diverse cells and molecules has become integrated into a coherent scientific discipline with major implications for many common and crippling diseases prevalent throughout the world.

Many of today's practitioners received little or no specific training in immunology and what was taught is very likely to have been overtaken by subsequent developments. This series of titles on IMMUNOLOGY AND MEDICINE is designed to rectify this deficiency in the form of distilled packages of information which the busy clinician, pathologist or other health care professional will be able to open and enjoy.

Professor W. G. Reeves, FRCP. FRCPath
Department of Immunology
University Hospital, Queen's Medical Centre
Nottingham

List of Contributors

N. C. M. ARMITAGE
Department of Surgery
University Hospital
Nottingham NG7 2UH
UK

R. W. BALDWIN
Cancer Research Campaign
Laboratories
University of Nottingham
Nottingham NG7 2RD
UK

R. C. BAST
Department of Medicine
Box 3898
Division of Hematology-Oncology
Duke University Medical Center
Durham, NC 27710
USA

K. BÖÖK
Department of Thoracic Surgery
Karolinska Hospital
104 01 Stockholm
SWEDEN

C. M. BOYER
Department of Medicine
Box 3898
Division of Hematology-Oncology
Duke University Medical Center
Durham, NC 27710
USA

V. S. BYERS
Xoma Corporation
2910 Seventh Street
Berkeley CA 94710
USA

A. CHACHOUA
Department of Medicine
Division of Oncology
New York University Medical Center
Old Bellevue Administration Building
462 First Avenue, Room 224
New York, NY 10016
USA

A. E. FRANKEL
Department of Medicine
Box 3898
Division of Hematology-Oncology
Duke University of Medical Center
Durham, NC 27710
USA

M. D. GREEN
Department of Hematology/Oncology
Royal Melbourne Hospital
Post Office
Victoria 3052
Australia

T. IVERT
Department of Thoracic Surgery
Karolinska Hospital
104 01 Stockholm
SWEDEN

E. KLEIN
Department of Tumor Biology
Karolinska Institute
104 01 Stockholm 60
SWEDEN

F. M. MUGGIA
Department of Medical Oncology
USC Comprehensive Cancer Center
1441 Eastlake Avenue
Los Angeles CA 90033
USA

R. ORATZ
Department of Medicine
Division of Oncology
New York University Medical Center
Old Bellevue Administration Building
462 First Avenue, Room 224
New York, NY 10016
USA

S. PAULIE
Department of Immunology
University of Stockholm
S-106 91 Stockholm
SWEDEN

P. PERLMANN
Department of Immunology
University of Stockholm
S-106 91 Stockholm
SWEDEN

A. PÉTERFFY
Department of Thoracic Surgery
Karolinska Hospital
104 01 Stockholm
SWEDEN

M. V. PIMM
Cancer Research Campaign
Laboratories
University of Nottingham
Nottingham NG7 2RD
UK

R. A. ROBINS
Cancer Research Campaign
Laboratories
Nottingham University
Nottingham NG7 2RD
UK

Ph. RÜMKE
Division of Immunology
The Netherlands Cancer Institute
Antoni van Leeuwenhoek Huis
Plesmanlaan 121
1066 CX Amsterdam
The Netherlands

F. VÁNKY
Department of Tumor Biology
Karolinska Institute
104 01 Stockholm 60
SWEDEN

B. M. VOSE
ICI Pharmaceuticals Division
Mereside, Alderley Park
Macclesfield
Cheshire SK10 4TG
UK

J. E. DE VRIES
Immunology Laboratories
Unicet
27 Chemin des Peupliers
BP 11
69572 Dardilly
FRANCE

J. WILLEMS
Department of Tumour Pathology
Karolinska Hospital
104 01 Stockholm
SWEDEN

1
Basic Tumour Immunology

R. A. ROBINS

INTRODUCTION

Although immunity has been shown to control the growth of a variety of experimental tumours, the question of whether the immune response participates in the relationship between tumour and host in human cancer remains controversial. The rejection of experimental tumours occurs as a result of immunological recognition of determinants that are present on the tumour cells, but not on normal tissues. A brief overview of the types of these neoantigens that are expressed following malignant transformation in experimental animal tumours will be given: this will then form the basis for consideration of the evidence for antigens which are capable of giving rise to autologous immunological recognition in human tumours. The possible role of oncogene activation in the development of human tumours will also be considered, paying particular attention to induced changes that may result in immunological recognition.

The nature of immune responses to tumours will then be considered, attempting to define the role of the various types of thymus-derived (T) cells, their possible interaction with other effector cell types such as natural killer (NK) cells and macrophages, as well as the possible contribution of antigen-specific and non-specific humoral factors such as antibodies, lymphotoxins, and interferons. An important aspect of tumour immune responses is the escape of tumour from immunological control; various mechanisms by which this can occur will be discussed.

ANTIGENS OF EXPERIMENTAL TUMOURS

The field of experimental tumour immunology has gone through several cycles of high optimism followed by disillusion. Early experiments to investigate the possibility that immunization with tumour cells might give rise to tumour immunity were conducted before the establishment of inbred strains of experimental animals. Rejection of tumours observed was due to

1

histocompatibility differences between the tumour donor and transplant recipient, rather than antigenicity of the tumour *per se*.

The initial high hopes that tumours give rise to a strong immune response were then replaced by a conviction that tumours did not have antigens giving rise to rejection responses, and that any rejection that was observed was due to residual genetic heterogeneity in the inbred animals used for experiment. Studies by Foley[1], Baldwin[2], and Prehn and Main[3], produced good evidence for tumour-specific transplantation antigens on chemically induced mouse and rat tumours, but it was not until the experiments of Klein and co-workers[4] that the existence of these antigens was fully accepted. These experiments involved the demonstration that a mouse in which a tumour was induced was able to reject viable cells of its own tumour when challenged after surgical removal of the primary tumour mass. In this case, there is no possibility of incompatibility between the mouse and its autochthonous tumour[4].

Developments of transplantation techniques to demonstrate tumour immunity and subsequently *in vitro* methods to detect cellular and antibody responses to tumours have led to the definition of a range of types of tumour antigen in different types of experimental tumour.

Rejection antigens

Chemically induced tumours

The most notable characteristic of rejection antigens on chemically induced tumours is their individual specificity. Thus if two tumours are induced by the same carcinogen in animals of the same strain, immunization of the group of recipients with one tumour will confer immunity to that tumour, but is unlikely to affect the growth of a challenge of viable cells from the second tumour. A large panel of this type of cross-immunization experiment has been done with a series of rat 3-methylcholanthrene induced tumours in order to determine the extent of the repertoire of individual antigens. Cross-reactions in transplantation tests were rarely found, and to extend the range of cross-testing, serological tests have also been performed. Here again, a high degree of individual specificity was found, so that in more than 100 tumour combinations, reproducible cross-reactions were not observed[5].

The nature of these highly polymorphic antigens has not been fully resolved, partly because of the difficulty in obtaining good serological reagents[6]. The origin of the diversity of these antigens is particularly intriguing; it has been suggested that they may represent the variable region of a family of molecular species involved in cellular interactions[7]. The basis for this hypothesis was the finding that antitumour antisera inhibited T-cell responses whose cellular interactions are restricted by determinants polymorphic at the immunoglobulin heavy chain complex.

A mechanism by which these antigens might become apparent is that the clonal expansion resulting from neoplastic transformation might make an antigen present on very occasional normal cells become well represented on the cells of the clone, and thus recognizable immunologically. Experiments

2

designed to investigate this point have involved the treatment *in vitro* of cells recently derived from a single untransformed clone with a chemical carcinogen, then testing resulting individual colonies of transformed cells for cross-reacting antigens[8]. The antigens found were generally not cross-reacting, indicating that it is likely that the antigens arose as a result of interaction of the carcinogen with the cell, although expansion of a rapidly diversifying determinant is difficult to rule out.

Although individual antigens are a frequent finding with tumours induced by a variety of chemical carcinogens (for example, 3-methylcholanthrene on the skin, azo dyes in the liver), some carcinogen-induced tumours are generally lacking in rejection antigens detectable by immunization and challenge with viable tumour. For example, liver tumours induced by acetyl-aminofluorene are frequently non-immunogenic by this criterion[9].

It should also be added that under particular circumstances, cross-reacting rejection responses can be elicited to methylcholanthrene-induced murine tumours. Thus Law[10] found that additional cross-reacting antigens were found on some, but not all, tumours adapted to ascitic growth. It is not yet clear how these antigens relate to the highly polymorphic determinants discussed above[11].

Tumours induced by physical agents

Tumours induced by ultraviolet irradiation in mice have been extensively investigated for rejection antigens, and have proved a particularly interesting system. This group of tumours are generally very immunogenic, to the extent that they may not be transplantable in normal syngeneic recipients. The growth of the tumour is dependent on the immunosuppressive effects of UV radiation.

The use of *in vitro* methods has allowed the typing of multiple antigens on the cells of UV-induced tumours, and in common with chemically induced tumours, a high degree of diversity in these antigens is observed (for example, see reference 12).

Virus-induced tumours

Oncogenic DNA viruses elicit consistent immune responses with a specificity related to the inducing virus. Thus polyoma virus induces a wide variety of tumours in different tissues, but these are able to cross-immunize. The oncogenic DNA viruses carry their own transforming gene, which has to be incorporated into the host genome during transformation, accounting for the consistent expression of virus related specificities[13].

The situation is less clear with the RNA viruses, where insertion of only a small part of the retrovirus genome is required for activation of the adjacent cellular oncogene (see below). It is possible for the protein coding regions of the viral genome to be lost whilst the transformed phenotype of the target cell is maintained: this will clearly allow the possibility of the development of malignant clones with little immunogenicity attributable to the viral genome[13].

3

Spontaneous tumours

Experimental tumours arising without deliberate inducement have been tested for immunogenicity in a number of laboratories. These tumours generally have weak or undetectable rejection responses[14], although occasional examples are moderately immunogenic[15].

When immunogenic examples of spontaneous tumours have been found, the rejection responses have been found to be individually specific, in common with the chemically induced tumours. The nature of the rejection antigens present on spontaneous tumours is unknown at present.

Tumour-associated antigens

Oncofetal antigens

In addition to antigens readily giving rise to rejection responses, there are other types of antigen associated with tumour cells. A major class of antigens of this type are oncofetal antigens, which are determinants expressed at some stage in fetal development, but not on normal adult cells.

For some of these determinants such as carcinoembryonic antigen[16] (CEA) or alpha-fetoprotein[17] (AFP), it has not been demonstrated conclusively that they elicit immune responses in the autologous tumour bearer: they have been demonstrated using antibodies raised in xenogeneic species. However, in experimental systems, tumours may express antigens recognized using antisera or immune cells raised against syngeneic fetal tissue (reviewed in reference 18) or teratocarcinoma cells[19].

Although it is possible to show *in vitro* reactivity with these antisera or immune cells against a range of syngeneic tumours that is shared with fetal cells at particular stages of development, it has proved much more difficult to demonstrate tumour rejection responses associated with these 'embryonic' antigens in, for example, rats[18] or mice[20]. A notable exception are tumours induced by SV40 virus in hamsters, where immunization with irradiated fetal tissue is protective against tumour challenge[21].

Differentiation antigens

This type of antigen appears on some tissues in the adult but not others, and may also be expressed as an abnormal product by a tumour cell. Depending on the distribution and accessibility to the immune system of the differentiation antigen involved, the antigen as expressed on tumour may be immunogenic. This category of antigen is most relevant in the diagnostic context, and xenogenic monoclonal antibodies to this type of determinant on human tumours are becoming increasingly useful (see below).

HUMAN TUMOUR ANTIGENS

It is clear that human tumours express oncofetal and differentiation antigens.

CEA and AFP have already been mentioned in the former category, and these determinants have proved useful for monitoring tumours expressing these antigens. A good example of the latter category is the epithelial membrane antigen found on breast cancer cells. Monoclonal antibodies to particular determinants of this antigen may be useful in determining the prognosis of breast cancer[22].

A much more vexed question is whether human tumours express antigens which are immunogenic in the patient, and following on from this, are any immune responses that may be induced capable of causing tumour rejection?

In vivo and ex vivo evidence

As outlined above, tumour rejection antigens on experimental animal tumours have been demonstrated by showing that immunization, for example by injection with attenuated tumour, suppresses the growth of a viable tumour cell inoculum. This approach is obviously not feasible in human cancer, although very occasional well documented spontaneous regressions of tumours have been taken as evidence of effective immune responses. However, particular tumour types predominate in these cases (melanoma, hypernephroma, choriocarcinoma and neuroblastoma), and although regression is accompanied by intense lymphocytic infiltration in some cases, non-immunological mechanisms may be operative in others. For example, induction of differentiation is known to occur in neuroblastoma.

Lymphocyte reactivity at the site of tumours has also been taken as evidence of an antitumour host response and this information has been gained from histopathological investigations on lymph nodes draining tumours, and mononuclear cell infiltration into tumours themselves. It is well established that mononuclear cell infiltration is a frequent occurrence in a variety of types of human cancer although in many cases the prognostic significance of such infiltration is controversial (for example, in breast cancer[23]): histological evidence of reactivity of lymph nodes draining breast tumours has been shown to carry a good prognosis[24].

In vitro evidence

The orginal evidence cited as identifying cell-mediated responses to human tumour associated antigens was derived primarily from studies showing that peripheral blood lymphocytes from tumour patients were cytotoxic when tested against cultured tumour cells from the lymphocyte donor, or patients with tumours of the same histological type[25]. This 'histological type' specificity was not observed in subsequent studies, and it was recognized that natural killer (NK) cells were an important contributor to the cytotoxic effects observed in these experiments.

Other tests for detecing T-lymphocyte responses to human tumours have been introduced, including leukocyte migration inhibition and leukocyte adherence inhibition tests[26]. These tests have been beset by many problems of standardization and interpretation, so, for example, whilst the leukocyte migration inhibition assay has provided some evidence for reactivity to

5

autologous and 'histological type' specific tumour-associated antigens, little progress has so far been made in the identification of these antigens, and the test is not considered to be useful for routine clinical investigation[27].

More recently, the reactivity of blood lymphocytes, or in some case tumour infiltrating lymphocytes, with freshly derived autologous tumour cells has been investigated[28,29] (see Chapter 7). This approach has the advantage of avoiding loss of tumour-associated antigens or acquisition of spurious antigens during prolonged target cell culture. The use of autologous combinations avoids problems of MHC antigen restriction which might limit the detection of reactions in allogeneic tests, and of course avoids reactions to alloantigens.

The T-cell responses investigated include short-term cytotoxicity (ALC, autologous lymphocyte cytotoxicity) and proliferative response measured by [³H]thymidine incorporation (ATS, autologous tumour stimulation). The relationship between these responses and the clinical course of disease has been investigated in lung carcinoma[28] and sarcoma[29].

Although these results suggest that recognition of tumour-associated antigens may be operative, it has also been shown that at least proliferative responses can be stimulated by autologous normal tissue, as well as by autologous tumour[30]. More detailed definition of the specificities involved may follow from investigations using T-cell lines and clones established from cancer patients[31].

Oncogene activation and human tumour antigens

The demonstration that specific cellular genes (oncogenes) are involved in the process of transformation to malignancy has become a very exciting aspect of our developing knowledge concerning the basic biology of cancer. A detailed discussion of the role of oncogenes in malignant transformation is not appropriate here: for a review see, for example, Cooper and Lane[32]. The point to be considered is by what mechanisms oncogene activation could result in neoantigen expression, allowing the transformed cell either to induce immune response which might result in its rejection, or at least provide a potential tumour-specific determinant that could be the point of attack for, for example, monoclonal antibody-directed therapy.

As indicated in the section on antigens on virus-induced tumours, transformation associated with DNA viruses is accompanied by viral antigen expression, because these viruses carry their own transforming genes. This means that these tumours are strongly antigenic, and only develop if the immune response is severely compromised. An example is the association of the Epstein–Barr virus with Burkitt's lymphoma, where chronic malaria may be the cause of immunosuppression[13].

Cellular oncogenes may also be activated by RNA virus promoter or enhancer insertion. These regulatory inserts do not code for a virus-related protein, but affect only the expression of cellular genes. It is therefore possible for oncogene activation to occur without virus antigen expression. Viral genome coding for viral proteins may also be inserted and expressed, and is thus a potential source of antigen recognizable by the host immune system.

However, as these additional genes are not required for oncogene activation, they will be an unreliable source of transformation-associated antigens.

Activation of cellular oncogenes by non-viral mechanisms is likely to account for a large proportion of spontaneously arising tumours. As this process may involve only modification of the expression of existing cellular genes, the possible sources of transformation-associated antigens in this case would appear to be limited.

Potential sites of recognition are the slight modifications that are known to occur in some oncogene products in tumour in comparison with their normal cell counterpart. Thus mutation at position 12 of the protein (p21) coded for by rasH oncogene appears to affect transformation strongly[32]. It is not known whether these modified products are sufficiently immunogenic to provide a target for immunological rejection of tumour.

A further point to be considered is what other changes in addition to oncogene activation are required for transformation. The most commonly used system to test for transforming gene sequences is the NIH/3T3 cell line, which on transfection with DNA containing activated oncogene shows phenotypic changes such as loss of contact inhibition and anchorage dependence. This cell line is not normal: indeed a recent report showed that the 'untransformed' line could give rise to tumours and even metastases at low frequency[33]. The process of oncogene activation is clearly very important in changing the behaviour of target cells, but these experiments emphasize that other changes are also required, and it is possible that some of these may involve expression of novel genes that could code for targets for immunological recognition.

The precise functions of oncogene products remain obscure, although intriguing relationships to cell growth factors are emerging (reviewed by Burgess[34]). Speculation in this area is limited by our restricted knowledge of how cellular growth control and differentiation are maintained in normal tissues. Perturbation of this control could arise at a variety of levels: modification of the production or activity of a growth factor (mutations such as those mentioned above may be important here); modification of its receptor; or disturbance of the interaction between the receptor/factor complex and other cell components.

The changes that occur during malignant transformation profoundly affect the behaviour of the cell and its interaction with surrounding normal cells. But, among the molecular events identified so far, there is no reliable theoretical source of novel determinants whose expression would be tightly linked to transformation, and would therefore be an ideal target for immunological recognition. However, because of the limitations on current knowledge of these processes, this question remains open.

IMMUNE RESPONSES TO TUMOURS

It has long been held that antibody-mediated effector mechanisms are not of primary importance in the rejection of 'solid' tumours (carcinomas and sarcomas), and that cell-mediated immune responses are principally involved.

7

This was demonstrated in transfer experiments, where non-immune recipients were injected with serum or lymphocytes from tumour immune donors, and an inoculum of viable tumour cells. This early work (for reviews see for example Hellstrom and Hellstrom[35], Baldwin and Robins[36]) has in general been confirmed by subsequent experience (reviewed by North[37], Robins and Baldwin[38]), and with the exception of some experimental leukaemias and lymphomas, the preoccupation of tumour immunologists has been with the nature and control of cellular responses to tumour-associated antigens.

In spite of these indications that antibodies may not contribute greatly in rejection responses developing after syngeneic tumour immunization, it is worthwhile considering antibodies binding to tumour-related determinants, and their possible usefulness for the control of tumours, especially in the context of the increasing availability of monoclonal reagents.

Antibody

There are two classic pathways by which antibodies to tumour-associated antigens could exert antitumour effects: in combination with fc receptor bearing effector cells in antibody-dependent cellular cytotoxicity (ADCC); and by fixation of complement. There are now examples of antitumour effects being obtained using monoclonal antibodies, and this approach is being subject to clinical trial in colon carcinoma[39] and melanoma[40].

Antitumour effects of monoclonal antibodies to human tumours were first observed in xenograft systems. Here, immunodeprived mice (congenitally athymic 'nude' mice, or thymectomized and irradiated mice) are implanted with human tumour cells, which grow progressively. Treatment of the mice with monoclonal antibody resulted in very marked reduction in tumour growth[41]. These effects are observed with antibodies of the IgG2a an IgG3 subclasses, and appear to be mediated by cellular mechanisms[42-44], although complement may play a role in some systems[45]. Human effector cells function with mouse monoclonal antibodies[46], and this interaction may also be subject to modulation by γ-interferon[47].

Treatment of human tumours in xenograft systems has also been attempted using 'armed' effector cells[44]. In this system, pretreatment of effector cells with monoclonal antibody, followed by their transfer to xenograft bearing 'nude' mice, proved more effective than treatment with monoclonal antibody directly.

In addition to these potentially beneficial effects, antibodies generated during the immune response to tumours might influence the effectiveness of the immune response in complex ways, and some of these aspects will be considered below. Negative effects include the blocking of cellular responses; positive effects might be obtained by the stimulation of anti-idiotypic responses[48].

Cell-mediated immunity

As indicated above, cell-mediated responses are of major importance in the immune response to tumours. The detail of precisely which cell types are involved, and how they interact and are controlled is still not fully understood. Thus, the relative importance of cytotoxic (CTL) and non-cytotoxic (delayed type hypersensitivity, DTH, inducing) subsets of T-cells is still controversial, as is the contribution of the less specific effector mechanisms such as macrophages, NK cells, and cells secreting cytotoxic factors. The case for each of these cell types will be considered, but it should be emphasized that many of these mechanisms are not mutually exclusive, and that multiple effector cell types may be involved in rejection responses, either simultaneously, or successively as the response develops.

T-cell responses

In view of the fine specificity of rejection responses to chemically induced tumours, a highly specific means of target cell destruction suggests itself, the obvious candidate being the cytotoxic T-cell (CTL). However, with the development of monoclonal antibodies which were thought to separate T-cells along functional lines into cytotoxic/suppressor and helper subsets, a more direct evaluation of the role of CTL became feasible.

Surprisingly, it was found that transfer of tumour immunity could be achieved with T-cells bearing the monoclonal antibody defined markers of helper cells in both rat[49,50] and mouse[51] tumour systems. This allowed the possibility that the specificity of the rejection response lay at the level of the helper cell, with a less specific mechanism controlled by helper cells being responsible for tumour cell destruction. Similar findings were reported in MHC incompatible allograft rejection systems, which suggested that T-cells of the helper subset were sufficient for the induction of rejection in T-cell depleted recipients[52,53].

More recently, this interpretation has been subject to a number of complications. These include the relationship between monoclonal antibody defined phenotype and cell function; the contribution of T-cell deficient recipients to tumour rejection in transfer experiments; and the variation and inducibility of antigens on target tissues.

In man as well as rats and mice, T-cell subsets have been conventionally defined as 'helper/inducer', bearing the OKT4 marker (W3/25 positive in rats, bearing L3T4 antigen in mice), and 'cytotoxic/suppressor', OKT8 positive cells (OX8 positive in the rat, Ly2 positive in the mouse). It now seems clear that these phenotypes relate to the class of major histo-compatibility complex (MHC) antigen restricting a response, rather than function *per se*. This was first described in the mouse, with the demonstration that, for example, helper responses restricted by class I MHC antigens were Ly2 positive (see Swain[54]).

There are strong homologies between these T-cell surface molecules in different species, and the terminology now commonly used[55] is CD4 (for cluster of differentiation 4) and CD8 for the molecules on T-cells restricted by class II and class I MHC antigens respectively. It is likely that these determinants function by recognizing non-polymorphic parts of MHC antigens during T-cell interactions.

From a practical point of view, this means that it is possible for the 'helper subset' separated by monoclonal antibody phenotype to function as a cytotoxic effector cell, albeit requiring class II MHC antigen expression on its target cell. This may occur after induction by lymphokines such as γ-interferon[56], which could be produced at the site of an antitumour immune response.

A further problem with T-cell subset separations in the mouse is that the Ly1 antigen has previously been used as a 'helper subset' marker. Unfortunately, this antigen is present at varying levels on most mouse T-cells, and under optimal conditions, anti-Ly1 antibody and complement can kill almost all T-cells: this may account for some discrepancies between different groups[57].

Having catalogued these complicating factors, it is not surprising that a very complex picture is emerging as to which T-cell subsets are required to transfer tumour immunity, and how the transfer of cells progresses to target cell destruction. There are clearly differences between different tumour systems, well exemplified in a recent comparative study[58]. Here, transfer of immunity to an immunogenic lymphoma was best achieved with a combination of $Ly1^+$, $Ly2^-$ and $Ly1^-$, $Ly2^+$ tumour immune T-cells, whereas sarcoma Meth A required cells bearing both markers. There are many examples of differing requirements for transfer of immunity, with some systems seemingly totally dependent on $Ly2^+$ cells or their equivalent in other species, some apparently totally independent of this subset, and as already indicated, some requiring a combination of subsets for optimum effects (see Robins and Baldwin[38,59]).

In order to obtain unambiguously uncontaminated effector cell populations, some groups have used clones of T-cells grown *in vitro*. Using this approach, it has been shown that cytotoxic clones are capable of destroying tumour cells[60] and normal tissues[61] in allogeneic models when in direct contact with target cells. When transferred systemically, however, cloned cytotoxic effectors cells are often disappointingly ineffective, possibly because they lack additional cell surface features necessary for recirculation and extravasation which would be required for effective *in vivo* function. Lymphokine dependence may also be a limiting factor, as some clones are highly dependent on exogenous supplies of interleukin-2; in this respect, 'helper independent' cytotoxic clones of the type originally described by Widmer and Bach[62] may be more effective[63]. This is not always the case, however, as in the transfer of immunity to Moloney leukaemia virus-induced tumour[63], where the effectiveness of particular clones could not be predicted from their *in vitro* dependence on IL-2.

Turning to the transfer of immunity by 'helper/inducer' T-cells, it is still not clear how these cells mediate tumour destruction. As indicated above, these cells could function as cytotoxic effector cells restricted by class II MHC antigens, although these antigens would need to be induced in most tumour systems. This point has been investigated[64] in a Friend virus-induced mouse tumour, the rejection of which appears to be independent of CTL. Thus, γ-interferon failed to induce the expression of class II antigen on this tumour, under conditions where the expression of class I antigen was augmented.

Another aspect of these studies is the possibility that T-cell deficient recipient animals may have significant cytotoxic precursor activity[65], which might be activated by the transferred helper T-cells. In the Friend virus tumour system, Greenberg et al.[64] used congenic recipients for transfer of tumour immunity, so that activated T-cells of recipient origin could be identified by their Thyl haplotype. No such cells were found, so transfer of immunity in this tumour system would appear to be independent of CTL.

In these circumstances, other candidate target cell destruction mechanisms include activation of less specific effector cell types, such as NK cells or macrophages, or the secretion of cytotoxic factors such as lymphotoxin. The participation of NK cells and macrophages in these T-cell-directed responses will be considered below together with a broader assessment of the participation of these cell types in the relationship between tumour and host. Characterization of lymphotoxins and evaluation of their antitumour effects have progressed rapidly recently, mainly because of the production of pure material by recombinant DNA technology[66]. These materials have allowed the unequivocal demonstration of the synergistic effects of various lymphokines (reviewed by Ruddle[67]). Lymphotoxin also appears to be related to tumour necrosis factor (TNF), a hitherto poorly defined activity induced in serum of experimental animals by endotoxin shock. As its names implies, this factor induces haemorrhagic necrosis of transplanted tumours when injected systemically[68]. Sequence data from TNF cDNA show considerable homology with lymphotoxin, although the two molecules are quite distinct[69]. It is not clear under what physiological conditions TNF might be produced, but it seems likely that this series of related factors, perhaps acting synergistically with γ-interferon, is produced in a DTH type response that results in tumour destruction.

NK cells

Natural killer cells are a subgroup of lymphocytes with in vitro cytotoxic activity against neoplastic cells. Cytotoxic activity is associated with cells of a distinct morphology, known as large granular lymphocytes (LGL). These cells are present and active without prior immunization, and have therefore been attractive candidates as effector cells that might recognize malignant cells early in their development, and thus act in a tumour surveillance role.

The beige mutation in the mouse results in very low levels of NK activity, whilst apparently not affecting T-cell and macrophage function; beige mice are therefore useful for investigating the in vivo role of NK cells in the resistance to tumours. Increased growth rates of NK sensitive tumours have in fact been observed in beige mice in comparison with heterozygous normal litter-mates[70]. This effect could be reversed by transfer of active NK cells, further supporting their in vivo role. More recently, the incidence of spontaneously arising and chemically induced tumours in beige mice has been investigated[71]. In comparison with their heterozygous (normal phenotype) litter-mates, the beige mice had a significantly higher probability of dying with a tumour. Such a clear-cut difference was not observed with carcinogen treatment, although this may be due to impairment of NK activity in the normal mice by the carcinogen, reducing the difference between the groups.

In view of the relatively high levels of NK cells in the blood, a role for these cells in the control of haematogenous metastasis has also been suggested. Recent studies have shown that in rats treated with anti-asialoGM1 antiserum, which selectively depletes NK activity, there was a reduced ability to eliminate mammary carcinoma cells injected into the circulation; this defect was reversed[72] by transfer of cell populations highly enriched for LGL. Resistance to experimental metastasis at other sites may be related to high local levels of NK activity[73].

These studies clearly show that NK cells can function *in vivo* in some circumstances, but these conditions may be strictly limited. For example, Zoller[74] showed that natural resistance to a spontaneously arising rat fibrosarcoma was limited to early stages after transplantation of tumour cells, and was restricted to sites with normally high NK activity.

As already indicated, the activity of NK cells is susceptible to modulation by lymphokines produced during T-cell responses, such as IL-2 and interferon. For example, NK cells are activated *in vitro* when T-cells from rats immune to Mycobacteria are stimulated with tuberculin purified protein[75]. This would fit in with the idea that NK cells could play a part in adaptive immune responses to tumour, responding at the tumour site to factors produced by T-cells sensitized to tumour antigens, and thus contributing to tumour cell elimination.

Activated killer cells

The activation of lymphoid cells to cytolytic activity by products of the immune response has been taken further by the use of lymphokines prepared from stimulated lymphocytes, and more recently using recombinant DNA technology derived material. Culture of murine splenocytes or human blood mononuclear cells with high levels of IL-2 results in the generation of large numbers of cytolytic cells known as lymphokine activated killer (LAK) cells[76]. In experimental tumour systems, these cells have been shown to have considerable therapeutic potential, especially when administered in combination with IL-2. The relationship of LAK cells to other forms of cytolytic effector cell is not clear, although it is important to note that the specificity of killing is much broader than, for example, NK cells[76].

Clinical experience with human LAK cells has given encouraging results, although the administration of large numbers of cells and IL-2 has given rise to considerable toxicity problems[77]. Studies developing methods for the production[78] and more effective clinical use[77] of LAK cells are continuing.

Macrophages

It has long been known that macrophages activated by a variety of specific and non-specific mechanisms can be highly cytotoxic for tumour cells *in vitro*. Moreover, is some tumours, *in vivo* activation of macrophages by products such as muramyl dipeptide[79] or killed *Corynebacterium parvum* organisms[74] can result in control of tumour growth. However, in some studies, there is a clear lack of correlation between the *in vitro* cytotoxic activity of activated macrophages and their ability to mediate tumour rejection *in vivo*[80]. This has been further explored in a chemoimmunotherapy model, where it was shown that effector cells from the site of a regressing tumour consisted of highly cytotoxic macrophages together with T-lymphocytes. However, the effectiveness of these cells in transfer of tumour immunity *in vivo* was completely dependent on the T-cell component[81].

Other evidence indicates that infiltration of macrophages may promote, or even be necessary for, tumour growth[82], and that macrophages present in tumour lesions after chemotherapy may stimulate the growth of residual malignant cells[83]. A further complicating factor is that macrophages may be attracted to the tumour site by factors released by malignant cells[84], so that the macrophage content of tumours may not necessarily be regulated by immune responses to that tumour. Taken together with the possible tumour growth stimulatory activity of macrophages, these findings indicated that the relationship between macrophages and malignant cells in tumours is a complex one, and that the presence of macrophages may not necessarily be beneficial.

ESCAPE FROM TUMOUR IMMUNITY

The possible basis for the persistent growth of tumours which are known to be immunogenic in the face of a host immune response has been widely investigated. Clearly, if the decisive factor(s) involved could be identified, their manipulation would obviously have major therapeutic implications. A variety of possible tumour escape mechanisms will be considered; as with effector mechanisms, however, it should be emphasized that different mechanisms are not necessarily mutually exclusive, and a combination of factors may be responsible for the failure of the immune response to control progressive tumour growth.

Kinetics of response

One of the simplest factors that should be considered is that with a replicating source of antigen stimulation, the immune response does not mobilize sufficiently rapidly to get on terms with the developing tumour. A manifestation of this problem may be the 'sneaking through' phenomenon, in which a low dose of immunogenic tumour cells may develop progressively, whereas a larger dose of cells does not. The larger number of cells are thought to provide sufficient antigen stimulation to provoke an immediate and sufficiently strong response to eliminate the tumour cells, but the lower number may not provide sufficient stimulus until already established. Suppression may also be involved in the escape of the low dose cells (see below) but clearly the kinetics of the response are important.

A recent approach to this aspect has been to model mathematically the kinetic interrelationships between tumour and various effector cell types that could be involved in tumour elimination[85]. This illustrates well the point that this kinetic argument can account for many of the features of tumour escape, at least in experimental systems, without invoking other escape mechanisms such as the development of cell-mediated suppression or soluble blocking factors (see below). In this model, the importance of the strength (i.e. specific precursor frequency) of the helper T-cell response was emphasized, so that the success of the response depended mainly on this factor, and tumour immunization could be accounted for by expansion of this helper cell compartment.

This fits in well with the demonstration in a number of tumour systems that augmentation of the helper T-cell response to tumour, by changing the genetic background for antigen presentation[86], or provision of additional antigenic determinants (for example, reference 87) can result in a much more effective antitumour immune response.

Antigen loss

Heterogeneity within tumours may present considerable problems to the immune system, and emergence of antigen-loss variants has been demonstrated to be a cause of failure of immunologically mediated tumour rejection[88].

Even with tumours that express multiple tumour-associated antigens such as UV light-induced tumours, this can be a problem. Thus these tumours seem to stimulate a response predominantly associated with one antigen[12]. This would tend to allow considerable time for the expansion of an antigen-loss variant even if still immunogenic, because the immune response to the variant's now dominant antigen would only be properly stimulated after the loss of the previously immunodominant antigen from these cells, perhaps allowing them to 'sneak through'.

The concept of antigen loss may also be applicable to self-MHC antigens which may be involved in the immunological recognition of the tumour. For example, with a spontaneously arising mouse tumour, lack of class I antigen coded at the H-2K locus has been associated with loss of immunogenicity. Thus, after transformation of the tumour cells *in vitro* with DNA from a cosmid coding for the H-2Kk gene, variants expressing the H-2K gene were rejected when transplanted *in vivo*. Interestingly, immunization with these variants[89] also conferred protection against the parent cell line lacking H-2K.

However, increased MHC expression is not always related to a beneficial outcome. Low levels of MHC antigens appear to be associated with a relative increase in susceptibility to natural cytotoxic mechanisms, and this has been proposed as a means for the elimination of 'not self' rather than 'altered self' cells[13,90]. This mechanism may be particularly important in tumours where T-cell recognition is not stimulated, and thus increased MHC gives NK resistance with no compensatory increase in the effectiveness of T-cell interactions.

Induction of suppression

There are many examples in the literature of experimental tumour immunology of the induction of suppressor cells by progressively growing tumour, and this aspect is well illustrated by the work of North and co-workers (reviewed by North[37,91]).

These studies show that as the tumour develops, a positive effector response is stimulated, measurable by *in vivo* transfer of immunity to tumour. However, a negative (suppressor cell) response soon becomes evident. In fact, the positive effector cells are only clearly demonstrable using cell populations from tumour bearing animals given sublethal irradiation. This is because the suppressor population is relatively radiosensitive, whereas the effector cells are radioresistant.

The development of suppression in the tumour system becomes critical as the tumour mass increases. Early surgical removal of the tumour results in the loss of suppression, and a strong positive antitumour response. When excision of tumour is left until later, the suppressor effect is not easily reversed. This would suggest that in immunotherapy, attempts to stimulate antitumour immunity where there is a large tumour burden, or even after 'tumour debulking' surgery, may be made ineffective by suppression.

Blocking factors

During early *in vitro* studies of the effects of tumour immune lymphocytes on target tumour cells, it was observed that serum from tumour bearing animals could block the cytotoxic activity of these effector cells[35]. Initially it was thought that antitumour antibody might be responsible for this activity, but immune complexes of tumour specific antibody and soluble tumour antigen were shown to be more important[92]. Anti-idiotypic antibodies, specifically reactive with the binding site of antitumour antigen recognition structures, have also been implicated in some systems.

Since these early studies, the nature of the effector mechanisms that were being blocked by serum factors has been called into question, because of the possible contribution of non-specific cytotoxic effector cells in these assays. Clearly, it is difficult to assess the relevance of the blocking response if the significance of the *in vitro* measurement being blocked is questionable[93].

However, this type of mechanism may still be important in the modulation of tumour immunity, but its precise definition awaits the development of more appropriate *in vitro* methods.

SUMMARY

Malignant transformation results in major changes in cellular growth control and interaction with surrounding cells. In many experimental systems, transformed cells are recognized specifically by the immune system, but in human cancer, evidence for such recognition remains equivocal. Rejection of experimental tumours depends primarily on cellular immune responses, although the relative importance of cytotoxic T-cells, helper/inducer T-cells, and less specific effector cells such as macrophages and NK cells varies between tumour systems. A variety of mechanisms by which tumours may escape immunological control have also been defined, including antigen loss,

15

suppression, and the development of factors which interfere with cellular immunity. Antibodies may be useful as agents of immunological attack against tumours, either functioning with effector cells or complement, or as the vehicle to carry drugs or toxins to the tumour.

References

1. Foley, E. J. (1953). Antigenic properties of methylcholanthrene induced tumours in mice of the strain of origin. *Cancer Res.*, **13**, 835–7
2. Baldwin, R. W. (1955). Immunity to methylcholanthrene induced tumours in inbred rats following atrophy and regression of implanted tumours. *Br. J. Cancer*, **9**, 652–7
3. Prehn, R. T. and Main, J. M. (1957). Immunity to methylcholanthrene induced sarcomas. *J. Natl. Cancer Inst.*, **18**, 769–78
4. Klein, G., Sjogren, H.O., Klein, E. and Hellstrom, K. E. (1960). Demonstration of resistance against methylcholanthrene induced sarcomas in the primary autochthonous host. *Cancer Res.*, **20**, 1561–72
5. Baldwin, R. W., Barker, C. R., Embleton, M. J., Glaves, D., Moore, M. and Pimm, M. V. (1971). Demonstration of cell surface antigens on chemically induced tumours. *Ann. N. Y. Acad. Sci.*, **177**, 268–78
6. De Leo, A. B., Jay, G., Appella, E., Dubois, G. C., Law, L. W. and Old L. J. (1979). Detection of transformation related antigen in chemically induced sarcomas and other transformed cells of the mouse. *Proc. Natl. Acad. Sci. USA*, **76**, 2420–4
7. Flood, P. M., DeLeo, A. B., Old, L. J. and Gershon, R. K. (1983). Relation of cell surface antigens on methylcholanthrene induced fibrosarcomas to immunoglobulin heavy chain complex variable region linked T cell interaction molecules. *Proc. Natl. Acad. Sci. USA*, **80**, 1683–7
8. Embleton, M. J. and Heidelberger, C. (1972). *Antigenicity of Clones of Mouse Prostate Cells Transformed In Vitro*. (New York: MSS Information Corporation)
9. Baldwin, R. W. and Embleton, M. J. (1971). Tumour specific antigens on 2-acetylamino-fluorene induced rat hepatomas and related tumours. *Israel. J. Med. Sci.*, **7**, 144–53
10. Law, L. W. (1984). Generation of crossreacting tumour antigens in ascitic derivatives from murine methylcholanthrene induced sarcomas. *Int. J. Cancer*, **33**, 547–51
11. Rodgers, M. J. (1984). Tumor associated transplantation antigens of chemically-induced tumors: new complexities. *Immunol. Today*, **5**, 167–8
12. Urban, J. L., Van Waes, C. and Schreiber, H. (1984). Pecking order among tumour specific antigens. *Eur. J. Immunol.*, **14**, 181–7
13. Klein, G. and Klein, E. (1985). Evolution of tumours and the impact of molecular oncology. *Nature (London)*, **315**, 190–5
14. Hewitt, H. B. (1979). The choice of animal tumours for experimental studies of cancer therapy. *Adv. Cancer Res.*, **27**, 149–200
15. Baldwin, R. W. and Embleton, M. J. (1969). Immunology of spontaneously arising rat mammary adenocarcinomas. *Int. J. Cancer*, **4**, 430–9
16. Gold, P. and Freedman, S. (1965). Specific carcinoembryonic antigens of the human digestive system. *J. Exp. Med.*, **122**, 467–81
17. Abelev, G. I. (1974). Alpha fetoprotein as a marker of embryo-specific differentiation in normal and tumour tissues. *Transplant. Rev.*, **20**, 1–37
18. Baldwin, R. W., Embleton, M. J., Price, M. R. and Vose, B. M. (1974). Embryonic antigen expression on experimental rat tumours. *Transplant. Rev.*, **20**, 77–99
19. Bartlett, P. F., Fenderson, B. A. and Edidin, M. (1978). Inhibition of tumour growth mediated by lymphocytes sensitized *in vitro* to a syngeneic murine teratocarcinoma 402AX. *J. Immunol.*, **120**, 1211–17
20. Ting, C.-C., Rodrigues, D. and Herberman, R. B. (1973). Expression of fetal antigens and tumour specific antigens on SV40 transformed cells. II. Tumour transplantation studies. *Int. J. Cancer*, **12**, 519–23
21. Coggin, J. H., Ambrose, K. R., Bellomy, B. B. and Anderson, N. G. (1971). Tumour immunity in hamsters immunized with fetal tissues. *J. Immunol.*, **107**, 526–33
22. Ellis, I. O., Hinton, C. P., NcNay, J., Elston, C. W., Robins, R. A., Owainati, A. A. R. S.,

Blamey, R. W., Baldwin, R. W. and Ferry, B. (1985). Immunocytochemical staining breast carcinoma with the monoclonal antibody NCRC 11: a new prognostic indicator. *Med. J.*, **290**, 881–3

23.   Morrison, A. S., Black, M. M., Lowe, C. L., MacMahon, B. and Yuasa, S. (1973). So international differences in histology and survival in breast cancer. *Int. J. Cancer*, 261–7

24.   Culter, S. J., Black, M. M., Mork, T., Harvei, S. and Freeman, C. (1969). Furt observations on prognostic factors in cancer of the female breast. *Cancer*, **24**, 653–67

25.   Hellstrom, I., Hellstrom, K. E., Sjogren, H. O. and Warner, G. A. (1971). Demonstrat of cell mediated immunity to human neoplasms of various histological types. *Int. Cancer*, **7**, 1–16

26.   Herberman, R. B. (1979). *Compendium of Assays for Immunodiagnosis of Hun Cancer.* (Amsterdam: Elsevier North Holland)

27.   Szigeti, R. (1985). Application of migration inhibition techniques in tumour immunolo *Adv. Cancer Res.*, **43**, 241–305

28.   Vanky, F., Petterffy, A., Book, K., Willems, J., Klein, E. and Klein, G. (1983). Correlat between lymphocyte-mediated auto-tumour reactivities and the clinical course. Evaluation of 69 patients with lung carcinoma. *Cancer Immunol. Immunother.*, **16**, 17

29.   Vanky, F., Willems, J., Kreicbergs, A., Aparasi, T., Andreen, M., Brostrom, L-Nilsonne, U., Klein, E. and Klein, G. (1983). Correlation between lymphocyte-media auto-tumour reactivities and the clinical course. I. Evaluation of 46 patients with sarcot *Cancer Immunol. Immunother.*, **16**, 11–16

30.   Grimm, E. A., Vose, B. M., Chu, E. W., Wilson, D. J., Lotze, M. T., Rayner, A. A. : Rosenberg, S. A. (1984). The human mixed lymphocyte-tumour cell interaction test Positive autologous lymphocyte proliferative responses can be stimulated by tumour c as well as by cells from normal tissues. *Cancer Immunol. Immunother.*, **17**, 83–9

31.   De Vries, J. E. and Spits, H. (1984). Cloned human cytotoxic T lymphocyte (CTL) li reactive with autologous melanoma cells. I. *In vitro* generation, isolation and analysi phenotype and specificity. *J. Immunol.*, **132**, 510–19

32.   Cooper, G. M. and Lane, M.-A. (1984). Cellular transforming genes and oncogene *Biochim. Biophys. Acta*, **738**, 9–20

33.   Greig, R. G., Koestler, T. P., Trainer, D. L., Corwin, S. P., Miles, L., Kline, T., Sweet, Yokoyama, S. and Poste, G. (1985). Tumorigenic and metastatic properties of 'normal' ras-transfected NIH/3T3 cells. *Proc. Natl. Acad. Sci. USA*, **82**, 3698–701

34.   Burgess, A. (1985). Growth factors and oncogenes. *Immunol. Today*, **6**, 107–12

35.   Hellstrom, K. E. and Hellstrom, I. (1974). Lymphocyte mediated cytotoxicity and blocl serum activity to tumour antigens. *Adv. Immunol.*, **18**, 209–77

36.   Baldwin, R. W. and Robins, R. A. (1976). Factors interfering with the immunolog rejection of tumours. *Br. Med. Bull.*, **32**, 118–23

37.   North, R. J. (1984). The murine antitumour immune response and its therape manipulation. *Adv. Immunol.*, **35**, 89–155

38.   Robins, R. A. and Baldwin, R. W. (1985). T cell subsets in tumour rejection respon *Immunol. Today*, **6**, 55–8

39.   Sears, H. F., Mattis, J., Herlyn, D., Hayry, P., Atkinson, B., Ernst, C., Steplewski, Z. Koprowski, H. (1982). Phase I clinical trial of monoclonal antibody in treatment of trointestinal tumours. *Lancet*, **1**, 761–5

40.   Houghton, A. N., Mintzer, D., Cordon-Cardo, C., Welt, S., Fleigel, B., Vadhan, Carswell, E., Melamed, M. R., Oettgen, H. F. and Old, L. J. (1985). Mouse monoclc IgG3 antibody detecting GD3 ganglioside: a phase I trial in patients with maligr melanoma. *Proc. Natl. Acad. Sci. USA*, **82**, 1242–6

41.   Herlyn, D. M., Steplewski, Z., Herlyn, M. F. and Koprowski, H. (1980). Inhibitio growth of colorectal carcinoma in nude mice by monoclonal antibody. *Cancer Res.* 717–21

42.   Herlyn, D. and Koprowski, H. (1982). IgG2a monoclonal antibodies inhibit hu tumour growth through interaction with effector cells. *Proc. Natl. Acad. Sci. USA* 4761–5

43.   Adams, D. O., Hall, T., Steplewski, Z. and Koprowski, H. (1984). Tumours underg rejection induced by monoclonal antibodies of the IgG2a isotype contain incre

85. De Boer, R. J., Hogeweg, P., Dullens, H. F. J., De Weger, R. A. and Den Otter, W. (1985). Macrophage T lymphocyte interactions in the antitumour immune response: a mathematical model. *J. Immunol.*, **134**, 2748–58

86. Bellgrau, D. and Zoller, M. (1983). Cytotoxic T lymphocyte response to spontaneously arising rat tumours: immunogenicity dependent on recognition of processed tumour antigens. *J. Immunol.*, **130**, 2005–7

87. Fujiwara, H., Aoki, H., Yoshioka, T., Tomita, S., Ikegami, R. and Hamaoka, T. (1984). Establishment of a tumour specific immunotherapy model utilizing TNP–reactive helper T cell activity and its application to the autochthonous tumour system. *J. Immunol.*, **133**, 509–14

88. Uyttenhove, C., Maryanski, J. and Boon, T. (1983). Escape of mouse mastocytoma P815 after nearly complete rejection is due to antigen loss variants rather than immunosuppression. *J. Exp. Med.*, **157**, 1040–52

89. Hui, K., Grosveld, F. and Festenstein, H. (1984). Rejection of transplantable AKR leukaemia cells following MHC DNA-mediated cell transformation. *Nature (London)*, **311**, 750–2

90. Karre, K., Ljunggren, H. G., Piontek, G. and Keissling, R. (1986). Selective rejection of H–2–deficient lymphoma variants suggests alternative immune defence strategy. *Nature (London)*, **319**, 675–8

91. North R. J. (1985). Down-regulation of the antitumour immune response. *Adv. Cancer Res.*, **45**, 1–43

92. Baldwin, R. W., Price, M. R. and Robins, R. A. (1972). Blocking of lymphocyte mediated cytotoxicity for rat hepatoma cells by tumour specific antigen–antibody complexes. *Nature New Biol.*, **238**, 185–7

93. Hellstrom, K. E., Hellstrom, I. and Nepom, J. T. (1978). Specific blocking factors – are they important? *Biochim. Biophys. Acta*, **473**, 121–48

2
Immunoscintigraphy:
Tumour Detection with Radiolabelled
Antitumour Monoclonal Antibodies

M. V. PIMM

INTRODUCTION

The feasibility of targeting specific agents both in malignant and other diseases has been a goal of medicine for over 2000 years. Paul Ehrlich, one of the pioneers of specific antibacterial agents, used the phrase 'the magic bullet' and this has recently been applied to possible targeting of antibodies to tumours. Although much pioneering work was carried out in this field with animal tumours by David Pressman and his colleagues in the early 1950s[1], it has been only in the last few years that major scientific, clinical and commercial attention has been focussed on this approach. This interest was revived firstly by the comparative ease of purification of polyclonal antibody to the carcinoembryonic antigen (CEA) and the influential studies by Goldenberg et al.[2] on the localization of such radiolabelled antibodies in colorectal and other carcinomas, and secondly by similar studies following the advent of monoclonal antibodies, initially to CEA[3] and later to a wider range of other tumour-associated antigens[4-21]. One aspect of this development is the clinical potential of monoclonal antibodies for the detection of primary, and probably more usefully, recurrent or metastatic tumours if these antibodies can 'localize' in tumour deposits and this can be visualized by external imaging following administration of suitably radiolabelled antibody. In addition these imaging studies could provide data on the biodistribution, pharmacokinetics and extent of tumour and normal tissue uptake of monoclonal antibodies which could be useful in designing therapeutic trials both with free antibody and drugs or isotopes conjugated to antibodies.

This chapter does not aim to review comprehensively the clinical findings with the variety of monoclonal antibodies which have been shown to localize the human tumours but rather to describe some of the fundamental aspects of this work, the criteria to be met for successful tumour localization and the problems potentially associated with this approach to diagnostic tumour imaging. Where appropriate, specific examples will be drawn from studies carried out by the author and his colleagues in Nottingham over the past few years.

MONOCLONAL ANTIBODIES AS RADIOPHARMACEUTICALS

Given that monoclonal antibodies are available to tumour-associated antigens in purified form, how can we study their biodistribution and tumour localization? Highly sophisticated medical physics procedures have been developed over the last few years for imaging the distribution of a wide range of diagnostic radiopharmaceuticals in patients. It is clearly appropriate to use this established expertise to examine tumour localization of monoclonal antibodies. In one sense these can be viewed as a new generation of radiopharmaceuticals, but it is important to appreciate not only their similarities to, but differences from, conventional agents. The majority of antibodies currently available are high molecular weight proteins (mouse immunoglobulins) and their response to radiolabelling, their *in vivo* fate, distribution and eventual catabolism will be unlike any other, conventional, radiopharmaceutical[20]. Moreover, since they are proteins foreign to man they can potentially act as immunogens, evoking, for example, the production of anti-mouse immunoglobulin antibodies in patients[20,22-24].

Radiolabelling of monoclonal antibodies

A number of radionuclides already widely used in nuclear medicine have been used to label monoclonal antibodies for clinical studies (Table 2.1) and all are gamma emitters since their biodistribution has to be imaged externally. The imaging of the distribution of radiolabelled antibody has been variously termed immunoscintigraphy, radioimmunoscintigraphy, radioimmunodetection or radioimmunolocalization.

Most of the early work with radiolabelled monoclonal antibodies used iodine-131 which has the advantage of low cost, ready availability and ease of attachment to proteins such as antibodies by oxidative incorporation into tyrosine amino acids within the protein structure (Figure 2.1A). Unreacted iodine-131 is removed by gel filtration chromatography. Iodine-131 has disadvantages, however, in that its high energy of gamma emission is not ideally suited to gamma cameras, and its long half-life and associated emission of β particles pose problems of radiation doses to the patients. Another radionuclide of iodine, iodine-123, has a lower energy of gamma emission more suitable for imaging, no β particle emission, and can be used to label antibodies in an identical fashion to iodine-131. Its disadvantages, however, include high cost, restricted availability and a half-life of only 13 hours. Since, as discussed below, most patient imaging is carried out 2-3 days after injection of labelled antibodies, high doses of ^{123}I-labelled antibody would be necessary for remaining radioactivity to be detected with a technically satisfactory count rate.

More recently, a radionuclide of the metal indium, indium-111, has been introduced for antibody labelling and used in a number of clinical trials. This has suitable physical characteristics but is expensive. In addition it cannot be simply attached directly to antibodies in the same way as radioiodine, and labelling requires preconjugation of the antibody to chelating agents which subsequently chelate indium-111 ions. Although a number of chelating agents

Table 2.1 Radionuclides used to label monoclonal antibodies for tumour immunoscintigraphy

Radionuclide	Half-life	Major energy of γ-emission (keV)	Practical mode of incorporation into antibody	Availability*	Cost†
[131]I	8 days	365+ β particles	Tyrosine iodination	Good	Moderate
[123]I	13 hours	159	Tyrosine iodination	Poor	Moderate
[111]In	1.8 days	171, 245	Chelation	Moderate	Expensive
[99m]Tc	6 hours	141	Chelation	Good	Cheap
[67]Ga	3.2 days	185, 300	Chelation	Moderate	Moderate

*Good – available any time; Poor – available only 1 day/week; Moderate – available at high specific activity only 2–3 days/week.
† Expensive > £50/patient; Moderate < £50/patient; Cheap < £5/patient

23

A

RADIOIODINE LABELLING

$$I^+ \ + \ HO - \bigcirc - ANTIBODY$$

Tyrosine

$$HO - \bigcirc - ANTIBODY$$
$$\underset{I}{|}$$

B

RADIOMETAL LABELLING

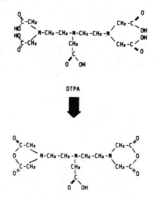

DTPA

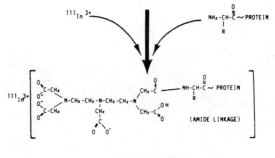

THE CYCLIC DIANHYDRIDE OF DTPA

CHELATION OF ^{111}In

Figure 2.1 Labelling of monoclonal antibody for tumour immunoscintigraphy. A. Labelling with radioiodine such as ^{131}I or ^{123}I is carried out by oxidation of iodide to I^+ with agents such as chloramine T or iodogen allowing simple incorporation into tyrosine groups of the antibody protein; B. Labelling with radiometals such as ^{111}In, ^{99m}Tc and ^{67}Ga is carried out by chelation to chelating groups such as DTPA previously linked to the antibody

have been investigated the one now most frequently used is diethylene-triamine pentaacetic acid (DTPA). This is usually converted initially to a bicyclic dianhydride which can react with antibody by the formation of stable amide bonds with amino groups. Subsequently its carboxyl groups are available to chelate indium-111 ions from a solution of [^{111}In]indium acetate (Figure 2.1B). (Unreacted indium is subsequently removed by gel filtration.) This reaction is clearly more complex than simple iodination of antibody protein, and unless carried out correctly can yield products containing either antibody molecules dimerized by DTPA linkages and/or free ^{111}In in the form of a colloid and both of these will cause unsatisfactory *in vivo* characteristics.

The radiometal gallium-67 is also a likely candidate for radiolabelling monoclonal antibodies for clinical imaging. It can be conjugated by the chelation techniques outlined above for indium-111. Although its use for tumour localization studies in animals has been reported there have, so far, been little or no reports of its clinical use. Gallium-67 injected in the form of gallium-citrate has been widely used as a tumour imaging agent. However, non-specific uptake in abscesses and inflammation have resulted in the continued search for more specific agents. Perhaps conjugation to monoclonal antibodies may provide even greater tumour discriminatory properties.

A fourth radionuclide which may be used for radiolabelling antibodies but not yet so widely used is technetium-99m. This is cheap, readily available and has an energy of gamma emission ideal for gamma camera detection and is the most widely used radiolabel for conventional radiopharmaceuticals. Its conjugation to antibody can be carried out by chelation to DTPA previously conjugated to antibody in the same way as for indium-111 labelling. However, with technetium labelling this is even more complex, involving an initial reduction of the pertechnetate ion (TcO_4^-) to the Tc^{4+} ion for chelation. Furthermore, one of the major disadvantages to technetium-99m is its short half-life of only 6 hours, which would require very large doses to be initially administered to give acceptable count rates at the usual time of imaging. As will be reviewed below, fragments of antibody, e.g. Fab and $F(ab')_2$ show more rapid discrimination between tumour and blood and other normal tissues allowing imaging within possibly 6–24 hours after injection. It is probably with these fragments that technetium-99m will gain greatest acceptability.

One factor to be considered in radiolabelling antibodies for tumour immunoscintigraphy, whichever radiolabel is used, is the effect on the immunological activity of the final product. If radiolabelling involves attachment of chelating agents to the antibody molecules these may be linked at or near the antigen combining sites and/or alter the secondary and tertiary structure of the molecule, reducing its ability to bind to antigen. Even with simple radioiodine incorporation, iodine may be introduced into critical parts of the molecule. The higher the substitution ratio of chelating groups or iodine atoms per antibody molecule the greater the potential damage. For example, Figure 2.2 illustrates the loss of immune function of one particular antibody as it was iodinated to increasing specific activities. This is probably an extreme example, and individual antibodies will very likely differ in their damage by labelling procedures, but each needs careful evaluation and optimization before it can be regarded as satisfactory for clinical use.

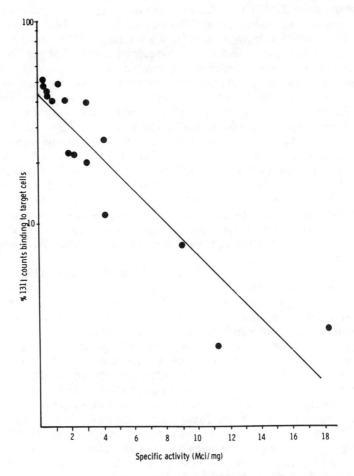

Figure 2.2 Loss of immunological function of an antitumour monoclonal antibody (791T/36) with increasing levels of labelling with [131]I. The preparations were evaluated by measuring the proportion of radioactive counts capable of binding, *in vitro*, to appropriate tumour cells

What happens to radiolabelled antibodies in the circulation?

Following intravenous injection, immunoglobulins distribute over a few hours between the intravascular and extravascular fluid compartments[20] (Figure 2.3). Thus a rapid initial drop in blood radioactivity is seen, followed by a slower decline[20]. For most intact antibodies the latter has a half-life between 1 and 3 days and this is similar to that seen when these mouse immunoglobulins are injected into mice, although it is much faster than the rate of catabolism of passively transferred human immunoglobulin.

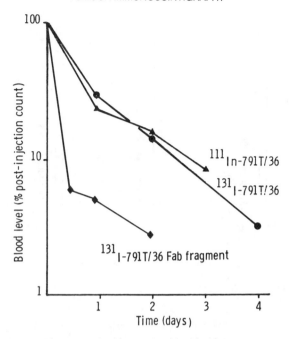

Figure 2.3 Blood levels of radioactivity following intravenous injection of ^{131}I or ^{111}In-labelled 791T/36 monoclonal antibody into patients with colorectal carcinoma. There is an initial rapid drop, followed by a slower decline as the antibody is catabolized. Note that ^{131}I-labelled Fab fragment is lost far more rapidly than intact antibody (3–6 patients/group)

Following catabolism of the antibody, radioiodide such as iodine-131 and iodine-123 is excreted predominantly in the urine, although some is taken up by the thyroid, and some secreted by the gastric mucosa. In contrast, indium-111 released *in vivo* from catabolized antibody is probably retained in most normal tissues, predominantly the liver, spleen and kidneys and is excreted only slowly both in urine and faeces. These differences in the biological fates of radioiodine and indium-111 account, at least in part, for the superiority of indium-111 as a radiolabel for antibody imaging. Thus retention of indium in tissues produces an *apparent* relative clearance from the blood, and this facilitates imaging of tumours, particularly in vascular regions such as the heart[25]. Moreover, indium deposited in tumour tissue is retained there following local catabolism of the antibody, and consequently much higher tumour levels of indium are attained and maintained. These properties of indium-111, together with its superior gamma emission, can produce markedly superior images of tumour localization of monoclonal antibodies compared with radioiodine-labelled preparations[25]. A major problem with indium-111, however, it its propensity to be taken up into liver tissue, and this can obscure localization of antibody in, for example, liver metastases. This is not such a problem with iodine-labelled antibody and clearly the choice of radiolabel is dictated, to some extent, by the investigation required.

A number of studies have shown that following administration of labelled

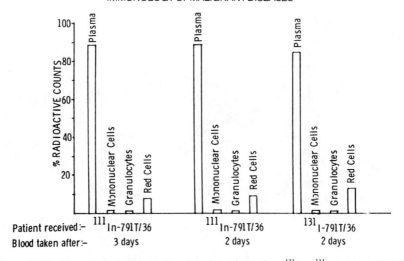

Figure 2.4 Profiles of blood-borne radioactivity in patients given ^{131}I or ^{111}In-labelled 791T/36 monoclonal antibody. Blood was fractionated into plasma, mononuclear cells, granulocytes and red cells and the radioactivity in each fraction counted. Plasma contains the vast majority of the circulating radioactivity

monoclonal antibodies the circulating radiolabel is still free in plasma and attached predominantly to the monoclonal antibody[20] as assessed by immune precipitation, chromatography and antigen binding tests (Figure 2.4. See also Figure 2.9A). The studies are an important part of the initial evaluation of a monoclonal antibody for imaging studies, since the efficient tumour localization of radiolabel requires effective delivery by the antibody. There are a number of potential problems which can arise here if labelled preparations are of poor quality, or if inappropriate antibodies are used:

(1)   The transfer of the radiolabel to other serum proteins may occur. This is certainly a possibility with ^{111}In-labelled antibody where any free indium-111 in the preparation can attach to serum transferrin which can persist in the circulation.

(2)   There may be formation of immune complexes with circulating tumour-derived antigen. This has been most widely documented with antibodies to CEA, where high molecular weight anti-CEA–CEA complexes have been shown in the circulation. Potentially the formation of such complexes could abrogate successful imaging, lead to erroneously false positive images in sites of immune complex deposition (e.g. the spleen), and be potentially deleterious to the patient. In practice, however, this has not been a problem with anti-CEA antibodies and patients with up to at least 5000 μg/L of CEA have been imaged successfully[3]. Presumably in this situation there is antibody equilibrium between plasma- and tumour-CEA and greater binding to the latter. This may not be the case with all monoclonal antibodies whose antigens are present in plasma at significant concentrations and this needs to be appreciated in evaluating new antibodies.

28

(3)   Binding of antibody to blood cells may occur. Anti-CEA antibodies have been prepared against several individual antigenic sites (epitopes) on the CEA molecule. However, not all of these epitopes are specific for CEA and some are expressed on other normal tissues. Most importantly, in the present context, granulocytes express some of these epitopes and there is at least one report of granulocyte depletion in patients given such an antibody with concomitant systemic toxicity including fevers, rigors and emesis[6]. Obviously epitope identification and assessment of granulocyte binding is an important part of the preclinical evaluation of such monoclonal anti-CEA antibodies.

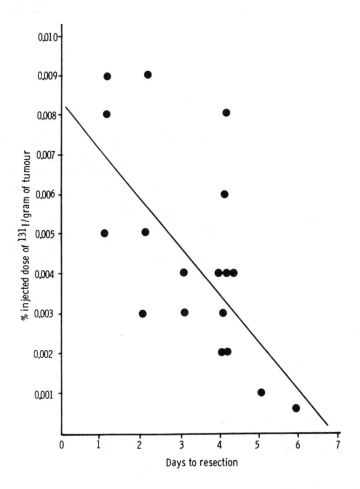

Figure 2.5 Tumour levels of radioactivity in colorectal carcinoma patients injected with ^{131}I-labelled 791T/36 monoclonal antibody. 1–6 days after administration of antibody resected tumour was counted for radioactivity and the level expressed as a percentage of the originally injected does of radiolabel

How much antibody localizes in tumours and what becomes of it?

A number of studies in which tumour has been resected from patients injected with radiolabelled antibodies have established that generally only very low proportions of the injected doses of antibody accumulate in tumour. This is generally of the order of less than 0.05% of the dose/gram[4,16] and tumour levels subsequently decline (Figure 2.5). The changing balance between tumour, normal tissue and blood levels of radiolabels results in optimum tumour detection by external imaging usually 2–3 days after administration. In relation to adjacent normal, non-malignant tissue this generally represents a tumour:non-tumour ratio of up to a maximum of 10:1, depending on the individual anitbody, and tumour type, although values are more generally[4,16,21] in the range of 3:1–5:1. Although these levels of radioactivity have proved viable in external imaging of tumour deposits, clearly higher ratios would further facilitate imaging. Theoretical considerations, from the characteristics of the particular radiolabel radiation and detector systems employed have been attempted to predict the detectability of different size tumours at different depths of the body and with different count rates for particular isotopes[26]. In practice the smallest tumour deposits generally visualized have been about 1–2 cm in diameter.

Although one might hope that antibody localized in tumour would 'coat' the surface of all malignant cells, analysis by autoradiography shows that deposition is far from uniform. Moreover, not all tumour-localized antibody may be in association with malignant cells and much may be associated with antigen as immune complex, for example in tumour acini or stroma[21]. Antibody fragments (see below) can theoretically give higher tumour to blood ratios, potentially improving tumour detection rates. In addition, at least from experimental animal studies, there is a probability that fragments penetrate more deeply into tumour tissue than intact antibody, possibly as a result of their greater rate and extent of extravasation.

A further point for consideration here is the heterogeneity of malignant cells within tumours, so that not all cells may be expressing the target antigen for the particular antibody[21]. Possibly improved imaging may result from combinations of antibodies and/or fragments[11] each to different antigen determinants although it may require a 'cocktail' of several antibodies to potentially react with all malignant cells.

The potential superiority of antibody fragments

Although immunoglobulins exist in five classes (IgA, IgD, IgE, IgG and IgM) the monoclonal antibodies which have been raised against human tumours and which are mostly available for immunoscintigraphy are IgG and IgM. A simplified structure of an IgG molecule is shown in Figure 2.6. It consists of two pairs of polypeptides, two of 23000 daltons molecular weight (light chains) and two of 53000 daltons (heavy chains). They are linked by interchain covalent disulphide bonds to form a 'Y'-shaped molecule with a total molecular weight of approximately 150000 daltons. IgG is bivalent, its two variable regions being the part of the molecule binding to specific antigen

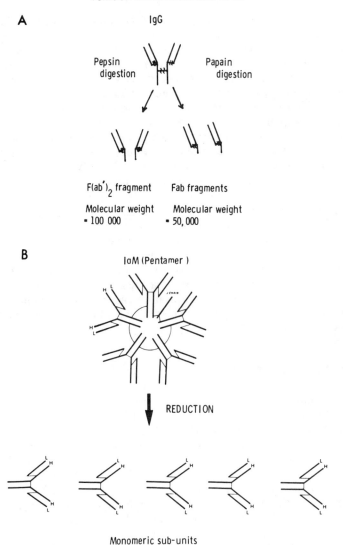

A

IgG

Pepsin digestion

Papain digestion

F(ab')₂ fragment   Fab fragments

Molecular weight   Molecular weight
≈ 100 000   ≈ 50,000

B

IgM (Pentamer)

REDUCTION

Monomeric sub-units

Figure 2.6 Schematic representations of structures of IgG and IgM antibodies. A. IgG can be broken down by enzyme treatments to Fab and F(ab')₂ fragments. Both retain antigen binding activity but the loss of the remainder of the molecule (the Fc portion) results in more rapid extravasation and catabolism *in vivo*; B. IgM can also be broken down to monomeric subunits and these too have altered *in vivo* distribution properties. It is also possible to fragment these subunits to Fab and F(ab')₂ fragments. Thus a range of subunits and fragments is potentially possible from IgM monoclonal antibodies

sites. Enzymic fragmentation of IgG with pepsin and papain can yield bivalent F(ab')₂ and univalent Fab fragments (Figure 2.6). In practice, mouse monoclonal antibodies are often more difficult to fragment in this way than immunoglobulin preparations of other species, and F(ab')₂ and Fab fragments cannot be readily prepared from all monoclonal antibodies. The importance of fragments in the present context is that, *in vivo*, they show altered pharmacokinetic properties compared with intact antibody (Figure 2.3). Both are more rapidly catabolized than free antibody and indeed Fab can undergo simple renal clearance and urinary excretion. In addition they extravasate more rapidly and to a greater extent than intact antibody[4,7,11,21]. The net consequence is that, compared with intact antibody, fragments can localize more rapidly, achieve higher tumour to blood ratios and possibly penetrate more deeply into tumour tissue. The absolute levels of tumour deposition, in relation to the injected dose are, however, lower than those with antibody. Since tumour localization can often be visualized earlier with fragments, acceptable count rates may still be present in tumour areas.

IgM antibodies consist, essentially, of a pentamer of IgG-like molecules with ten possible antigen binding sites (Figure 2.6). Although there are some reports of tumour imaging with IgM antibodies they have the disadvantage, compared with IgG antibody, of rapid catabolism but slow and poor extravasation. In some cases IgM antibodies can be broken down to IgG-like subunits. Although these are still rapidly catabolized (a feature dependent on the μ heavy chain of the molecule) they may be more suitable than intact IgM in relation to extent and rate of extravasation and their ease of radiolabelling, but this area has as yet been poorly explored, at least in the clinical evaluation of IgM fragments.

IMMUNOSCINTIGRAPHY

For most tumour imaging studies patients have been given intravenously between 0.1 mg and 10 mg of monoclonal antibodies labelled with usually 2, but sometimes up to 6 millicuries (222 MBq) of iodine-131, iodine-123, indium-111 or technetium-99m. Usually a small sample of the material is used as a skin test dose to test patients' hypersensitivity to mouse immunoglobulins before injection of the bulk of the material. Hypersensitivity is occasionally seen in previously uninjected patients and here it is clearly inappropriate to proceed with the investigation. Following repeated imaging investigations, patients can become sensitized to the monoclonal antibody[20,22-24] and this restricts the feasibility of more repeat investigations. At the time of writing, monoclonal antibodies for clinical imaging are not generally commercially available. If they were they would obviously need to satisfy legislative criteria of purity, sterility, lack of toxicity, etc. However, since all such antibody investigations are currently carried out only on a trial basis, standards to be met are only locally determined, but have generally involved at least sterility and lack of pyrogenicity before clinical evaluation.

Imaging the tumour localization of radiolabelled monoclonal antibodies

Imaging of patients is usually carried out 2–3 days after intravenous injection of radiolabelled antibody using either gamma cameras or rectilinear scanners to produce planar images, or tomographic cameras allowing construction of

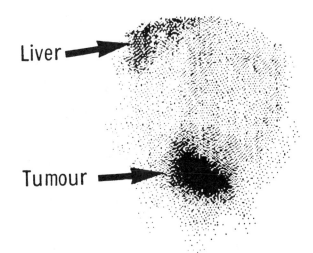

Liver

Tumour

Figure 2.7 Anterior view of the pelvis of a patient with ovarian carcinoma 48 hours after intravenous administration of 80 MBq of [^{111}In]791T/36 monoclonal antibody. Tumour localization of ^{111}In is clearly visible with some ^{111}In also in the liver

image 'slices' similar to X-ray CT. The quality of images obtained is dependent in great part on the radionuclide used to label the antibody. With indium-111 and iodine-123, planar images can generally be viewed directly on film and both provide adequate count rates for tomographic data collection (Figure 2.7). With iodine-131 due to poor resolution and gamma camera detection, tomography is poor. In addition, because of the high proportion of circulating radioiodine a process of 'image enhancement' needs to be used for tumour detection from planar images. In this case, in addition to acquiring an image of the iodine-131 distribution, an injection of another radiotracer is given before the time of the imaging session to simulate the blood pool distribution. This second tracer is usually technetium-99m given in a form to remain in the circulation as labelled albumin or labelled onto the patient's red blood cells and also as free pertechnetate to simulate extravascular activity. The technetium-99m image is then subtracted by computer from the iodine-131 image thus enabling visualization of areas of increased radioactivity which are not simply due to blood-borne iodine-131 or areas of increased tissue vascularity (Figure 2.8). This procedure is not without problems, however, since differences in energies of the gamma emissions of iodine-131 and technetium-99m produce different degrees of scatter and subtraction of a relatively 'sharp' ^{99m}Tc image from a relatively 'fuzzy' ^{131}I image can give artefacts which could, in inexperienced hands, be thought to represent specific iodine-131 accumulation. A further disadvantage of iodine-131 and also of iodine-123 is the high amount of urinary excretion of radioactivity in the bladder which can mask uptake into tumours within this region.

An additional possibility for 'image enhancement', particularly applicable to investigations with radioiodine, is to remove 'excess' circulating radio-

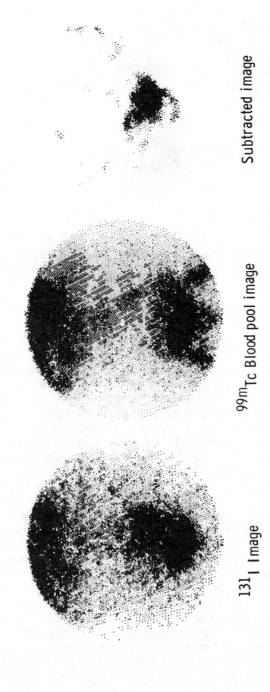

^{131}I Image ^{99m}Tc Blood pool image   Subtracted image

Figure 2.8 Anterior views of the pelvis of a patient with ovarian carcinoma 48 hours after intravenous administration of 70 MBq of [^{131}I]791T/36 monoclonal antibody. Tumour localization of ^{131}I is not convincingly seen without computer subtraction of a ^{99m}Tc blood pool image. Note radioactivity in the bladder in the ^{131}I image, which is simulated in the ^{99m}Tc image

labelled antibody by a subsequent injection of a second anti-mouse immuno-globulin antibody[27], for example made in goats. This has been reported to improve tumour imaging, the immune complexes formed being rapidly cleared to the liver and spleen with subsequent catabolism and clearance of radiolabel. However, it does have the added problem of possibly deleterious effect to patients following rapid immune complex formation. Moreover, as will be discussed below, patients are already potentially capable of making antibodies to the mouse immunoglobulin of the monoclonal antibody, and this situation could be worsened by the production also of the immune response to the second, goat antibody.

In some studies it has been found that increasing the dose of antibody increases tumour detection rates[28]. This could, in some circumstances, be due to increasing reduction in the specific activity of the labelled antibody with concomitant increase in its immunological activity. With some antibodies, however, it is probable that, while the antigen is expressed in high levels in tumour, the antibodies are not absolutely tumour-specific and a low level of antigen expression may occur in some normal tissues[28]. A consequence of this would be that increasing the dose of antibody would saturate this low level of expression in normal tissues, while localization in tumour tissue would continue to increase; discrimination between normal and tumour tissues would progressively increase and tumour detection by external imaging would become more efficient.

Clinical success of tumour imaging

Table 2.2 summarizes a representative sample of imaging studies with radiolabelled monoclonal antibodies reported over the last 4 years. These cover IgG and IgM antibodies and their fragments labelled with iodine-131, iodine-123, indium-111 or technetium-99m in malignancies of colon, rectum, breast, lung, ovary, thyroid, uterus and bone and melanoma, teratoma, neuroblastoma, glioma and meningioma. It is not possible here to describe any of these trials in detail but rather to indicate the diversity of malignant diseases in which antibody imaging is being evaluated.

Although a number of these studies report 100% tumour detection rates, an overall average is nearer 70% and the smallest tumours visualized have generally been of the order of 1–2 cm in diameter. It should be borne in mind, however, that this is a rapidly developing area and as antibodies, labelling techniques and expertise are improved so detection rates and size of tumours detected will improve. To take one example, Perkins et al. (personal communication, Table 2.2) imaging primary lung carcinoma showed positive imaging in only 3 out of 8 (37%) cases using ^{131}I-labelled antibody and planar imaging. With ^{111}In-labelled antibody, 7 out of 12 (67%) of tumours were visualized by planar imaging, but with ^{111}In-labelled antibody and tomography 6 of 6 (100%) of tumours were seen. Probably the further use of antibody fragments, and indium-111 and technetium-99m labels and tomoscintigraphy can be expected to lead to overall increase in detection rates. In some cases previously unsuspected tumour deposits (e.g. metastases or new primary tumours) have been detected during immunoscintigraphy, but

Table 2.2 Clinical imaging with radiolabelled monoclonal antibodies

Author	Antibody designation/antigen	Antibody class	Tumour type	Radiolabel/imaging	No. lesions examined	Positive rate %	Smallest lesion found
Smedley et al.[5]	YPC/121/CEA	IgG2a	Colorectal, breast, lung carcinoma, teratoma	^{131}I with ^{99m}Tc blood pool subtraction	28	60	–
Davies et al.[14]	NDOG2/Placental alkaline phosphate	IgG	Ovarian carcinoma	^{123}I	15	73	–
Thompson et al.[13]*	3E1.2/Breast carcinoma	IgM	Primary/metastatic breast carcinoma	^{131}I	9	100	Lesions detected in two patients with impalpable nodes
Berche et al.[3]	–/CEA	IgG	Gastrointestinal, Medullary thyroid	^{131}I with ^{99m}Tc blood pool subtraction	17	94	4 cm^2
Pateisky et al.[17]	HMFG-2/Milk fat globulin membrane	IgG	Ovarian carcinoma	^{123}I	18	90	1.5 cm diameter
Rainsbury[9]	M8/Milk fat globule membrane	IgG1	Primary/metastatic breast carcinoma	^{111}In	Multiple skeletal secondaries,	100	–
					Soft tissue secondaries	0	–
				^{123}I	Skeletal metastases	0	–
Perkins et al. 1986†	79IT/36/p72 glycoprotein	IgG2b	Primary lung carcinoma	^{131}I with ^{99m}Tc blood pool subtraction	8	37	–
	"	"	"	^{111}In	12	67	2 cm diameter
				^{111}In/tomoscintigraphy	6	100	

Reference	Antibody/antigen	Isotype	Tumour type	Radiolabel		%	Notes
Armitage et al.[18]	791T/36 p72 glycoprotein	IgG2b	Osteosarcoma primary/recurrent	^{131}I with ^{99m}Tc blood pool subtraction ^{111}In	} 5	100	–
Goldman et al.[8]	UJ13A/ Fetal brain	IgG	Primary neuroblastoma	^{123}I or ^{131}I	17	88	1.7cm (Two previously unsuspected secondaries detected)
Kemshead et al.[12]	UJ13A/ Fetal brain	IgG	Glioma and meningioma	^{131}I	4⁻	100	–
Chatal et al.[11]	17–1A/ colon carcinoma	IgG/ F(ab')₂	Primary/metastatic colorectal carcinomas	^{131}I with ^{99m}Tc blood pool subtraction	46	59	–
"	19-9/ colon carcinoma	IgG1/ F(ab')₂	"	"	29	66	–
Morrison et al.[10]	–/ HCG-Beta	IgG1 Fab and F(ab')₂	Uterus, lung, etc.	^{99m}Tc	28	64	–
Buraggi et al.[7]	225–285/ melanoma antigen	IgG/ F(ab')₂	Metastatic melanoma	^{123}I, ^{111}In, ^{99m}Tc	38	68	0.7cm
Larson et.[4]	8.2/p72 Melanoma	IgG1/ Fab	"	^{131}I with ^{99m}Tc blood pool subtraction	25	88	<1.5cm
Armitage et al.[16]	791T/36 p72 glycoprotein	IgG2B	Primary/metastatic colorectal carcinoma	^{111}In	16	75	–
Symonds et al.[15]	791T/36 p72 glycoprotein	IgG1b	Primary/recurrent ovarian carcinoma	^{131}I with ^{99m}Tc blood pool subtraction	12	91	–

* Antibody injected into web of hand to drain to lymph node metastases. All other injections intravenously

† Personal communication

NB This is intended to be a representative example of studies with various antibodies, tumours and radiolabels reported in the literature. It is not intended to be comprehensive.

37

it does not follow of course that these might not have been detected by other techniques if these had been included in the investigation.

The role of immunoscintigraphy in complementing other diagnostic imaging procedures such as X-ray computed axial tomography and NMR will only emerge from further study and prospective studies to determine the usefulness of immunoscintigraphy are now being carried out. For example, multicentre and prospective trials are on going with an anti-melanoma[7,29] and anti-colorectal carcinoma[11] antibodies and with ^{131}I and ^{111}In-labelled 791T/36 antibody a trial is under way to evaluate prospectively the use of this antibody in the detection of suspected recurrent and metastatic colorectal cancer[19]. 46 patients (25 men, 21 women) have undergone 52 immunoscintigraphy investigations. Of these, 42 had ^{99m}Tc liver scintigraphy, 28 abdominal ultrasonography, 28 computerized axial tomography and 17 laparotomy. The indications for investigation were pain (46%), a mass (27%), hepatomegaly (13%) and elevated carcinoembryonic antigen (CEA) (65%). In 19% patients elevated CEA was the only detectable abnormality. 57 sites of recurrent diseases were detected in 37 patients; 37 of these sites were positively identified by immunoscintigraphy, giving a sensitivity of 64%. Nine patients remain disease-free with a median follow-up of 12 months (9–27 months). 13 had false positive images giving a specificity of 70%, but the conclusion so far is that immunoscintigraphy is a clinically useful imaging modality in the detection of recurrent and metastatic colorectal cancer, and is likely to prove of particular value where computerized tomography is not available. The same antibody (791T/36) successfully images primary and recurrent ovarian carcinoma and is viewed as a 'possible alternative to second look surgery in these patients'[15].

One point to emerge from these studies is that some radiolabelled antibodies are proving capable of imaging more than one type of malignancy. This is clearly the case with anti-CEA antibodies. To take some other examples, antibodies to antigens associated with human milk fat globule membranes have been used to image both breast and ovarian carcinomas[9,17]. The 791T/36 antibody, originally raised against osteogenic sarcoma, identifies an antigen expressed in other, quite diverse malignancies, such as colorectal[16], ovarian[15], breast and lung carcinoma and has been used in imaging all of these diseases. In addition a number of trials are now ongoing to evaluate immunoscintigraphy with mixtures of antibodies potentially to overcome some of the problems of heterogeneity of antigen expression in tumours. For example, there are now reports of both the simultaneous use of two anti-colorectal carcinoma antibodies (17–1A and 19–9) showing improved detection rates, and the 19–9 antibody $F(ab')_2$ fragment together with an anti-CEA antibody[11] $F(ab')_2$.

The problems of patients' antibody responses to murine monoclonal antibodies

Because monoclonal antibodies currently being evaluated for immunoscintigraphy are mouse immunoglobulins, they could potentially evoke patients' production of antibodies to mouse immunoglobulin. This has now been

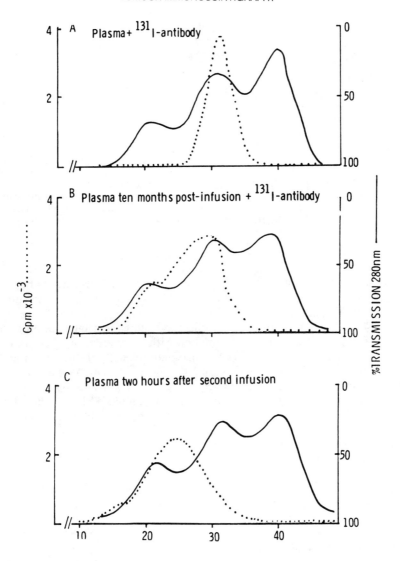

Figure 2.9 The effect of a patient's antibody response to an antitumour monoclonal antibody (791T/36). A. Radiolabelled antibody was mixed with plasma from the patient before the investigation and fractionated by gel filtration chromatography (Sephacryl S300 column) which separated plasma proteins into high, medium and low molecular weights, monitored by absorption of ultraviolet light at 280 nm. Radiolabel is present only in the second plasma protein peak corresponding to the molecular weight (150 000 daltons) of the antibody; B. Plasma from the same patient 10 months after the first investigation added to labelled monoclonal antibody. The presence of antibody to the monoclonal antibody forms high molecular weight immune complexes and the radioactivity is now eluted earlier from the column; C. Plasma from the patient 2 hours after a second injection of radiolabelled monoclonal antibody. *In vivo* formation of immune complexes has now taken place and circulating radiolabel is in high molecular weight form

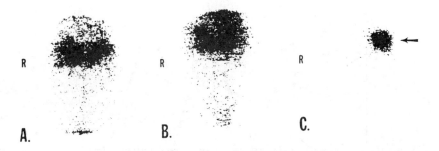

R

R

R

A.   B.   C.

Figure 2.10 The effect of a patient's antibody response to an antitumour monoclonal antibody (791T/36) on imaging the distribution of radiolabelled 791T/36. Anterior views of the upper abdomen of a 68-year-old female patient with carcinoma of the endometrium. A. 48 hours after first injection of [^{131}I]791T/36; B. 3 weeks later and 48 hours after a second injection of [^{131}I]791T/36; C. 6 months following the first injection and 48 hours after a third injection of ^{131}I-labelled 791T/36 showing intense uptake in spleen (arrow). The site of the tumour was not shown without blood pool subtraction and the final study was unsatisfactory

reported from a number of trials[4,20,22-24] and an example is illustrated in Figure 2.9. Although repeat investigations are possible in many patients, by the time three or four administrations of antibody have been given often patients' antibody levels are sufficient to neutralize the subsequent imaging doses[20]. This results in immune complex formation with subsequent rapid clearance from the blood, appearance of radiolabel predominantly in the spleen and abrogation of tumour imaging (Figure 2.10). There are a number of ways in which it might be possible to circumvent this problem. For example, antibody fragments might be less immunogenic than intact antibody. Thus removal of the Fc part of the molecule removes one of its more highly immunogenic regions and also hampers immune recognition and processing which could lead to antibody formation against the rest of the immunoglobulin molecule. There are, however, now some reports of antibody responses to Fab fragments, albeit in patients given large doses of fragments. Furthermore, there is some evidence that the antibody responses in patients given mouse monoclonal antibodies are not the result only of primary immune responses to mouse immunoglobulin but represent secondary responses to antigenic determinants common to mouse immunoglobulins and, for example porcine and bovine immunoglobulins, to which low levels of sensitization had already occurred from food[22]. However, patients' antibody responses have been shown to include, at least in part, antibodies against the unique antigen binding part of the monoclonal antibody molecule (the idiotope) and so some primary sensitization is also occurring[23,24]. These anti-idiotypic antibodies could also be produced against Fab and F(ab')$_2$ fragments and this is another reason why use of these fragments may not entirely circumvent the problem of immunogenicity in patients. Human, rather than mouse monoclonal antibodies are now being produced against some tumour-associated antigens. If these were used for immunoscintigraphy they would probably be less immunogenic than mouse immunoglobulin, but may still evoke at least the production of anti-idiotypic antibodies.

40

SUMMARY AND CONCLUSIONS

Monoclonal antibodies can be made to antigens preferentially associated with, even if not totally specific for, human tumours. These antibodies can be purified and radiolabelled and, *in vivo*, can be seen to accumulate preferentially in tumour deposits, both primary and secondary in a wide variety of malignancies. It can be envisaged that development of further antibodies, radiolabelling procedures and imaging equipment will refine this technique to give greater sensitivity and specificity. Obviously this development will take place alongside progress in other imaging and diagnostic modalities and the final place of immunoscintigraphy as an alternative or complementary procedure cannot yet be assessed. It seems likely, however, that it will find a role in clinical practice.

ACKNOWLEDGEMENTS

The author's work is supported by the Cancer Research Campaign. He thanks his colleagues in the Cancer Research Campaign Laboratories and Departments of Medical Physics, Surgery, and Obstetrics and Gynaecology, Queen's Medical Centre, University of Nottingham for extensive collaboration and particularly Dr A. C. Perkins, Medical Physics, for provision of several figures and critical reading of the manuscript.

References

1. Pressman, D. and Korngold, L. (1953). The *in vivo* localization of anti-Wagner-osteogenic sarcoma antibodies. *Cancer*, **6**, 619–23
2. Goldenberg, D. M., Deland, F., Kimm, E. E., Bennett, S., Primus, F. J., Vannagell, J. R., Estes, N., Desimone, P. and Rayburn, P. (1978). Use of radio-labeled antibodies to carcinoembryonic antigen for the detection and localization of diverse cancers by external photoscanning. *N. Engl. J. Med.*, **298**, 1384–8
3. Berche, C., Mach, J. -P., Lumbroso, J. -D., Langlais, C., Aubry, F., Buchegger, F., Carrel, S. Rougier, P., Parmentier, C. and Tubiana, M. (1982). Tomoscintigraphy for detecting gastrointestinal and medullary thyroid cancers: first clinical results using radiolabelled monoclonal antibodies against carcino-embryonic antigen. *Br. Med. J.*, **285**, 1447–51
4. Larson, S. M., Brown, J. P., Wright, P. W., Carrasquillo, J. A., Hellstrom, I. and Hellstrom, K. E. (1983). Imaging of melanoma with I-131-labeled monoclonal antibodies. *J. Nucl. Med.*, **24**, 123–9
5. Smedley, H. M., Finan, P., Lennox, E. J., Ritson, A., Takei, F., Wraight, P. and Sikora, K. (1983). Localization of metastatic carcinoma by a radiolabelled monoclonal antibody. *Br. J. Cancer*, **47**, 253–9
6. Dillman, R. O., Beauregard, J. C., Sobol, R. E., Royston, I., Bartholomew, R. M., Hagan, P. S. and Halpern S.E. (1984). Lack of radioimmunodetection and complications associated with monoclonal anticarcinoembryonic antigen antibody cross reactivity with an antigen on circulating cells. *Cancer Res.*, **44**, 2212–18
7. Buraggi, G. L., Callegaro, L., Turrin, A., Cascinelli, N., Attili, A., Emanuelli, H., Gasparini, M., Deleide, G., Plassio, G., Dovis, M., Mariani, G., Natali, P. G., Scassellata, G. A., Rosa, V. and Ferrone, S. (1984). Immunoscintigraphy with ^{123}I, ^{99m}Tc and ^{111}In-labelled F(ab')$_2$ fragments of monoclonal antibodies to a human high molecular weight, melanoma associated antigen. *J. Nucl. Med. Allied Sci.*, **28**, 283–95
8. Goldman, A., Vivian, G., Gordon, I., Pritchard, J. and Kemshead, J. (1984). Immunolocalization of neuroblastoma using radiolabelled monoclonal antibody UJ13A. *J. Paediatrics*, **105**, 252–6

9. Rainsbury, R. M. (1984). The localization of human breast carcinomas by radiolabelled monoclonal antibodies. *Br. J. Surg.*, **71**, 805–12
10. Morrison, R. T., Lyster, D. M., Allcorn, L., Rhodes, B. A., Brescon, K. and Burchell, S. (1984) Radioimmunoimaging with ^{99m}Tc monoclonal antibodies: clinical studies. *Int. J. Nucl. Med. Biol.*, **11**, 184–8
11. Chatal, J. -F., Saccavini, J. -C., Fumoleau, P., Douillard, J. -Y., Curtet, C., Kremer, M., Le Mevel, B. and Koprowski, H. (1984). Immunoscintigraphy of colon carcinoma. *J. Nucl. Med.*, **25**, 307–14
12. Kemshead, J. J., Jones, D. M., Goldman, A., Richardson, R. B. and Coakham, H. B. (1984). Is there a role for radioimmunolocalization in diagnosis of intracranial malignancies? *J. R. Soc. Med.*, **77**, 847–54
13. Thompson, C. H., Lichtenstein, M., Stacker, S. A., Leyden, M. J., Saleri, N., Andrews, J. T. and McKenzie, I. F. C. (1984). Immunoscintigraphy for detection of lymph node metastases from breast cancer. *Lancet*, **2**, 1245–7
14. Davies, J. D., Davies, E. R., Howe, K., Jackson, P. C., Pitcher, E. M., Sadowski, C. S., Stirrat, G. M. and Sunderland, C. A. (1985). Radionuclide imaging of ovarian tumours with ^{123}I-labelled monoclonal antibody (NCOG$_2$) directed against placental alkaline phosphatase. *Br. J. Obstet. Gynaecol.*, **92**, 277–86
15. Symonds, E. M., Perkins, A. C., Pimm, M. V., Baldwin, R. W., Hardy, J. G. and Williams, D. A. (1985). Clinical implications for immunoscintigraphy in patients with ovarian malignancy: a preliminary study using monoclonal antibody 791T/26. *Br. J. Obstet. Gynaecol.*, **92**, 270–6
16. Armitage, N. C., Perkins, A. C., Pimm, M. V., Wastie, M. L., Baldwin, R. W. and Hardcastle, J. D. (1985). Imaging of primary and metastatic colorectal cancer using an ^{111}In-labelled anti-tumour monoclonal antibody (791T/36). *Nucl. Med. Commun.*, **6**, 623–31
17. Pateisky, N., Philipp, K., Skodler, W. D., Czerwenka, K., Hamilton, G. and Burchell, J. (1985). Radioimmunodetection in patients with suspected ovarian cancer. *J. Nucl. Med.*, **26**, 1369–76
18. Armitage, N. C., Perkins, A. C., Pimm, M. V., Wastie, M., Hopkins, J. S., Dowling, F., Baldwin, R. W. and Hardcastle, J. D. (1986). Imaging of bone tumours using a monoclonal antibody raised against human osteosarcoma. *Cancer*, **58**, 37–42
19. Ballantyne, K. C., Armitage, N. C., Perkins, A. C., Pimm, M. V., Wastie, M. L., Baldwin, R. W. and Hardcastle, J. D. (1986). Monoclonal antibody 791T/36 imaging in the detection of recurrent colorectal cancer. *Eur. J. Surg. Oncol.*, in press
20. Pimm, M. V., Perkins, A. C., Armitage, N. C. and Baldwin, R. W. (1985). The characteristics of blood-borne radiolabels and the effect of anti-mouse IgG antibodies on localization of radiolabeled monoclonal antibody in cancer patients. *J. Nucl. Med.*, **26**, 1011–23
21. Armitage, N. C., Perkins, A. C., Pimm, M. V., Farrands, P. A., Baldwin, R. W. and Hardcastle, J. D. (1984) The localization of an anti-tumour monoclonal antibody (791T/36) in gastrointestinal tumours. *Br. J. Surg.*, **71**, 407–12
22. Schroff, R. W., Foon, K. A., Bearry, S., Oldham, R. K. and Morgan, A. (1985). Human anti-murine immunoglobulin responses in patients receiving monoclonal antibody therapy. *Cancer Res.*, **45**, 879–85
23. Rowe, R. E., Pimm, M. V. and Baldwin, R. W. (1985). Anti-idiotype antibody responses in cancer patients receiving a murine monoclonal antibody. *IRCS Med. Sci.*, **13**, 936–7
24. Jaffers, G. J., Colvin, R. B., Cosimi, A. B., Giorgi, J. V., Goldstein, G., Fuller, T. C., Kurnick, J. T., Lillenhei, C. and Russell, P. S. (1983). The human immune response to murine OKT3 monoclonal antibody. *Transplant. Proc.*, **15**, 646–8
25. Perkins, A. C. and Pimm, M. V. (1985). Differences in tumour and normal tissue concentrations of iodine and indium-labelled monoclonal antibody. I. The effect on image contrast in clinical studies. *Eur. J. Nucl. Med.*, **11**, 295–9
26. Rockoff, S. D., Goodenough, D. J. and McIntire, K. R. (1980). Theoretical limitations in the immunodiagnosis imaging of cancer with computed tomography and nuclear scanning. *Cancer Res.*, **40**, 3054–8
27. Begent, R. H. J., Keep, P. A., Green, A. J., Searle, F., Bagshawe, K. D., Jewkes, R. F., Jones, B. E., Barratt, G. M. and Ryman, B. E. (1982). Liposomally entrapped second

antibody improves tumour imaging with radiolabelled (first) anti-tumour antibody. *Lancet*, **2**, 739–42

28. Halpern, S. and Hagan, P. (1985). Effect of protein mass on the pharmacokinetics of murine monoclonal antibodies. *J. Nucl. Med*, **26**, 818–19

29. Buraggi, G. L., Turrin, A., Cascinelli, N., Ferrone, S., Callegaro, L., Attili, A., Bombardieri, E., Scassellati, G. A., Gaspatrini, N. and Seregni, E. (1985). Radioimmuno-detection with an anti-melanoma monoclonal antibody. *Cancer Detec. Prevent.*, **8**, 575

3
Monoclonal Antibody Targeting of Cytotoxic Agents for Cancer Therapy

R. W. BALDWIN AND V. S. BYERS

INTRODUCTION

The technique of immortalizing individual clones of antibody secreting cells by fusing them with cultured myeloma cells to form hybridomas which continuously secrete antibody has for the first time made possible the reproducible production of antitumour antibodies[1-3]. Typically these are murine monoclonal antibodies produced by hybridomas formed by fusing splenocytes from mice immunized with human tumour cells or cell fractions. These hybridomas are maintained continuously either in culture or as ascites in mice so allowing production of monoclonal antibodies in multigram amounts. The repertoire of murine monoclonal antibodies which react with human tumours is now quite extensive and preparations are available which recognize almost all of the major types of human cancer[1-4]. These include antibodies reacting with carcinomas of colon, rectum, breast, ovary, lung and bladder as well as malignant melanoma and bone and soft tissue sarcomas. It is important to recognize, however, that these antibodies generated by immunizing mice with human tumour cells do not recognize tumour specific antigens. Rather, they react with normal or modified tissue antigens which are either preferentially or inappropriately expressed upon malignant cells. One class of antigens, the so-called oncofetal antigens, are tumour cell products which are associated with fetal and malignant tissues[5]. These include carcinoembryonic antigen (CEA) widely associated with colonic carcinomas[6] and α-fetoprotein secreted by hepatocellular carcinomas[7]. Other tumour-associated antigens against which monoclonal antibodies have been generated are probably differentiation antigens. These include a range of protein antigens on malignant melanoma cells[8] as well as glycolipid antigens in colorectal cancer[9,10]. Likewise monoclonal antibodies have been produced against human milk fat globule membrane which recognize carbohydrate antigens expressed upon carcinomas of breast and ovary[11].

Although the monoclonal antibodies produced against these antigens are not strictly tumour specific, they are being examined for drug targeting[1,4,12]. This application is based upon extensive related studies where it has been shown that radiolabelled antibodies preferentially localize in human tumours (see Chapter 2). Based upon these findings it is proposed that antibody-targeted cytotoxic agents may have more effective antitumour activities and/or reduced toxicity for normal tissues.

IMMUNOTOXINS

Ribosome-inactivating proteins represent a class of highly cytotoxic agents being used to construct immunotoxins by linking to monoclonal anti-bodies[13-16]. It has been calculated that one molecule of these toxins entering the cytoplasm of a cell is sufficient to produce a lethal response. Therefore, they have considerable appeal for antibody targeting, since the amount of antibody which can bind to a target cell is limited by the number of antigen receptors expressed.

One type of toxin typified by ricin toxin (from castor beans) consists of two polypeptide chains (A-chain and B-chain) joined by a disulphide bond. In the natural course of events, the toxin binds through a site on the B-chain to receptors which are expressed upon essentially all cells in a susceptible host. The A-chain then penetrates into the cytoplasm, probably following internal-ization via the endosome and produces cell kill following inactivation of protein synthesis[13,14].

Immunotoxins constructed by linking whole toxin to antibody are highly toxic and their activity may even exceed that of the native toxin. But because of the presence of the B-chain component, which binds to most cells, they lack specificity. One approach to this problem is to 'block' the B-chain reaction with cell receptors by, for example, including galactose or lactose in the reaction mixture. This blocking is effected since the cell receptor for B-chain recognizes oligosaccharides. This is readily feasible *in vitro* but less easily achieved *in vivo*. A preferred approach, therefore, is to separate the A-chain and B-chain polypeptides following enzymic cleavage of the whole toxin. The isolated A-chain is then linked to antibody to form an A-chain immunotoxin (Figure 3.1). The coupling is generally produced by introducing an activated disulphide residue (e.g. dithiopyridine) into the antibody which then is reacted with free sulphydryl groups of the A-chain. This forms a conjugate in which the A-chain toxin is linked to antibody through a disulphide bond.

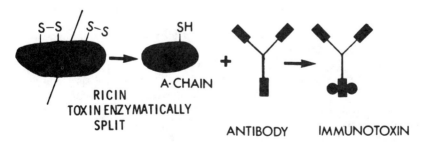

Figure 3.1 Synthesis of ricin A-chain antibody conjugates

There is now a considerable range of immunotoxins produced by linking ricin A-chain to antibody[13-16]. These include immunotoxins cytotoxic for many types of solid tumour including carcinoma of colon, breast, lung and ovary, malignant melanoma and bone sarcomas[16-19]. Immunotoxins cytotoxic for leukaemic cells have also been synthesized[4,16,20]. When tested *in vitro* these immunotoxins are exquisitely specific for target cells which express the antigen recognized by the antibody component. They lack the very high cytotoxicity of immunotoxins constructed with whole toxins since the B-chain also plays an important role in the internalization of the A-chain component. This is well illustrated by the enhancement of A-chain immunotoxin cytotoxicity with so-called potentiating agents[21]. For example, the *in vitro* cytotoxicity of one immunotoxin for leukaemic cells is potentiated some 6700 times by the inclusion of ammonium chloride in the incubation medium[21]. Even more pronounced potentiation is achieved with carboxylic ionophores and with monensin a 50000 fold increase in cytotoxic potency has been reported. These potentiating agents probably function by modifying the fate of immunotoxins following their entry into the cell, although their exact mechanism of action is still unresolved[22]. Even with these limitations, however, immunotoxins have high potency when compared with antibody conjugates with cytotoxic drugs. This is illustrated by comparing the *in vitro* cytotoxicity of conjugates constructed by linking one monoclonal antibody (791T/36) to methotrexate and ricin A-chain for a standard tumour target cell[17]. When assessed by the dose in terms of methotrexate or ricin A-chain producing 50% cell kill (IC_{50}) the RTA conjugate (1.4×10^{-10} mol/L) was some 100-fold more cytotoxic than the methotrexate conjugate (1.5×10^{-8} mol/L).

Other naturally occurring ribosome–inactivating proteins (RIP) are being investigated for immunotoxin synthesis[23]. These include RIPs which occur naturally as single polypeptide chains such as gelonin, saporin and pokeweed antiviral peptide (PAP). Although these natural A-chain RIPs are less cytotoxic than two-chain RIPs like ricin, they can be readily linked to antibody.

The *in vivo* efficacy of a number of immunotoxins has been demonstrated by showing that they suppress growth of human tumour xenografts in immunodeprived (athymic) mice[15,16,19]. Active products include immunotoxins containing antibodies reacting with carcinomas of colon, breast and ovary and malignant melanoma and osteogenic sarcoma. In addition, immunotoxins reacting with T-cell leukaemias have been developed and these are also being utilized for T-cell depletion in allogeneic bone marrow transplanation (see Chapter 4).

Based upon the *in vitro* assay data and efficacy trials with human tumour xenografts, immunotoxins are being evaluated for clinical trials. Initially it was felt that because of their high potency immunotoxins might have associated side-effects which would preclude their clinical use. A phase I clinical trial in malignant melanoma patients with a ricin A-chain immunotoxin constructed with an anti-melanoma antibody has established that this is not the case[18].

Immunotoxin was administered daily for 5 days to 22 patients with metastatic malignant melanoma. Side-effects observed were a transient fall in serum albumin with an associated fall in serum albumin, weight gain and fluid shifts resulting in oedema and mild hypovolaemia. Encouraging clinical results were reported and on the basis of these studies a phase II clinical trial is in progress.

The toxicity of immunotoxins will be dependent upon the reactivity of the antibody component with normal tissues and will have to be assessed with each new product. This is an important point since, as already referred to, the monoclonal antibodies being used for immunotoxin construction are not completely tumour specific, but do show some, albeit low, cross-reactivity with some normal tissues. Related to this is the powerful influence of the RIP component upon the biodistribution *in vivo* of immunotoxins. Thus several trials with ricin A-chain immunotoxins have shown that there is rapid liver uptake and detoxification[24,25]. This is because the RTA moiety contains an oligosaccharide structure which is recognized by receptors on the Kupffer cells in the liver. On one hand this may be viewed as a disadvantage in that it leads to rapid loss of available immunotoxin for targeting to a tumour site. On the other hand it does provide a rapid means for detoxifying immuno-toxin and this may be advantageous in the clinical trials with immunotoxins which are now being initiated in the treatment of malignant melanoma and colorectal cancer.

Monoclonal antibody drug conjugates

Targeting of 'conventional' cytotoxic drugs conjugated to monoclonal anti-bodies is being developed as a means of improving their therapeutic efficacy. This may result either from improved localization and/or retention of drug in tumours, especially metastatic deposits or by reducing normal tissue toxicity, this being a major limitation in cancer therapy with cytotoxic drugs. There are several pathways which can be exploited for antibody-mediated delivery of drugs (Figure 3.2). Drugs may be targeted to tumour cells following anti-

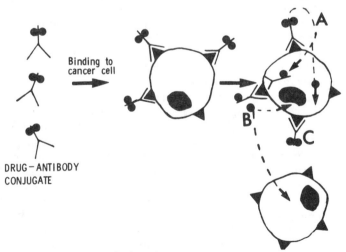

Figure 3.2 Cell attack of drug–antibody conjugate

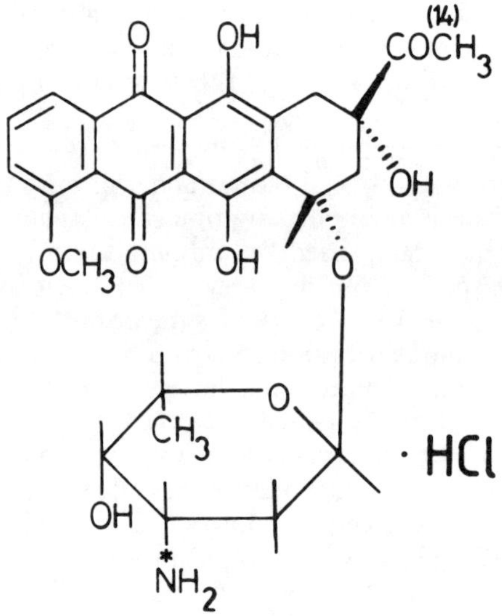

Figure 3.3 Chemical stucture of daunomycin (Dau)

body-conjugate binding to tumour antigen expressed upon the tumour cell surface and, as with immunotoxins, exert their effects following internalization and intercellular release of drugs. This is the preferred pathway of action, but requires that sufficient drug can be targeted to the tumour, that the drug–antibody conjugate is stable and that the conjugate is efficiently internalized and can undergo intracellular release of drug in an active form.

A cytotoxic drug may also be released extracellularly following antibody conjugate localization in tumours and thereafter function as free drug. In this case, conjugates can be targeted to tumour cell antigens as well as to extracellular antigens, and it also requires that the drug–antibody linkage should be cleaved, e.g. through the action of enzymes present in tumour tissue. Finally, drug–antibody conjugates may localize at the tumour cell surface and thereafter function by producing cell membrane damage.

Chemical conjugation of drugs to antibody requires the availability of a reactive functional group in the drug such as amino, hydroxyl or carboxyl group. These reactive groups should also not be required for drug action unless it is envisaged that they will become available following intracellular release after internalization of the conjugate. For example, the sugar amino group of daunomycin (Figure 3.3) is required for drug action and so it is not an appropriate site for antibody linkage. In this particular case, this has led to the synthesis of antibody conjugate through the carbon-14 position[26].

Cytotoxic drugs are also much less potent than the plant toxins used to construct immunotoxins. It is thus necessary to introduce the maximum number of drug residues whilst ensuring adequate retention of antibody reactivity. This will be influenced by a number of factors still not very well defined which include the size and charge of the conjugated drug and the site(s) of chemical conjugation in the antibody molecule. But in general, substitution of more than ten drug residues/antibody molecules will produce an unacceptable degree of antibody damage. In some examples, e.g. methotrexate linked to monoclonal antibody 791T/36, only as few as 3/4 drug group/antibody molecules could be introduced[27]. In comparison, conjugation of the vinca alkaloid analogue vindesine (desacetyl vinblastine amide) to an anti-melanoma antibody (96.5) at drug:antibody ratios up to 10:1 yielded conjugates with adequate antibody reactivity[28].

Drug carrier systems are being developed in order to increase drug–antibody levels[27,29,30]. This involves first linking drug to carrier molecule which has multiple combining sites and then the drug–carrier conjugate is linked to antibody. Several 'carriers' have been used for drug conjugation including human serum albumin, dextran and poly-L-lysine but all have limitations and research is now being directed towards the design of more

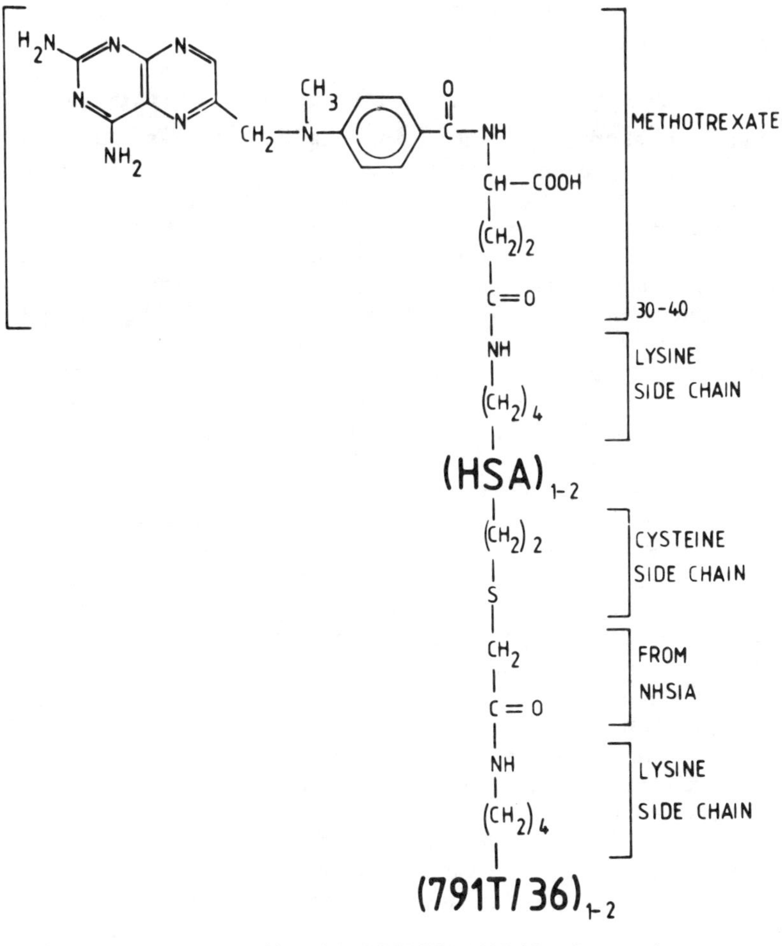

Figure 3.4 General composition of the MTX-HSA-791T/36 antibody conjugate

49

appropriate carriers. Nevertheless, these approaches have led to the construction of drug conjugates with therapeutic potential. This is exemplified by the design of methotrexate conjugates where methotrexate (MTX) was first coupled to human serum albumin (HSA)[26]. The MTX-HSA conjugate was then linked to antibody to yield products with the general composition shown in Figure 3.4 containing 30–40 moles MTX/mole antibody. These conjugates are cytotoxic *in vitro* for tumour cells binding the antibody and they suppress growth of human tumour cells. Based upon the laboratory studies the MTX-HSA-791T/36 antibody conjugate is being entered into clinical trial in colorectal cancer.

The vinca alkaloid analogue vindesine (desacetyl vinblastine amide) has also been used to construct antibody conjugates, in this case by directly linking drug to antibody for clinical trial. Conjugates prepared by linking to anti-CEA monoclonal antibody inhibit growth of xenografts of human colon carcinoma xenografts[31] and a product constructed using a monoclonal antibody reacting with 'adenocarcinoma-associated' antigen has been designed for clinical trial in lung carcinoma.

Tumour localization of monoclonal antibodies and drug conjugates

In vivo localization of monoclonal antibodies in human tumours has been well documented in tumour imaging trials where patients injected with antibody preparations labelled with γ-emitting radioisotopes such as ^{131}I and ^{111}In have been imaged on a gamma camera[1] (see Chapter 2). Antibody distribution in resected tumour and adjacent normal tissue in patients injected with radiolabelled antibody for imaging studies prior to surgery also demonstrated preferential antibody localization in tumour. For example, the tumour to non-tumour ratio of radioactivity in colorectal cancer in patients injected with ^{131}I-labelled monoclonal antibody 791T/36 ranged[32] from 2:1 to 10:1. This approach has been used also to show that methotrexate monoclonal antibody 791T/36 conjugates localize in tumour. In ten patients with primary colorectal cancer injected with ^{131}I-labelled MTX-791T/36 conjugate[33] the tumour to non-tumour ratio of ^{131}I was 3.9–2.1:1.

For effective delivery of agents linked to monoclonal antibodies the conjugates should ideally uniformly penetrate regions of the tumour contributing to its progressive growth and bind to most if not all individual tumour cells. As already described, immunotoxins are only effective where the toxin moiety is internalized and so tumour cell binding is obligatory in this approach. Similarly, the most effective pathway of drug delivery is via drug–antibody conjugate binding to tumour cells.

Autoradiography of tumour tissue sections obtained following injection of radioisotope-labelled antibodies has revealed considerable variation in their deposition. For example, in one study with monoclonal antibody 791T/36, localization in human tumour xenografts was predominantly at the periphery of the tumour with only low levels of penetration[34]. Each monoclonal antibody will probably have a characteristic tissue distribution pattern. So, for example, an anti-CEA monoclonal antibody was shown to localize on tumour cells when injected into mice bearing colon carcinoma xenograft[35] (Figure 3.5). Another monoclonal antibody B72-3 produced a relatively

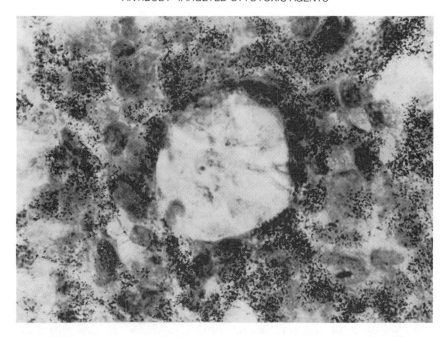

Figure 3.5 Anti-CEA monoclonal antibody localized on tumour cells after injection into a mouse bearing colon carcinoma xenograft

homogeneous staining of cells with antibody also being mucin-associated[36].

Vascularization of the tumour and rate of extravasation spread of antibody are important factors in penetration into tumours and the use of antibody F(ab′)₂ and Fab fragments may aid extravasation. For example, tumour localization tests with an anti-CEA monoclonal antibody (MAb35) in human colon carcinoma xenografts showed that F(ab′)₂ and Fab fragments gave 3.5 and 11.7 times higher tumour to non-tumour ratios[37]. Heterogeneity of antigen expression in tumour cell populations is a more fundamental problem. Immunohistological staining of tumour with many antitumour monoclonal antibodies shows that tissue staining is usually quite variable with regions of intense antibody localization through to areas showing no detectable reactivity. This heterogeneity of tumour antigen expression is further illustrated by flow cytometry tests in which monoclonal antibodies have been reacted with tumour cells derived from primary and metastatic colorectal carcinomas[38]. For example, positive binding with an anti-CEA monoclonal antibody (C24) was observed with 92% of the cell preparations isolated from 47 primary colorectal carcinomas. But the intensity of antibody binding within tumour cell populations was quite variable, so that 8% did not show significant reactivity, 11% showed weak reactivity, and 81% showed moderate or strong reactivity. A similar degree of variability in reactivity has been observed with other monoclonal antibodies reacting with colorectal carcinomas[38]. This has led to a further analysis aimed at defining the numbers of monoclonal antibodies required in 'cocktails' to essentially 'recognize' all of the malignant cells. Thus in one trial on primary colon carcinomas 98% reacted with at least two of a panel of five antibodies.

CONCLUSIONS

The potential of monoclonal antibodies for targeting cytotoxic molecules to tumour cells has been substantiated and clinical trials under way will determine the efficacy of drug and toxin conjugates in cancer treatment. Even so there are many features of this approach which require further investigation in order to optimize *in vivo* efficacy of immunoconjugates. The design of antibody conjugates has often been pursued on an empirical basis but one now anticipates that attention will be given to the design of more appropriate cytotoxic agents. These developments have to take into account the mode of action of immunoconjugates following binding to tumour cell membrane antigens. Immunotoxins are thought to enter cells by endocytosis through smooth microinvaginations or coated pits of the plasma membrane. Endocytosis of the methotrexate–antibody conjugates has been reported and is thought to involve adsorptive endocytosis. A clearer understanding of immunoconjugate internalization followed by release of cytotoxic agents from lysosomes is required.

One of the most important aspects of this approach to cancer treatment with murine monoclonal antibodies is the design of protocols which will minimize the development of anti-mouse antibodies, since once this occurs further therapy will be ineffectual. This is evident from imaging trials where patients receiving multiple, but interrupted, injections of radiolabelled antibody have developed anti-mouse antibody which has interfered with tumour localization (see Chapter 2). The generation of anti-mouse antibody will probably restrict treatment to a single course of antibody conjugate treatment designed so as to minimize host responses to mouse immunoglobulin. Alternatively, procedures will be required which prevent the generation of antibodies to mouse monoclonal antibodies.

References

1. Baldwin, R. W. and Byers, V. S. (eds.) (1985). *Monoclonal Antibodies for Cancer Detection and Therapy.* (London: Academic Press)
2. Springer, T. A. (ed.) (1985). *Hybridoma Technology in the Biosciences and Medicine.* (New York: Plenum Press)
3. Reisfeld, R. A. and Sell, S. (eds.) (1985). *Monoclonal Antibodies and Cancer Therapy.* Vol. 27. (New York: Alan R. Liss)
4. Baldwin, R. W. and Byers, V. S. (1986). Monoclonal antibodies in cancer treatment. *Lancet*, **1**, 603–5
5. Sells, S. (ed.) (1980). *Cancer Markers. Diagnostic and Developmental Significance.* (Clifton, NJ: Humana Press Inc.)
6. Shively, J. E. and Todd, C. W. (1980). Carcinoembryonic antigen A: chemistry and biology. In Sell, S. (ed.) *Cancer Markers, Diagnostic and Developmental Significance.* Ch. 11, pp. 295–314. (Clifton, NJ: Humana Press)
7. Sell, S. (1982). Hepatocellular carcinoma markers. In Sell, S. and Wahren, B. (eds.) *Human Cancer Markers.* Ch. 6, pp. 133–64. (Clifton, NJ: Humana Press)

8. Hellstrom, K. E. and Hellstrom, I. (1985). Monoclonal anti-melanoma antibodies and their possible clinical use. In Baldwin, R. W. and Byers, V. S. (eds.) *Monoclonal Antibodies for Cancer Detection and Therapy*. pp.17–51. (London: Academic Press)
9. Hakomori, S. (1984). Tumor-associated carbohydrate antigens. *Ann. Rev. Immunol.*, **2**, 103–26
10. Feizi, T. (1985). Demonstration by monoclonal antibodies that carbohydrate structures of glycoproteins and glycolipids are onco-developmental antigens. *Nature (London)*, **314**, 53–7
11. Burchell, J. M. and Taylor-Papadimitriou, J. (1985). Monoclonal antibodies to breast cancer and their application. In Baldwin, R. W. and Byers, V. S. (eds.) *Monoclonal Antibodies for Cancer Detection and Therapy*. Ch.1, pp. 1–15. (London: Academic Press)
12. Foon, K. A. and Morgan, A. C. Jr. (eds.) (1985). *Monoclonal Antibody Therapy of Human Cancer*. (Boston: Martinus Nijhoff)
13. Vitetta, E. S. and Uhr, J. W. (1985). Immunotoxins. *Ann. Rev. Immunol.*, **3**, 197–212
14. Frankel, A. E. and Houston, L. L. (1986). Immunotoxin therapy of cancer. In Carlo, D. (ed.) *Immunoconjugates and Cancer*. (Orlando: Academic Press). In press
15. Baldwin, R. W. and Byers, V. S. (1986). Immunotherapy of cancer. In Pinedo, H. M. and Chapner, B. A. *Cancer Chemotherapy Annual 8*. Ch. 13. pp. 209–23
16. Baldwin, R. W. and Byers, V. S. (1986). Monoclonal antibody targeting of cytotoxic agents for cancer therapy. *Progress in Immunology VI*. (*Academic Press*). In press
17. Embleton, M. J., Byers, V. S., Lee, H. M., Scannon, P., Blackhall, N. W. and Baldwin, R. W. (1986). Sensitivity and selectivity in ricin toxin A chain – monoclonal antibody 791T/36 conjugates against human tumor cell lines. *Cancer Res.*, **46**, 5524–8
18. Spitler, L. E., del Rio, M., Kentigan, A., Wedel, N. I., Brophy, N. A., Miller, L. L., Harkonen, W. S., Rosendorf, L. L., Shannon, C. E., Lee, H. M., Mischak, R. P., Kawahata, R. T., Stoudemire, J. B., Fradkin, L. B., Bautista, E. E., Dellio, C. L., Mendell, S. C. and Scannon, P. J. (1986). Therapy of patients with malignant melanoma using a monoclonal antimelanoma antibody-ricin A chain immunotoxin. *Cancer Res.*, submitted
19. Frankel, A. E. (1985). Antibody-toxin hybrids: a clinical review of their use. *J. Biol. Resp. Modif.*, **4**, 437–46
20. Jansen, F. K., Laurent, G., Liance, M. C., Blythman, H. E., Berthe, J., Canat, X., Carayon, P., Carriere, D., Casellas, P., Derocq, J. M., Dussossoy, D., Fauser, A. A., Gorin, N. C., Gros, O., Gros, P., Laurent, J. C., Poncelet, P., Remandet, B., Richer, G. and Vidal, H. (1985). Efficiency and tolerance of the treatment with immuno-A-chain-toxins in human bone marrow transplantations. In Baldwin, R. W. and Byers, V. S. (eds.) *Monoclonal Antibodies for Cancer Detection and Therapy*. pp. 224–48. (London: Academic Press)
21. Casellas, P., Bourrie, B. J. P., Gros, P. and Jansen, F. K. (1984). Kinetics of cytotoxicity induced by immunotoxins. Enhancement by lysosomotropic amines and carboxylic ionophores. *J. Biol. Chem.*, **259**, 9359–64
22. Carriere, D., Casellas, P., Richer, G., Gros, P. and Jansen, F. K. (1985). Endocytosis of an antibody ricin A-chain conjugate (Immuno-A-toxin) adsorbed on colloidal gold. *Exp. Cell Res.*, **156**, 327–40
23. Stirpe, F. and Barbieri, L. (1986). Ribosome-inactivating proteins up to date. *FEBS Letters*, **195**, 1–8
24. Thorpe, P. E., Detre, S. I., Foxwell, B. M. J., Brown, A. N. F., Skilleter, D. N., Wilson, G., Forrester, I. A. and Stirpe, F. (1985). Modification of the carbohydrate in ricin with metaperiodate-cyanoborohydride mixtures. *Eur. J. Biochem.*, **147**, 197–206
25. Bourrie, J. P., Casellas, P., Blythman, H. E. and Jansen, F. K. (1986). Study of the plasma clearance of antibody-ricin-A-chain immunotoxins. *Eur. J. Biochem.*, **155**, 1–10
26. Garnett, M. C. and Baldwin, R. W. (1986). An improved synthesis of a methotrexate-albumin-791T/36 monoclonal antibody conjugate cytotoxic to osteogenic sarcoma cell lines. *Cancer Res.*, **46**, 2407–12
27. Baldwin, R. W., Durrant, L., Embleton, M. J., Garnett, M., Pimm, M. V., Robins, R. A., Hardcastle, J. D., Armitage, N. and Ballantyne, K. (1985). Design and therapeutic evaluation of monoclonal antibody 791T/36-methotrexate conjugates. In Reisfeld, R. A. and Sell, S. (eds.) *Monoclonal Antibodies and Cancer Therapy*. pp. 215–31. (New York: Alan R. Liss)
28. Rowland, G. F., Axton, C. A., Baldwin, R. W., Brown, J. P., Corvalan, J. R. F., Embleton, M. J., Gore, V. A., Hellstrom, I., Hellstrom, K. E., Jacobs, E., Marsden, C. H., Pimm, M. V., Simmonds, R. G. and Smith, W. (1986). Anti-tumor properties of vindesine–monoclonal antibody conjugates. *Cancer Immunol. Immunother.*, **19**, 1–7

29. Baldwin, R. W. (1985). Design and development of drug–monoclonal antibody 791T/36 conjugate for cancer therapy. In Foon, K. A. and Morgan, A. C. Jr. (eds.) *Monoclonal Antibody Therapy of Human Cancer.* pp. 23–56. (Boston: Martinus Nijhoff)

30. Arnon, R. and Hurwitz, E. (1985). Monoclonal antibodies as carriers for immunotargeting of drugs. In Baldwin, R. W. and Byers, V. S. (eds.) *Monoclonal Antibodies for Cancer Detection and Therapy.* pp. 367–83. (London: Academic Press)

31. Rowland, G. F., Simmonds, R. G., Gore, V. A., Marsden, C. H. and Smith, W. (1986). Drug localisation and growth inhibition studies of vindesine–monoclonal anti-CEA conjugates in a human tumour xenograft. *Cancer Immunol. Immunother.*, **21**, 183–7

32. Armitage, N. C., Perkins, A. C., Pimm, M. V., Farrands, P. A., Baldwin, R. W. and Hardcastle, J. D. (1984). The localisation of an anti-tumour monoclonal antibody (791T/36) in gastrointestinal tumours. *Br. J. Surgery*, **71**, 407–12

33. Ballantyne, K. C., Perkins, A. C., Pimm, M. V., Garnett, M. C., Armitage, N. C., Baldwin, R. W. and Hardcastle, J. D. (1986). Biodistribution and tumour localisation of a monoclonal-antibody drug conjugate (791T/36-methotrexate). *Nucl. Med. Comm.*, **7**, 310

34. Pimm, M.V., Embleton, M. J., Perkins, A. C., Price, M. R., Robins, R. A., Robinson, G. R. and Baldwin, R. W. (1982). *In vivo* localization of anti-osteogenic sarcoma 791T monoclonal antibody in osteogenic sarcoma xenografts. *Int. J. Cancer*, **30**, 75–85

35. Pimm, M. V., Perkins, A. C., Armitage N. C. and Baldwin, R. W. (1985). Localization of anti-osteogenic sarcoma monoclonal antibody 791T/36 in a primary human osteogenic sarcoma and its subsequent xenograft in immunodeprived mice. *Cancer Immunol. Immunother.*, **19**, 18–21

36. Jones, P. L., Gallagher, B. M. and Sands, H. (1986). Autoradiographic analysis of monoclonal antibody distribution in human colon and breast tumor xenografts. *Cancer Immunol. Immunother.*, **22**, 139–43

37. Buchegger, F., Haskell, C. M., Schreyer, M., Scazziga, B. R., Randin, S., Carrel, S. and Mach, J-P. (1983). Radiolabeled fragments of monoclonal antibodies against carcinoembryonic antigen for localization of human colon carcinoma grafted into nude mice. *J. Exp. Med.*, **158**, 413–27

38. Durrant, L. G., Robins, R. A., Armitage, N. C., Brown, A., Baldwin, R. W. and Hardcastle, J. D. (1986). Association of antigen expression and DNA ploidy in colorectal tumors. *Cancer Res.*, **46**, 3543–9

4
Bone Marrow Transplantation

V. S. BYERS

INTRODUCTION

Over the last 15 years, a number of congenital and acquired disorders of the haematopoietic and lymphoid system have been demonstrated to benefit from allogeneic bone marrow transplantation (BMT). These diseases include varying kinds of leukaemias, aplastic anaemia, and congenital immunodeficiency disorders such as severe combined immunodeficiency syndrome (SCIDS) and the Wiskott–Aldrich syndrome. BMT is also beneficial in diseases with abnormalities in other haematopoietic progenitor cells such as hereditary platelet defects, abnormalities in macrophages or osteoclasts (Gaucher disease and osteopetrosis), or in diseases where a missing enzyme may be provided to the tissues, e.g. mucopolysaccharidoses.

Bone marrow transplantation takes advantage of the fact that under proper *in vivo* conditions the progenitor cells in the donor bone marrow will develop into mature haematopoietic cells in the recipient. Under certain conditions, it can be demonstrated that the circulating granulocytes, erythrocytes, platelets and lymphoid elements are derived from the donor bone marrow, and that neither the host lymphoid cells nor the donor lymphoid cells recognize the other as foreign. The actual transplant procedure is fairly standard. Heparinized marrow is harvested from an anaesthetized donor by multiple aspirations from the anterior and posterior iliac crests of the pelvis and the resultant 500–1000 cc of marrow (5×10^{10} cells) is pooled, heparinized, filtered, and subsequently administered intravenously. Most recipients must be intensively immunosuppressed prior to bone marrow transplantation. The purpose of the immunosuppression is to ablate host immunocompetent cells which could reject the graft, and to produce 'room' for the graft by myeloablation. No preparatory regimen is required in transplants between identical twins, nor in diseases such as SCIDS where the host immune reponse is already compromised. However, in other diseases the preparatory regimen, usually done during the week prior to transplant, must be intense enough to produce pancytopenia involving all the haematopoietic elements. Cytotoxic agents such as cyclophosphamide or total body irradiation are

the patients treated with BMT compared with 90% in those treated with conventional chemotherapy. However, the overall increased survival at 3 years was not improved to a statistically significant extent in the BMT group in any study because of complications associated with BMT such as GvHD and infectious disease[4]. Also the performance status in the BMT group was compromised by chronic GvHD. Nevertheless, all studies showed a trend to improved long-term survival with BMT, and BMT is certainly indicated for patients who have relapsed and who have suitable donors. BMT can also be justified over conventional therapy for those patients in first remission at high risk for leukaemic relapse or at low risk for GvHD. At present it can not be stated that BMT is preferred over chemotherapy for other AML patients in first remission but if the incidence of GvHD can be reduced, the potential of this modality can be fully realized.

Chronic myelogenous leukaemia (CML)

Although conventional chemotherapy may improve the quality of life of patients with CML, it does not delay or prevent blast crises or prolong life. Median survival is about 3 years; less than 20% of patients are alive at 5 years and there are no cures. The Philadelphia chromosome marks a clone of cells that are very resistant to chemotherapy, and after transition into blast crises only short remissions are attained with chemotherapy. The only chance of cure for such patients is allogeneic BMT.

Initial studies on allogeneic BMT in CML patients with accelerated phase or blast crises were very disappointing due to infection, leukaemic relapse, and incomplete engraftment. However, the results of BMT in chronic phase have been much more encouraging. Analysis of results submitted to an international registry by 23 centres, published in 1984[5] concluded that although transplant-related mortality of such patients was 30–35%, of those surviving, the risk of relapse within 2 years after BMT was only 5–10%. Recently, a study of allogeneic BMT for CML was performed comparing in a single centre BMT in chronic with that in accelerated phase, and the results were similar to those cited above. The survival rate among those transplanted in chronic phase (median follow-up of 25 months) was 72%; among those transplanted in advanced phase it was 18%. The probability of remaining in remission among these survivors was 93% in those transplanted in chronic phase as opposed to 58% in those transplanted in advanced phases[6].

Aplastic anaemia

Severe aplastic anaemia (granulocyte count less than 500 per mm^3, platelets less than 20000 per mm^3) is lethal for over 75% of patients, more than half of whom die within 6 months of diagnosis. Bone marrow transplantation can improve survival from 23% to 57%. Although GvHD and infection, usual complications of BMT, are seen here, graft rejection is a particular problem in aplastic anaemia. It has been documented that the graft rejection is characterized by initial successful engraftment followed by the replacement of donor-derived haematopoietic and lymphoid elements with presumably cyclophosphamide-resistant host lymphocytes. The cellular characteristics of graft rejection in patients with aplasia rejecting HLA-identical marrow transplants are not known, and the donor alloantigens against which these cells react are not defined. Graft rejection is significantly higher in patients who have been tranfused extensively, suggesting that the sensitization has occurred through prior blood transfusions .

Other indications

Bone marrow transplantation has long been the treatment of choice for SCIDS. This uniformly fatal disease responds to BMT with a 50–90% survival rate, particularly if transplantation occurs before the onset of debilitating pulmonary infections. The Wiskott–Aldrich syndrome, a sex-linked disorder affecting the life span and/or function of platelets and lymphocytes and manifested by recurrent sino-pulmonary infections with pyrogenic bacteria, herpes virus infections, eczema, and thrombocytopenia, is also amenable to BMT after cytoreduction.

Other immunodeficiency disorders for which there is no current therapy and which are candidate diseases for bone marrow transplantation include ataxia-telangiectasia, bare lymphocyte syndrome, nucleoside phosphorylase deficiency and chronic granulatomous disease[8].

HLA ANTIGENS

The antigen(s) involved in transplantation have been intensely studied. The strongest of the alloantigens are those coded by the major histocompatibility complex (MHC) locus on human chromosome 6. There are four clusters of human leukocyte antigens (HLA) which are coded by this chromosome: HLA-A, B, C, and D. The antigens are polymorphic and codominant; since a given individual has two number 6 chromosomes he will express two different sets of HLA antigens. The HLA antigens represent the major barrier to tissue transplantation and, until recently, if this barrier were crossed, as in HLA-mismatched donor–recipient pairs, the resultant GvHD was uniformly lethal. For this reason acceptable donors for conventional (non-depleted) marrows are HLA-matched siblings. Because one chromosome 6 is usually inherited *in toto* from each parent, the HLA region is also usually inherited as an intact HLA-A, B, C, and D haplotype. Thus, a patient with only one sibling has a one in four chance that that sibling will be HLA identical. In practice, most patients have more than one sibling so 40% of candidates have a suitable donor.

GRAFT-VERSUS-HOST DISEASE

Graft-versus-host disease (GvHD) has been recognized for many years as being initiated by engrafted immunocompetent donor T-lymphocytes reacting against alloantigens expressed on host cells, particularly cells of a haematopoietic system. GvHD is most commonly manifested by a maculo-papular rash, hepatitis, and diarrhoea. These symptoms are accompanied by

Table 4.1 Severity of individual organ involvement in graft versus host disease

---

Skin

+1	A maculopapular eruption involving less than 25% of the body surface
+2	A maculopapular eruption involving 25–50% of the body surface
+3	Generalized erythroderma
+4	Generalized erthyroderma with bullous formation and often with desquamation

Liver

+1	Moderate increase of SGOT (150–750 IU) and bilirubin (2.0–3.0 mg/100 ml)
+2	Bilirubin rise (3–5.9 mg/100 ml) with or without an increase in SGOT
+3	Bilirubin rise (6–14.9 mg/100 ml) with or without an increase in SGOT
+4	Bilirubin rise to >15 mg/100 ml with or without an increase in SGOT.

Increases in SGOT were temporarily related to either the onset or worsening of the skin rash

Gut

Diarrhoea, nausea, and vomiting were graded +1 to +4 in severity, and the severity of gut involvement was assigned to the most severe involvement noted. It was difficult to quantitate most of these manifestations except for diarrhoea

Diarrhoea

+1	>500 ml of stool/day
+2	>1000 ml of stool/day
+3	>1500 ml of stool/day
+4	>2000 ml of stool/day

---

lymphocytic infiltrates into periarteriolar regions and into the dermal-epidermal junction of the skin, epithelium at the base of the tongue, oesophagus, pharynx, and the crypts and villi of the small or large intestine, with necrosis of host cells in involved tissues.

GvHD is graded according to clinical and histopathological parameters (see Tables 4.1 and 4.2). When mild, GvHD can be manifested only by a

Table 4.2 Staging of graft versus host disease

Based on the severity and number of organ systems involved, patients are placed into four categories

Grade 1   is +1–+2 skin rash without gut involvement with more than +1 liver involvement, and no decrease in performance status or fever.

Grade 2   is +1–+3 skin rash with either +1–+2 gastrointestinal involvement or +1–+2 liver involvement, or both. All grade 2 patients exhibit a mild decrease in performance status and some have fever.

Grade 3   is +2–+4 skin rash with +2–+4 gastrointestinal involvement with or without +2–+4 liver involvement. All patients exhibit a marked decrease in performance status and many have fever.

Grade 4   is pattern and severity of GvHD similar to grade 3 with extreme constitutional symptoms.

---

transient skin rash; when more severe, the manifestations may directly lead to death or so compromise immunologic and haematologic reconstitution as to foster infectious complications causing increased morbidity or death.

Experiments in numerous rodent models have demonstrated that mature T-lymphocytes cause GvHD after allogeneic marrow or spleen cell grafting. GvHD does not occur in irradiated animals when the graft is devoid of mature T-cells. Transplanted fetal liver cells or spleen cells from neonatally thymectomized mice can reconstitute normal haematopoiesis without causing acute GvHD. Furthermore, removal of mature T-cells from allogeneic donor spleen cells with the use of anti-Thy-1 heteroantisera, or monoclonal antibodies, can prevent GvHD. As few as 3×10^4 total T-cells can cause GvHD in recipient mice with disparity only for non-H-2 minor histocompatibility antigens. Prevention of lethal GvHD by removal of mature T-cells has also been demonstrated in other species, specifically the rat, dog and primates.

The aetiology of GvHD when it involves T-cell reaction against HLA antigens is clear; however, acute GvHD also develops in 30–70% of patients transplanted with HLA-matched bone marrow and may be a direct or indirect cause of death in 20–40% of these affected individuals. It is generally accepted that the reaction is initiated by the donor T-cells[1], although the antigens with which they react still remain unclear. Since the donors and recipients are HLA-matched, the reactivity is probably directed against non-HLA antigens.

The development of grade II–IV GvHD after BMT is associated with decreased survival. Roughly 40% of patients with grade II disease die or develop chronic GvHD, and about 80% of those with grade III/IV disease die. Death may be either from GvHD or from infection, usually interstitial pneumonia. The infectious deaths may be indirectly due to GvHD. Processes such as virus-induced pneumonias are increased in patients with GvHD, and rare in patients transplanted with an identical twin.

In the majority of patients, acute GvHD begins within 30 days posttransplant. The incidence and severity increase with age, as well as among individuals prepared for transplant with total body irradiation. Marrow transplants for older patients with chronic myelogenous leukaemia are associated with an incidence of GvHD approaching 70%, and an increased frequency of severe grade III/IV disease. Recent analysis from the International Bone Marrow Transplant Register of 1871 patients receiving HLA-identical sibling donors BMT indicated the overall incidence of GvHD grade II or greater was 44%.

Apart from recipient age the risk was highest when female donors were used for male recipients, especially if the donors had undergone pregnancy or transfusion, increasing their risk of being sensitized to cell antigens.

Therapy of GvHD has included prophylactic methotrexate (MTX), antithymocyte globulin (ATG), cyclosporin, or steroids. Although these agents continue to be used, controlled studies have not demonstrated the superiority of a particular treatment over another or that any of these agents improve survival. ATG carries the additional significant risk of anaphylaxis in patients, particularly those with aplastic anaemia who have received it before.

It also exhibits significant cytotoxicity to progenitor cells. However, most centres include prophylactic MTX in their conventional (non-T-cell depleted) allogeneic HLA-identical BMT regimens because of its relatively low toxicity and the belief that it does help in preventing this complication. Most centres are now increasing the mean age of their patients undergoing BMT and the search continues for newer agents which will decrease the high incidence of GvHD in these older populations. Recently Storb et al.[10] completed a randomized trial of prophylactic MTX and cyclosporin A compared with cyclosporin A alone in HLA-matched BMT. All patients engrafted, and there was a significant decrease in grade II–IV GvHD in patients receiving both drugs.

For established GvHD, steroids, ATG or both remain the standard therapy. In a comparative study, both agents improved skin and gut manifestations but liver involvement remained untouched. Overall there was no difference between the two modalities. Other modalities are now being evaluated, such as anti-T-lymphocyte immunotoxin, discussed later.

Bone marrow recipients are also at risk for a chronic form of GvHD, which is clinically akin to scleroderma, with characteristic changes of the skin, xerostomia, xerophthalmia, and malabsorption. This chronic GvHD with associated infection is observed in 25–40% of long-term survivors of allogenic BMT. Older patient age and prior acute GvHD increase risk of developing this complication. Two forms of the disease are noted: those with disease of skin and/or liver only where the outcome may be favourable even without treatment; and those with extensive (multi-organ) disease where there is only 20% survival without therapy. Prednisone and trimethoprim-sulphoxazole is the usual treatment. Morbidity is due to contractures and pulmonary obstructive disease. It is now being realized that GvHD is a disease of immune dysregulation and death is usually due to bacterial infection.

BMT FROM NON-HLA-IDENTICAL SIBLINGS

Because about 60% of BMT candidates lack HLA-identical siblings, other methods are under investigation to expand the donor population. These include haploidentical related donors, and HLA-matched non-related donors. In one recent study with haploidentical donors it was found that such grafts were associated with delayed engraftment and an increase in graft failure, as well as acute GvHD. There was, however, no increase in leukaemic relapse over patients given HLA-identical sibling grafts and there was no difference in survival[11]. These data are encouraging since they suggest that if GvHD and graft rejection can be controlled, such grafts may be suitable for BMT.

T-CELL-DEPLETED MARROW TRANSPLANTS

Since GvHD is initiated by mature T-cells in the donor bone marrow, attention has been focussed on selectively depleting the marrow of such cells.

This technique has reduced the incidence of GvHD in HLA-matched sibling BMT, and for the first time, allowed the HLA barrier to be crossed, so that HLA non-identical BMT can be accomplished.

In human transplantation, donor bone marrow usually contains about 10^{10} nucleated cells of which 10–20%, or 10^9, represent mature T-cells. These mature T-lymphocytes probably originate from blood co-aspirated with the marrow. Since the entire marrow is transfused into recipients a substantial number of mature T-lymphocytes are also infused. If 99% depletion of these cells can be attained this could substantially reduce the donor cell burden. Various methods have been used to deplete T-cells from bone marrow, and those currently in clinical trials use soybean lectin/sheep red cells, or monoclonal antibodies.

Much clinical experience has been gained with the serial use of soybean lectin agglutin and E rosette formation both of which remove mature T-lymphocytes. It has reduced clinically significant (grade II+) acute GvHD in acute leukaemics from an incidence of 50–70%, to one of less than 5% among HLA-matched sibling donor recipient pairs. It has virtually eliminated the risk of chronic GvHD, and permits the use of HLA-haplotype mismatched marrow grafts without risk of severe or lethal GvHD[12].

Early investigations demonstrated that treatment of marrow with unmodified murine monoclonal antibodies in the absence of exogenous complement did not prevent GvHD, presumably because it did not produce adequate depletion of T-cells. Several centres have demonstrated that complement fixing monoclonal anti-T-lymphocyte monoclonal antibodies in the presence of exogenous rabbit complement does produce depletion, and cocktails of such antibodies are now being used. These are either complement fixing murine monoclonal antibodies directed against one of the pan T-lymphocyte antigens which are used with rabbit complement, or rat IgM antibodies such as CAMPATH 1, which fix human complement and can be used in combination with the donor's own serum. A third type of depletion is attained by anti-pan T immunotoxins which consist either of conjugates of the plant toxin ricin, or of A-chain coupled to anti-T-lymphocyte antibodies.

Table 4.3 summarizes recently published reports from six centres. Depletion of progenitor cells as measured by *in vitro* assays is not a problem with any of the techniques, and most studies demonstrated a significant decrease in incidence and severity of GvHD if the depletion is at least 99%.

There is probably a threshold of the number of mature T-lymphocytes which may be transplanted with bone marrows; and above this number the incidence of GvHD is markedly increased. One centre reports that of 25 patients engrafted with HLA-identical sibling marrows, those receiving less than 1×10^5 T-lymphocytes/kg did not develop GvHD, while 50% of those receiving $1–4 \times 10^5$ T-cells/kg developed skin GvHD[13]. This suggests that 99% T-cell depletion is necessary to prevent GvHD in HLA-matched BMT.

T-cell depletion methods have, for the first time, allowed the use of HLA-mismatched transplants without the high incidence of GvHD which characterizes non-depleted marrows. Non-matched donor–recipient pairs have seldom been used in the past. With T-cell depletion from familial marrows,

conventionally transplanted group. In another study with CAMPATH-1 depleted BMT in CML, the incidence of GvHD was substantially reduced in T-cell depleted BMT patients but leukaemic relapse was increased[16].

AUTOLOGOUS BMT (ABMT)

Leukaemias

Even with depletion procedures, allogeneic BMT is limited by GvHD and infection. These problems increase with age so patients over 40 years of age, as well as those with no suitable donors, are ineligible for this modality. One alternative is to treat those patients with autologous BMT using marrow obtained during remission and stored until relapse or until elective intensive chemo/radiotherapy is completed. Experience with BMT between identical twins has shown that both GvHD and infection are reduced with this modality. If autologous marrow could be obtained free of tumour cells, similar results might be obtained. The results of initial trials have not been encouraging, however. Thus, for example, one study treated AML patients in relapse with chemo/radiotherapy and autologous BMT collected from marrows when patients were in first or second remission. Only 5% showed long-term survival as compared to 24% of similar patients treated with BMT from identical twins[21]. This underscores the additional problem with such techniques: one does not know if the relapse was peripheral or from tumour cells infused with the BMT. For this reason, attention was turned to purging autologous BMT with monoclonal antibodies directed against antigens on the tumour cells but which spare the progenitor cells. Several studies have used monoclonal antibodies (mabs) directed against the common acute lymphocytic leukaemia antigen (CALLA) present on about 70% of the patients with ALL. Such mabs do not destroy the progenitor cells and allow effective engraftment. However, the long-term survival of such patients was relatively poor[22], and lack of randomized studies make it difficult to compare long-term survival with that of patients treated with allogeneic BMT. The central problem with this modality remains the difficulty of determining if relapse is due to inadequate chemo/radiotherapy, inadequate BMT purging, or the loss of an antileukaemic effect which would be produced by allogeneic BMT.

Solid tumours

Several solid tumours are being considered for autologous BMT with purged bone marrows. One of these is small bronchogenic carcinoma. This tumour is quite responsive to chemotherapy with approximately 60% complete remission rate, but few of these are durable. There is a dose–response effect of most of the drugs active in this disease, and the drugs are also predominantly toxic to bone marrow. This suggests that supratoxic drug therapy with autologous BMT could improve survival in the disease. Since the tumour is haematogenously spread and a large number of patients have contaminated marrows at presentation, *in vitro* purging should be beneficial. One study carried out with non-purged bone marrow did indicate haematopoietic recovery was attained but the rate of long-term survival was disappointing[21]. Nevertheless, this approach with mab purged marrows continues under investigation in solid tumours including breast and neuroblastoma.

CONCLUSION

Allogeneic BMT is now an established modality in acute leukaemias and chronic mylogenous leukaemia at certain phases. It is at least as good as conventional chemotherapy at producing long-term survivals in acute leukaemia. Chronic myelogenous leukaemia is still under investigation but since the Philadelphia chromosome-bearing cells are very refractory to chemotherapy, it is anticipated that CML in first remission may prove to be the clearest indication of all the leukaemias for BMT. BMT has been the primary therapeutic modality in aplastic anaemia and immunodeficiency disorders for several years, and its benefit in these diseases is clear.

Since only 40% of candidates for BMT have suitable HLA-matched related donors, attention has turned to other methods by which this pool can be expanded. These include HLA-haploidentical related donors (matched at only one of HLA genomes), HLA-matched non-related donors, and HLA-mismatched non-related donors whose marrows are depleted of T-cells prior to transplant. It is probable that any of these donor pools will prove suitable once adequate T-cell depletion methods are established.

The complications of T-cell depleted BMT are increased leukaemic relapse and graft failure/rejection. In part these are probably an inevitable result of decreased GvHD since it is known that syngeneic BMT also has an increased incidence of leukaemic relapse. However, there is hope that more selective removal of T-cells, or exogenous addition of soluble factors may ameliorate graft failure/rejection and leukaemic relapse. T-cell depletion is the most important advance in BMT for many years. Its importance has already been demonstrated and it is hoped that additional refinements will occur in the next several years that will allow the technique to be expanded to additional patients both by establishment of new clinical centres with experience in this modality and by recruitment of additional (non-HLA-matched) donors.

References

1. O'Reilly, R. J. (1983). Allogeneic bone marrow transplantation: current status and future directions. *Blood*, **62**, 941–64
2. Buckner, C. D. and Clift, R. A. (1984). Marrow transplantation for acute lymphoblastic leukaemia. *Semin. Hematol.*, **21**, 43–7
3. Powles, R. L., Morgenstern, G., Clink, M., Hedley, D., Bandini, G., Lumley, H., Watson, J. G., Lawson, D., Spence, D., Barrett, A., Jameson, B., Lawler, S., Kay, H. E. M. and McElwain, T. J. (1980). The place of bone marrow transplantation in acute myelogenous leukaemia. *Lancet*, **1**, 1047–50
4. Champlin, R. E. and Golde, D. W. (1985). Chronic myelogeneous leukaemia: recent advances. *Blood*, **65**, 1039–47
5. Speck, B., Gratwohl, A., Osterwalder, B. and Nissen, C. (1984). Bone marrow transplantation for chronic myeloid leukaemia. *Semin. Hematol.*, **21**, 48–52
6. Goldman, J. M., Apperley, J. F., Jones, L., Marcus, R., Goolden, A. W. G., Batchelor, R., Waldmann, H., Reid, C. D., Hows, J., Gordon-Smith, E., Catovsky, D. and Galton, D. A.

G. (1986). Bone marrow transplantation for patients with chronic myeloid leukaemia. *N. Engl. J. Med.*, **314**, 202-7

7. Storb, R., Prentice, R. L. and Thomas, E. D. (1977). Marrow transplantation for treatment of aplastic anaemia: an analysis of factors associated with graft rejection. *N. Engl. J. Med.*, **296**, 61-6

8. O'Reilly, R. J., Brochstein, J., Dinsmore, R. and Kirkpatrick, D. (1984). Marrow transplantation for congenital disorders. *Semin. Hematol.*, **21**, 188-222

9. Glucksberg, H., Storb, R., Fefer, A., Buckner, C. D., Neiman, P. E., Clift, R. A., Lerner, K. G. and Thomas, E. D. (1974). Clinical manifestations of graft-versus-host disease in human recipients of marrow from HL-A-matched sibling donors. *Transplantation*, **18**, 295-304

10. Storb, R., Deeg, H. J., Whitehead, J., Appelbaum, F., Beatty, P., Bensinger, W., Buckner, C. D., Clift, R., Doney, R., Farewell, V., Hansen, J., Hill, R., Lum, L., Martin, P., McGuffin, R., Sanders, J., Stewart, P., Sullivan, K., Witherspoon, R., Yee, G. and Thomas, E. D. (1986). Methotrexate and cyclosporine compound with cyclosporine alone for prophylaxis of acute graft versus host disease after marrow transplantation for leukaemia. *N. Engl. J. Med.*, **314**, 729-35

11. Beatty, P. G., Clift, R. A., Mickelson, E. M., Nipersos, B. B., Flournoy, N., Martin, P. J., Sanders, J. E., Stewart, P., Buckner, C. D., Storb, R., Thomas, E. D. and Hansen, J. A. (1985). Marrow transplantation from related donors other than HLA-identical siblings. *N. Engl. J. Med.*, **313**, 765-71

12. O'Reilly, R. J., Collins, N. H., Kernan, N., Brochstein, J., Dinsmore, R., Kirkpatrick, D., Siena, S., Keever, C., Jordan, B., Shank, B., Wolf, L., Dupont, B. and Reisner, Y. (1985). Transplantation of marrow-depleted T-cells by soybean lectin agglutination and E-rosette depletion: major histocompatibility complex-related graft resistance in leukaemic transplant recipients. *Transplant. Proc.*, **17**, 455-9

13. Kernan, N. A. (1986). A direct relationship between clonable T lymphocytes in a T-cell depleted bone marrow transplant and the subsequent development of graft versus host disease. *Blood*, In press

14. Martin, P. J., Hansen, J. A., Buckner, C. D., Sanders, J. E., Deeg, H. K., Stewart, P., Applebaum F. R., Clift, R., Fefer, A., Witherspoon, R. P., Kennedy, M. S., Sullivan, K. M., Flournoy, N., Storb, R. and Thomas, E. D. (1985). Effects of *in vitro* depletion of T cells in HLA-identical allogeneic marrow grafts. *Blood*, **66**, 664-72

15. Mitsuyasu, A., Champlin, R. W., Ho, W. G., Sinston, D., Feig, S., Wells, J., Terasaki, P., Billing, R., Weaver, M. and Gale, R. P. (1985). Prospective randomized controlled trial of *ex vivo* treatment of donor bone marrow with monoclonal anti-T cell antibody and complement for prevention of graft-versus-host disease: a preliminary report. *Transplant. Proc.*, **17**, 482-5

16. Apperley, J. F., Jones, L., Hale, G., Waldmann, H., Hows, J., Rombos, Y., Tsatalas, C., Marcus, R. E., Goolden, A. W. G., Gordon-Smith, E. C., Catovsky, D., Galton, D. A. G. and Goldman, J. M. (1986). Bone marrow transplantation for patients with chronic myeloid leukaemia: T-cell depletion with Campath-1 reduces incidence of graft-verus-host disease but may increase risk of leukaemic relapse. *Bone Marrow Transplant.*, **1**, In press

17. Filopovich, A. H., Vallera, D. A., Youle, R. J., Neville, D. M. Jr. and Kersey, J. H. (1985). *Ex vivo* T cell depletion with immunotoxins in allogeneic bone marrow transplantation: the pilot clinical study for prevention of graft-versus-host disease. *Transplant. Proc.*, **17**, 442-4

18. Martin, P. J., Hansen, J. A., Storb, R. and Thomas, E. D. (1985). A clinical trial of *in vitro* depletion of T cells in donor marrow for prevention of acute graft-versus-host disease. *Transplant. Proc.*, **17**, 486-7

19. Prentice, H. G., Blacklock, H. A., Jovossy, G., Gilmore, M. J. M. L., Price-Jones, L., Tidman, N., Trejdosiewicz, L. K., Skeggs, D. B. L., Panjwani, D., Balls, S., Graphakos, S., Patterson, J., Ivory, K. and Hoffbrand, A. V. (1984). Depletion of T lymphocytes in donor marrow prevents significant graft-versus-host disease in matched allogeneic leukaemic marrow transplant recipients. *Lancet*, **1**, 472-6

20. Waldmann, H., Polliak, A., Hale, G., Or, R., Cividalli, G., Weiss, L., Weshler, Z., Samuel, J. S., Mannor, D., Brautbar, C., Rachmilewitz, E. A. and Slavin, S. (1984). Elimination of graft-versus-host disease by *in vitro* depletion of alloreactive lymphocytes with a

monoclonal rat anti-human lymphocyte antibody (Campath-1). *Lancet*, **2**, 483–6

21. Dickie, K. A., Jagannath, S., Spitzer, G., Poynton, C., Zander, A., Vellekoop, L., Reading, C. L., Jehn, U. W. and Tindle, S. (1984). The role of autologous bone marrow transplantation in various malignancies. *Semin. Hematol.*, **21**, 109–22

22. Bast, R. C. Jr., Sallan, S. E., Reynolds, C., Lipton, J. and Ritz, J. (1986). Autologous bone marrow transplantation for CALLA-positive acute lymphoblastic leukaemia: an update. *Autologous Bone Marrow Transplantation. Proceedings First International Symposium*, pp. 3–6

5
Immunomodulating Agents

B. M. VOSE

A major factor limiting the eradication of malignant disease from cancer patients is the early appearance of metastatic foci. While surgical and radiological intervention can be used to treat the primary tumour, it is these secondary deposits which are the targets for systemic therapeutic modalities. The finding that metastases show considerable phenotypic variation, including the evolution of clones which are resistant to available chemo-therapeutic drugs, has had an impact on drug scheduling and has altered the direction of research in this area. In addition to programmes seeking new, more effective or less toxic cytotoxic agents exploiting differences between normal and tumour cells, considerable interest has been shown in the possibility that augmentation of the immunological host defence against cancer could lead to therapeutic benefit. The spectacular accumulation of knowledge of the molecular mechanisms controlling the immune system and the description of a variety of different effector cells in the antitumour response engender great optimism that immunotherapy will become a fourth arm of cancer treatment in addition to surgery, radiation and chemotherapy. A major research effort is being applied to the search for immunomodulating agents which seek to alter the balance of the tumour–host interaction.

At least three routes to effective manipulation of the immune system can be considered:

(1) Defined small molecular weight chemical entities,
(2) Microbial products, a category including Bacille Calmette Guérin (BCG) and *Corynebacterium parvum* which have been widely tested for their effects in cancer patients and which brought about much of the early optimism for an immunological approach to cancer treatment, and
(3) Lymphokines and cytokines – the products of the immune cells themselves.

Each of these different approaches may yield products with influence parti-cular parts of the antitumour response. Before reviewing the different

70

approaches which may yield therapeutically useful agents, it is appropriate to consider the nature of the defence mechanisms which will be the targets for immunomodulators.

THE IMMUNE RESPONSE AGAINST HUMAN CANCER

There is an undoubted role for the immune system in protection against some induced malignancies in experimental animals as evidenced by the resistance of animals to tumour challenge following immunization (see Chapter 1). It has, however, proved more difficult to obtain definitive data showing the capacity of spontaneous animal tumours and human cancer to evoke an effective, specific host response. In spite of these problems, there is now sufficient information from many sources to conclude that human tumours can be subject to attack by a variety of different cell types including cytotoxic T-cells, macrophages, natural killer cells and the more recently described lymphokine activated killers (LAK). Each of these effectors employs different lytic mechanisms so that the cells of different tumours may show susceptibility to a spectrum of killer cells. While there appears to be no universally effective surveillance system against the initiation of the malignant process, the possibility is high that augmentation of at least some of these functions by immunomodulators will lead to clinical benefit. In addition, the finding that many of these effector cells secrete proteins which are themselves lytic for transformed cells such as tumour necrosis factor, lymphotoxin and natural killer cytotoxic factor offers the possibility that these molecules may also be clinically useful as they become available as recombinant DNA products.

Two important factors influencing the feasibility of an immunological approach to cancer therapy must be that the antitumour effector cells identified in *in vitro* studies are present at the tumour site or can be induced to localize there and that the phenotypic variability among metastases mentioned above does not lead to loss of the critical surface determinants which the effectors recognize. The major emphasis of the published work has centred on the investigation of antitumour effectors in the blood, spleen or peritoneal cavity. The data obtained have revealed an impressive array of cells with the ability to lyse tumour cells, but are of limited value in predicting the relative importance of different immunological components in cancer control since sequestration of reactive cells in the tumour may lead to a corresponding depletion in the periphery. Conversely, cells in the circulation or resident if different organs could, because they do not enter the tumour, have little relevance to the therapy of established disease (though they may have considerable efficacy against blood-borne metastases). Increasingly, studies are directed towards measurement of effector function at other, less easily sampled compartments[1].

The nature of the *in situ* antitumour response has been reviewed recently[2]. Monoclonal antibodies have allowed the immunohistological detection of macrophages and T-lymphocytes in many neoplasms. A limited number of observations, suggesting that the presence of inflammatory infiltrates is a favourable prognostic sign in some tumour types, testifies to their biological significance. There have also been functional studies which point to the effector role of the cells infiltrating both human and experimental tumours. Cytotoxic T-lymphocytes and their precursors and cytolytic macrophages have been isolated from malignant tissue and have the capacity to kill autologous tumour cells. Surprisingly, cells of the NK phenotype, which have been the subject of much recent discussion, have been found only rarely in human tumours and isolated cells express poor lytic activity against susceptible cell lines. This, together with the low susceptibility of freshly isolated tumour cells to lysis by blood effectors, argues against a major role for NK in control of established cancer and their true biological importance awaits definition.

The immunological response to malignancy, as evidenced by the finding of different effector cell types, encourages consideration of immunotherapy even though the nature of the cancer cell surface determinants, critical for effector cell recognition, remain unknown. However, it is also clear that, by a number of criteria, the immune system of cancer patients can become increasingly compromised with progressive disease. This diminished responsiveness has been attributed to the appearance of cells which down-regulate the immune system (suppressor cells) and which have the phenotype of monocytes/macrophages or T-lymphocytes. This, together with other mechanisms by which tumours may escape the effects of the immune system (antigen shedding or modulation, tumour heterogeneity) means that the goal of the cancer immunotherapist will not be easy and any attempt to intervene in the complex pattern of the host–tumour relationship will be successful only when the critical effectors are identified. The simplistic view that a general boost of the immune system with all its interactive components will lead to arrest of tumour growth seems naive.

TARGETS FOR IMMUNOMODULATION

Consideration of the host response to tumour suggests several targets of immunomodulation. These include the macrophage, cytotoxic and helper T-cells, suppressor cells and natural killer cells. The evidence for a role of these cells in the reaction against cancer and means by which their activity might be increased or controlled will now be considered.

Macrophages

There is evidence that both animal and human tumours contain significant numbers of macrophages recognizable cytochemically, immunologically and functionally (reviewed in ref. 2).

An increasing number of studies have reported that these cells, at an appropriate stage of activation, show selective and efficient lytic activity against tumour cells while leaving non-transformed cells intact. They may also inhibit cell division without inducing lysis (cytostasis). The cytolytic process is mediated only after cell–cell contact but proceeds via the secretion of a multiplicity of soluble products including cytolytic proteases, oxygen radicals, arginase and complement breakdown products as well as tumour necrosis factor. Activation to the tumoricidal state involves two separate signals – lymphokines derived from T-lymphocytes and endotoxin[3]. Responsive macrophages, after treatment with lymphokine, are primed to respond to endotoxin and express their full cytolytic potential. One of the lymphokines involved in this activation process is γ interferon but evidence is emerging that other macrophage activating factors are also effective[4].

The potent and antitumour-selective effector function of activated macrophages has made them prime candidates for immunomodulation and several groups have now shown that it is possible to induce increased tumour protection in animal models by this route. Much of the attention has focussed in two areas – natural products of bacterial fermentation and macrophage activating lymphokines. However, it is important to recognize that macrophages may also have the capacity to down-regulate immune reactivity and act as suppressors of NK and lymphocyte function and may induce other effects such as intravascular aggregation of neutrophils or production of neutral proteases such as collagenase, which actually increase the metastatic spread of tumour cells. This adverse activity of transferred macrophages is exemplified in recent studies of Gorelik *et al.* in which transfer of macrophages elicited by thioglycollate medium increased the number of metastatic foci of B16 melanoma in the lungs of injected mice[5]. Thus, activation protocols need to be monitored to ensure that cytolytic and not suppressor functions are increased. An imporant marker of this process may be decreased RNA synthesis and imbalanced accumulation of ribosomal RNA which occurs as cytotoxic but not suppressor functions are increased[6].

A leading group in the studies of macrophage activators in cancer treatment is that led by Isiah Fidler. In a series of elegant studies this group has been able to obtain impressive therapeutic benefit in animal models by inclusion of a variety of activators in liposomes. The *in vitro* activation of human monocytes to a tumoricidal state has also been described[7,8]. Two critical points emerge from these data:

(1) That a variety of agents derived from bacterial fermentation including muramyl dipeptide (MDP the minimal material of BCG which has adjuvant activity) and its lipophilic derivatives as well as lymphokines such as γ interferon, which augment macrophage activity *in vitro* induce antitumour effects in different animal models, and

(2) That incorporation of material in multi-lammelar vesicles leads to a considerable increase of the efficacy of these activators by targeting the molecule to the reticuloendothelial system and by prolonging the persistence of the stimulator in the body.

These findings, together with those of other authors using different agents, clearly point to the potential of macrophage activators in tumour therapy and work is proceeding towards the enhancement or prolongation of activity. The findings that lipophilic muramyl peptide derivatives such as MTP-PE [N-acetylmuramyl-L-alanyl-D-isoglutamy l-L-alanyl-2-(1',2'-dipalmitoyl-sn-glycero-3' phosphoryl)-ethylamide] show more potent effects and that they

T-cell and the natural killer cells, a further lymphoid cell population can manifest potent lytic activity against tumour target cells – the lymphokine-activated killer cells[25]. The precursors of LAK can be induced to lytic activity by exposure to the T-cell-derived lymphokine interleukin-2 and are then able to lyse a range of NK resistant targets including freshly isolated tumour cells but not normal cells. These precursors can be distinguished from both T-cells and NK cells on the basis of surface phenotype and are found in several sites including bone marrow, thoracic duct and within the tumour mass[26]. Evidence[27] now points to the fact that these LAK cells can mediate potent antitumour effects in animal models when co-administered with recombinant interleukin-2. More importantly, therapeutic effects have now been seen in a preliminary trial in man with objective remission observed in 11 of 25 patients with a variety of different tumour types previously shown to be resistant to conventional therapy[28].

The protocol used in this trial involved stimulation of large numbers of patients' leukocytes obtained by repeated leukophoresis with recombinant IL-2 for 3 days. Stimulated cells were then reinfused together with IL-2. While the possibility of passive cell therapy of cancer has been discussed for several years[29] this report is, to my knowledge, the most dramatic example of its successful application and clearly indicates the high potential for immunotherapy of a broad spectrum of human malignancy. Much remains to be done to optimize the treatment but, for the first time, we have an example of successful therapy by a defined effector mechanism of experimental and clinical cancer. It should do much to encourage further effort in the search for alternative immunologically-based therapeutic modalities.

DIFFERENT CATEGORIES OF IMMUNOMODULATORS

It is clear from the foregoing discussion that many products have been developed which show immunomodulating activity. It is outside the scope of this report to detail the studies which have been performed with them to identify their activity profile. The interested reader is referred to a recent publication[30]. As stated previously, the search for active agents has concentrated on products of biological origin such as micro-organisms (BCG and *C. parvum*) and extracts at various stages of purification, on natural products and their analogues (retinoids, lentinen) or on synthetic compounds (levamisole, cimetidine, isoprinosine). A further compound group which has come to the fore since the introduction of molecular biology has been the products of the immune system such as lymphokines and cytokines. Several of these molecules are now available in amounts which enable investigation of their clincal efficacy. Amongst these are interleukin-2 which has potent stimulatory activity on T-cells, NK cells and B-cells and which is the inducer of LAK activity, and γ-interferon which is a potent macrophage activator and B-cell differentiation inducer, and colony stimulating factors which expand different populations with the granulocyte/macrophage series and may be useful as promoters of bone marrow proliferation, so overcoming the depletion of neutrophils induced by conventional tumour therapy protocols.

In addition, protein products directly toxic for tumour cells – lymphotoxin and tumour necrosis factors – are now available and undergoing clinical trial.

The interferons were the first of this type of product to undergo extensive testing. From the beginning it was unclear which of the several properties of the interferons was of major importance in any antitumour effects – antiproliferative or immunomodulating. It was for this reason that testing of interferons escalated to the maximum tolerated dose as would be appropriate for a standard cytotoxic rather than the determination of an immunomodulating dose. Indeed, the efficacy of the interferons as immunomodulators in man must still remain in doubt since few studies have addressed the problem. This raises the whole question of what would constitute a satisfactory trial of immunomodulators given that, with the majority of defined chemical entities tested to date, the window of dose giving effects on the immune system has been small. The testing of new classes of anticancer agents will require re-evaluation of trial design if meaningful data are to be obtained. Certainly the determination of maximum tolerated doses in advanced cancer patients, in whom the immunological apparatus is already compromised, appears questionable. The known species differences in response to some immunomodulators and the species specificity of products of the immune system further complicate this situation.

The testing of products in animal models of dubious relevance to the human disease must be of limited value in study design although it may give information on efficacy and delineate the potential sites of action of the agent. The trials in animals of the LAK system had a major impact on the development of the clinical protocol. The process of trial design must then involve careful evaluation of the effects of treatment on immunological activity of the critical effector system. There is a widely held opinion that immunomodulators are likely to be effective only in the presence of limited residual disease or as adjuvant therapy with or without contemporaneous treatment with more conventional agents. Their testing as single agents in advanced cancer patients who have failed to respond to other treatment modalities appears therefore to be unnecessarily restrictive.

IMMUNOMODULATORS – A PERSPECTIVE

Modification of the immune response of the host against his cancer to obtain therapeutic benefit can be viewed either with an optimism based on the efficacy of many of the agents described above on cancer in animals or with a pessimism based on the failure of tumour immunology to identify the critical immunogenic moieties on the cancer cells recognized by the effectors which would offer scientific rationale to the approach. What is clear already is that there is no simple approach to the identification of effective treatments.

A major limitation to study design is that the critical effector mechanisms by which the host immune system attempts to reduce the neoplastic burden have yet to be defined. Work over the last several years has identified a multiplicity of immunological effector systems which show *in vitro* activity against cancer cells. It is likely that different tumours may evoke qualitatively different patterns of response. Studies have also revealed that in the presence of malignancy there is compromise of the immune apparatus to the extent that the antitumour response is down-regulated.

The search for immunomodulating drugs is not helped by a plethora of quite inappropriate animal models which bear little resemblance to the human disease. In the absence of any clear consensus on the nature of the antitumour response in man (if it exists at all) immunotherapy has failed to make an impact on cancer treatment.

In the last few years there have been advances which allow the possibility of intervention in the immune system and the identification of the important decision points in assessment of the feasibility of the therapy of cancer by immunomodulation. Thus, there are now clear demonstrations of the presence of active T-cells and macrophages at the tumour site and of the underlying mechanisms by which these cells can be (a) expanded, and (b) activated to a lytic state. There are also descriptions of the immunological controls of these effector elements. The search for effective immunomodulators should now be specifically directed against these targets and seek to exploit the molecular mechanisms for activity which are now emerging. It is not enough to seek means of a general augmentation of the immune response. Rather, the goal must be to intervene specifically at defined points of the host–tumour relationship. It would seem appropriate at present to direct the search towards agents which augment macrophage or LAK activation, increase helper T-cell activity or decrease suppressor T-cell responses. In each of these areas model systems are available which appear to sensibly match the situation in human tumours.

There must also be the realization that clinical trials need to be designed to take into account the limitations of the immune response. New trials need to determine the optimal immunomodulating dose rather than the maximum tolerated dose of the selected agent in man and to accept that these molecules are unlikely to have an effect in individuals with advanced disease in whom the essential immune system has been compromised or eliminated by tumour burden or previous treatment. Strenuous efforts must be made to determine how agents can be delivered to the tumour site or to the immune system to induce the influx of effectors.

It seems unlikely that the available agents will revolutionize cancer treatment. Collectively they support the feasibility of the approach but without a major improvement in efficacy and targeting of immunomodulatory agents they may remain of limited usefulness to the oncologist.

ACKNOWLEDGEMENTS

The author is grateful to Dr J. E. Holmes for critical reading of this report and to Mrs J. Appleton for preparation of the manuscript.

References

1. Zhang, R. -R., Salup, R. R., Urias, P. E., Twilley, T. A., Talmadge, J. E., Herbernan, R. B. and Wiltrout, R. H. (1986). Augmentation of NK activity and/or macrophage-mediated cytotoxicity in the liver by biological response modifiers including human recombinant interleukin 2. *Cancer Immunol. Immunother.*, **21**, 19-25
2. Vose, B. M. and Moore, M. (1985). Human tumour-infiltrating lymphocytes: a marker of host response. *Semin. Hematol.*, **22**, 27-40
3. Ruco, L. P. and Meltzer, N. S. (1978). Macrophage activation for tumour cytotoxicity: development of macrophage cytotoxic activity requires completion of a sequence of short-lived intermediary reactions. *J. Immunol.*, **121**, 2035-42
4. Kleinerman, E. S., Wiltrout, R. H., Zicht, R. and Fidler, I. H. (1985). Human lymphokine preparations which generate tumoricidal properties of human monocytes *in vitro* may be distinct from gamma interferon. *Cancer Immunol. Immunother.*, **20**, 151-7
5. Gorelik, E., Wiltrout, R. H., Copeland, D. and Herberman, R. B. (1985). Modulation of formation of tumour metastases by peritoneal macrophages elicited by various agents. *Cancer Immunol. Immunother.*, **19**, 35-42
6. Varesio, L. (1985). Imbalanced accumulation of ribosomal RNA in macrophages activated *in vivo* or *in vitro* to a cytolytic stage. *J. Immunol.*, **134**, 1262-7
7. Fidler, I. J., Barnes, Z., Fogler, W. E., Kirsh, R., Bugelski, P. and Poste, G. (1982). Involvement of macrophages in the eradication of established metastases following intravenous injection of liposomes containing macrophage activators. *Cancer Res.*, **42**, 469-501
8. Koff, W. C., Fogler, E. W., Gutterman, J. and Fidler, I. J. (1985). Efficient activation of human blood monocytes to a tumoricidal state by liposomes containing human recombinant gamma interferon. *Cancer Immunol. Immunother.*, **19**, 85-9
9. Brownhill, A. F., Braun, D. G., Dukor, P. and Schumann, G. (1985). Induction of tumouricidal leucocytes by the intranasal application of MTP-PE, a lipophilic muramyl peptide. *Cancer Immunol. Immunother.*, **20**, 11-17
10. Maluish, A. E., Ortaldo, J. R., Conlon, J. C., Sherwin, S. A., Leavitt, R., Strong, D. M., Wernick, P., Oldham, R. K. and Herberman, R. B. (1983). Depression of natural killer cytotoxicity after *in vivo* administration of recombinant leukocyte interferon. *J. Immunol.*, **131**, 503-7
11. Saito, T., Ruffman, R., Walker, R. D., Herberman, R. B. and Chrigos, M. A. (1985). Development of hyporesponsiveness of natural killer cells to augmentation of activity after multiple treatments of biological response modifiers. *Cancer Immunol. Immunother.*, **19**, 103-5
12. Kallend, T., Alm, G. and Stolhandske, T. (1985). Augmentation of mouse natural killer cell activity by LS 2616, a new immunomodulator. *J. Immunol.*, **134**, 3956-6
13. Hewitt, H. B., Blake, E. R. and Walder, A. (1976). A critique of the evidence for active host defence against cancer, based on personal studies of 27 murine tumours of spontaneous origin. *Br. J. Cancer*, **33**, 241-59
14. Vanky, F., Withems, J., Kreubergs, A., Aparisi, T., Andreen, M., Brostrom, L.-A., Nilsonne, V., Klein, E. and Klein, G. (1983). Correlation between lymphocyte-mediated auto-tumour reactivities and clinical course. 1. Evaluation of 46 patients with sarcoma. *Cancer Immunol. Immunother.*, **16**, 11-16
15. Vankey, F., Klein, E., Willems, J., Brook, K., Ivert, T., Peterffy, A., Nilsonne, V., Kreicbergs, A. and Aparisi, T. (1986). Lysis of autologous tumour cells by blood lymphocytes tested at the time of surgery. Correlation with the postsurgical clinical course. *Cancer Immunol. Immunother.*, **21**, 69-76
16. Cheever, M. A., Greenberg, P. D. and Fefer, A. (1980). Specificity of adaptive chemo-immunotherapy of established syngeneic tumours. *J. Immunol.*, **125**, 711-14
17. Renoux, G. (1978). Modulation of immunity by levamisole. *Pharm. Ther.*, **2**, 397-423
18. Eccles, S. A., Purvies, H. P., Barnett, S. C. and Alexander, P. (1985). Inhibition of growth and metastasis of syngeneic transplantable tumours by an aromatic retinoic acid analogue. 2. T cell dependence of retinoids effects *in vivo*. *Cancer Immunol. Immunother.*, **19**, 115-20
19. Hadden, J., Hadden, E., Spira, T., Settineri, R., Simon, L. and Giner-Sorella, A. (1982).

81

Effects of NPT 15392 *in vitro* on human leukocyte functions. *Int. J. Immunopharm.*, **4**, 235–42

20. Umezawa, H. (1983). Studies of microbial products in rising to the challenge of curing cancer. *Proc. R. Soc. Lond.*, **217**, 357–76
21. Bruley-Rosset, M., Florentine, I., Kiger, N., Schuly, J. and Mathe, G. (1979). Restoration of impaired immune function of aged animals by chronic bestatin treatment. *Immunology*, **38**, 75–83
22. Beer, D. J. and Rocklin, R. E. (1984). Histamine induced suppressor cell activity. *J. Allergy Clin. Immunol.*, **73**, 439–52
23. Armitage, J. O. and Sidner, R. D. (1979). Antitumour effect of cimetidine. *Lancet*, **1**, 882–3
24. Flodgren, P., Borgstrom, S., Jonsson, P. E., Lindstrom, C. and Sjogren, H. O. (1983). Metastatic melanoma: regression induced by combined treatment with interferon [HuIFN-α(Le)] and cimetidine. *Int. J. Cancer*, **32**, 657–65
25. Grimm, E. A., Mazumder, A., Zhang, H. Z. and Rosenberg, S. A. (1982). Lymphokine-activated killer cell phenomenon: lysis of natural killer resistant fresh solid tumour cells by interleukin 2-activated autologous human peripheral blood lymphocytes. *J. Exp. Med.*, **155**, 1823–41
26. Grimm, E. A., Ramsey, K. M., Mazumder, A., Wilson, D. J., Djen, J. Y. and Rosenberg, S. A. (1983). Lymphokine-activated killer cell phenomenon. II. Precursor phenotype is serologically distinct from peripheral T lymphocytes, memory cytotoxic thymus-derived lymphocytes and natural killer cells. *J. Exp. Med.*, **157**, 884–97
27. Mule, J. J., Shu, S. Rosenbuerg, S. A. (1985). The anti-tumour efficacy of lymphokine-activated killer cells and recombinant interleukin 2 *in vivo*. *J. Immunol.*, **135**, 646–52
28. Rosenberg, S. A., Lotze, M. T., Muul, L. M., Leitman, S., Chang, A. E., Ettinghausen, S. E., Matory, Y. L., Skibber, J. M., Shiloni, E., Vetto, J. T., Seipp, C. A., Simpson, C. and Reichert, C. M. (1985). Observations on the systemic administration of autologous lymphokine-activated killer cells and recombinant interleukin 2 to patients with metastatic cancer. *N. Engl. J. Med.*, **313**, 1485–92
29. Vose, B. M. and Howell, A. (1983). Cultured human antitumour T cells and their potential for therapy. In Herberman, R. B. (ed.) *Basic and Clinical Tumour Immunology. pp. 129–57.* (Boston: Martinus Nijhoff)
30. Fenichel, R. L. and Chirigos, M. A. (1984). *Immune Modulation Agents and their Mechanisms.* (New York: Marcel Dekker)

6
Immunology in Bowel Cancer

N. C. ARMITAGE

IMMUNOLOGICAL RESPONSE TO COLORECTAL CANCER

The immunological response to colorectal cancer may be thought of as the systemic response and the response at the tumour site, both of which may be related[1]. There is evidence that some patients with colorectal cancer are immunosuppressed. It has been demonstrated that patients with depressed peripheral blood lymphocyte counts have a tendency towards a poorer prognosis[2,3] and this may be related to the tumour lymphocyte infiltration. Bone and Lauder[4] have also reported a relationship between advanced stage, depressed peripheral blood lymphocyte count and poor response to dinitro-chlorobenzene (DCNB). The DCNB reaction involves a skin test to this chemical and is a sensitive test of the integrity of the cell-mediated immunological response. This observation of depression of DCNB response in colorectal cancer and increasing depression with advancing disease has been made by other authors[5,6]. *In vitro* tests of cell-mediated immunocompetence have also shown depression in patients with colorectal cancer. A common test is the induction of lymphocyte blastogenesis by the mitogen phytohaemagglutinin (PHA). The dose–response curves of normal lymphocytes to the mitogen can be depressed by culture in sera from colon cancer patients[7]. There is also a lower response to PHA than expected from the lymphocytes of patients with colorectal cancer[8]. It has been shown that migration of normal subjects' leukocytes could be inhibited by serum from patients with colorectal cancer. Other workers, however, have found no difference of PHA response from control in colorectal cancer[9].

It is known, however, that peripheral blood mononuclear cells from patients with colorectal cancer are capable of destroying cultured colorectal cancer cells[10]. This cytotoxicity is depressed in lymphocytes derived from tumour regional lymph nodes[11]. Baldwin *et al.* showed that blood lymphocyte cytotoxicity could be inhibited by treatment with solubilized tumour membrane fractions[12]. These findings indicate that tumour antigen may be implicated in the local immune paralysis. So it would seem that there is both local and general suppression of immunity of colorectal cancer.

With regard to local tumour immunological response it has been shown that tumour lymphocyte infiltration may impart an improved patient

is a false negative rate of 54% in established metastatic disease[31,32]. Similarly the antigen Ca-50 is a tumour-associated carbohydrate antigen recognized by the monoclonal antibody C50, raised against a colorectal adenocarcinoma cell line[33]. This antigen has been detected in the serum of patients with colorectal cancer. However, although 27/36 (75%) of patients with advanced disease had elevated levels only 9/18 (50%) with early disease had elevated levels[34].

It has been suggested that if tumours shed antigens these may be detected in the serum bound to antibody as circulating immune complexes (CIC). These CIC have been shown to be present in serum but their role in diagnosis suffers from non-specificity as do the other previously described tests based on antigens[35,26]. Thus in terms of primary diagnosis these serum tests have proved disappointing and their role appears to be in follow-up.

Faecal tests

Just as substances may be shed into the bloodstream by colorectal cancers so they may be shed into the lumen of the bowel and be detected in the faeces. Most colorectal cancers bleed in small amounts and tests for this faecal occult blood are mostly based on simple chemical tests such as the guaiac reaction. These suffer from a number of disadvantages in that they may not be sufficiently sensitive to detect the minute amounts of blood shed by some tumours and they will cross-react with animal haemoglobin and vegetable peroxidases. A test based on an antibody to human haemoglobin should overcome these problems. Several such tests have been developed using immunofluorescence[37], immunodiffusion[38] and solid phase enzyme linked immunoassay (ELIZA)[39] based on polyclonal antisera. These tests have been shown to detect small quantities of faecal blood but only one has been tested in a population screening situation. If was found that, although the test was more sensitive than the simple chemical test, large numbers of false positive reactions made the test unsuitable in its present form[40]. Tests based upon monoclonal antibodies to human haemoglobin are currently being developed and may produce a test nearer to the ideal (Baldwin, 1986, personal communication).

These tests depend upon the tumours bleeding, which may only happen intermittently. Thus tests for other faecal products such as shed antigens may be of some value. Mucus distal to colorectal cancers has been shown to contain raised levels of CEA compared with normals[41]. Similar raised levels may also be found in perfusates when colorectal tumours are irrigated[42]. A recent report, using a monoclonal anti-CEA antibody showed elevated levels in faeces of patients with colorectal cancer compared with controls[43]. However, CEA can also be demonstrated in normal gastrointestinal secretions and thus an assay for faecal tumour products may be faced with the problem of a cut-off limit between normal and abnormal levels of marker. However, it is hoped that a combination of faecal tests will be developed based on the newer antitumour antibodies previously described.

CHARACTERIZATION OF COLORECTAL CANCERS USING MONOCLONAL ANTIBODIES

Antibodies can be shown to bind to sections of colorectal cancer by various immunohistological techniques. CEA was initially shown to be present using polyclonal sera and more recently using monoclonal antibodies. Indeed Primus et al. were able to demonstrate that monoclonal antibodies defining different epitopes of CEA have distinct patterns of staining in CEA-producing tumours[17]. A differential expression has also been suggested between vital and necrotic tumour[44].

Immunohistology has assumed an important place in the screening and work-up of new antitumour antibodies in defining patterns of expression in a wide variety of tumours and normal tissues. The great majority of the antibodies mentioned previously have been characterized by immuno-histology.

Immunohistological diagnosis

It has been shown in the lymphomas and leukaemias that more precise definition of the antigenic phenotype will help to distinguish one type of tumour from another with implications for patient outcome[45]. In straight-forward colorectal cancer diagnosis there are limited applications for such antigenic determinants. However, antigenic expression or cytokeratin production as defined by monoclonal antibodies may be of value in the cytology of ascites, pleural aspirates and in anaplastic tumours where the cell of origin is in doubt[46].

One potential application, that of improving the detection of micro-metastases in lymph nodes by staining the CEA, has been tested and found not to increase the number of positive nodes when compared with good conventional histopathology[47].

Markers for prognosis

It was shown using polyclonal antisera to CEA that there was a relationship between antigen expression as shown by immunohistological staining and tumour grade. Goslin et al.[48] showed that even in poorly differentiated cancers some could be shown to express CEA and that these patients had elevated CEA serum levels.

In other tumour types differential antigen expression is related to prognosis. Staining of breast cancer with a membrane antigen, NCRC11, has been shown to be directly related to survival[49]. Also in breast cancer, receptors for human growth factor have been demonstrated by monoclonal antibody[50]. In bladder cancer the same receptor expression is related to a worse stage of disease with little or no expression in disease confined to the epithelium and increase of expression in tumours which have penetrated the bladder wall[51].

In the large bowel there has been interest in the expression of blood group antigens (BGA). These substances are present throughout the fetal colon but are lost from the left side of the large bowel[52,53]. With the onset of neoplasia there is reacquisition by some tumours. In adenomas expression of BGA is related to a worse type (tubular, tubulo-villous to villous adenoma) and increasing dysplasia[54]. Wiley *et al.* showed that cancers of the left side of the colon and rectum which expressed BGA had significantly fewer metastases (2/13) compared with those not expressing them[55]. Recently it has been shown that expression of BGA H – the blood group substance expressed by erythrocytes of blood group O individuals – by the cancer conferred a significant survival advantage. This survival advantage was almost confined to blood group O individuals with 12/27 (44%) patients with positive staining cancers living 5 years compared with only 1/18 (5%) with negative staining cancers[56]. Currently these and other monoclonal antibody markers are being investigated as prognostic indicators.

Expression of these antigens may be considered as indicating the degree of differentiation of aggressiveness of the tumour and thus an indicator of likely outcome. The other side of the equation which must be considered is the reaction of the body's tissues to the tumour or host response. This has already been discussed in part previously with regard to systemic effects. However, at the tumour site the lymphocytes involved with cell-mediated immunity (thymus derived or T-lymphocytes) have been postulated to be involved in tumour surveillance or rejection. A quantitative analysis of lymphocyte infiltration at the periphery of colorectal cancer has shown a significant difference between tumours without lymph node involvement (Stage B) compared to tumours with nodal metastases (Stage C), the latter having little or no lymphocyte infiltration[57]. The importance of lymphocyte infiltration in determining prognosis has recently been highlighted by Jass[58]. However, other authors have found no correlation between lymphocyte infiltration and survival[59].

RADIOIMMUNOLOCALIZATION

The first studies of the localization of tumours by radiolabelled antibodies were done using labelled polyclonal antibodies raised against specific rodent tumours[60,61]. The first localization of a human colorectal tumour was reported by Goldenberg *et al.*[62] who used human colorectal cancer xenografts in golden hamsters. The group showed that a polyclonal anti-CEA antibody could be demonstrated by external gamma camera imaging. Dissection showed a preferential uptake into tumour compared with other organs with an uptake ratio of 5–20:1.

These animal observations were followed up by patient studies and in 1978 they reported the successful localization of colorectal cancers in seven patients using a polyclonal antiCEA antibody[63]. This was followed up in 1980 and localization was reported in nine out of ten primary sites and 26 of 31 sites of recurrent colorectal cancer[64]. A similar experience was reported by Dykes *et al.*[65] using a polyclonal anti-CEA antibody raised in sheep. As has been discussed elsewhere, monoclonal antibodies have several advantages over polyclonal antibodies which include increased specificity and reduced cross-reactions.

Table 6.1 Monoclonal antibodies used for tumour imaging

Author	Antibody	Immunogen	Patient imaging	Measured tumour: non-tumour
Mach et al.[66]	Anti-CEA	CEA	18/28 +ve	3.7:1
Epenetos et al.[118]	HMFG 1+2	Human milk fat globule membrane	2/4 +ve	ND
Farrands et al.[67]	791T/36	Osteosarcoma cell line	10/11 +ve	2.8:1
Berche et al.[75]	Anti-CEA	CEA	6/7 +ve	ND
Smedley et al.[119]	YPC2/12.1	Colorectal cancer membrane prep.	13/16 +ve	ND
Moldofsky et al.[78]	17–1AF(ab)₂	Colorectal cancer cell line	22/32 +ve	ND
Mach et al.[120]	17–1A intact + F(ab)₂	Colorectal cancer cell line	34/63 +ve	3.0:1
Chatal et al.[121]	17–1A intact + 19–9 + 171AF(ab)₂	Colorectal cancer cell line	27/46 +ve	ND
	Anti-CEA + 19–9	Colorectal cancer cell line	10/13 +ve	2.6–3.0:1
Armitage et al.[68]	791T/36	Osteosarcoma cell line	26/38 +ve	2.5:1
Allum et al.[122]	Anti-CEA	CEA	–	3.1:1
Finan et al.[123]	YPC2/12.1	Colorectal cancer membrane prep.	1/12 +ve	1.3:1
Delaloye et al.[124]	Anti-CEA Fab F(ab)₂	CEA	28/31 +ve	4.2:1
Leyden et al.[125]	250.36	HT29 cell line	9/10 +ve	ND
Schlom[126]	B72.3	Breast cancer membrane prep.	14/27 +ve	>3.0:1

The first study to report the localization of a monoclonal antibody in colorectal cancer was that reported by Mach et al.[66]. A monoclonal anti-CEA antibody was shown to give positive images when labelled with ^{131}I and injected into patients with colorectal cancer. Since that time several antibodies have been shown to localize in colorectal cancer (Table 6.1). The monoclonal antibody 791T/36 was raised against a human osteosarcoma cell line 791T and initial *in vitro* studies showed binding to several different malignant cell lines, including colorectal cancer[24]. A pilot study showed successful localization in four of five patients with primary tumours and six patients with disseminated disease[67]. The follow-up study reported successful imaging of eight of 11 colonic primary cancers (Figure 6.1) and of five of 13 rectal or rectosigmoid cancers. When these tumours were resected and samples of tumour and normal colon counted for radioactivity a tumour: non-tumour (T:NT) ratio of 2.5:1 was found with no significant difference in uptake between rectal and colonic tumours[68]. The difference in sensitivity of the imaging of colonic and rectal tumours is the proximity of the latter to the bladder. Metabolized iodine is excreted through the urinary tract and the presence of ^{131}I in the bladder masks many lesions. [131]I has a high energy of gamma emission and is thus inefficiently imaged by the gamma camera with the majority of the gamma particles passing through rather than being detected by the crystal. This means that in studies using ^{131}I as the radiolabel a subtraction technique must be employed[69]. For this technique the distribution of a different radionuclide – ^{99m}Tc-labelled red blood cells or [113m]In-labelled transferrin – is acquired to simulate distribution of ^{131}I-labelled antibody in the circulation. This blood pool image is subtracted from the ^{131}I image by a computer technique to leave a resultant antibody image. Most of the studies have employed this technique to localize primary and secondary colorectal cancers (Table 6.1). One of the features of colorectal cancer is that most primary tumours are resected giving an opportunity to directly measure the uptake of radiolabelled antibody. The resultant preferential uptake may be expressed as a tumour:non-tumour ratio and the results of various studies using ^{131}I-labelled antibodies are shown in Table 6.1. It is surprising that with the wide variety of immunogens there is not a wider range of T:NT ratios with these all about 2.5–3.0:1. Using active monoclonal antibody labelled with one radionuclide and an irrelevant antibody labelled with a different radionuclide it is possible to show that the localization of the monoclonal antibody is a specific antibody/antigen reaction rather than non-specific accumulation[68].

[^{131}I]791T/36 (osteosarcoma antibody) was shown to have a T:NT of 3:1 compared with [^{123}I]normal immunoglobulin which had a T:NT of 1.1:1 (Figure 6.2). Similar specific uptake has also been shown using other monoclonal antibodies[66].

The antibody/antigen complexes have been extracted from resected specimens from patients injected with [^{131}I]791T/36. The antibody was found complexed with a 72000 dalton molecular weight protein identical to that found on the cell surface of osteosarcoma and colorectal cancer cell lines[70].

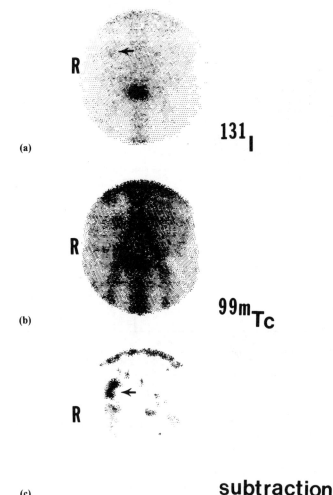

(a)

131I

(b)

99m Tc

(c)   **subtraction**

Figure 6.1 Anterior abdominal images of patient with a carcinoma of the ascending colon. (a) [^{131}I] antibody image, (b) [^{99m}Tc] blood pool image; (c) subtraction image. From Armitage *et al.* (1985). *Monoclonal Antibodies for Cancer Detection and Therapy,* London: Academic Press, reproduced with permission

Improvement of imaging

The methods of improving imaging quality using monoclonal antibodies are shown in Table 6.2 and some will also be relevant for optimizing the targeting potential of these antibodies. As has been discussed, ^{131}I is far from ideal as a radiolabel and the metal ^{111}In has many advantages which include a half-life of 2.8 days, little urinary excretion and two peaks of gamma emission which are more efficiently detected by the gamma camera. Since it is a metal labelling has to be through a chelating agent. A number of workers have

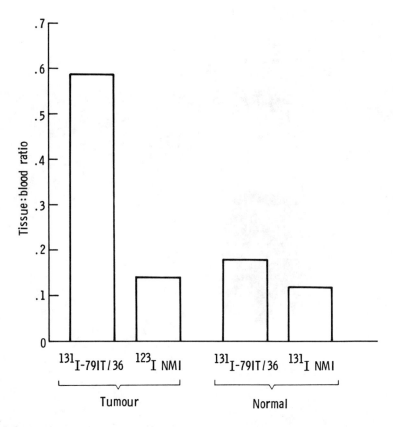

Figure 6.2 Tumour/blood ratios for [^{131}I]791T/36 and [^{123}I]normal mouse immunoglobulin. From Baldwin, R. W. *et al.* (1984). Cancer Invasion and Metastasis, *Biologic and Therapeutic Aspects,* New York: Raven Press, reproduced with permission

Table 6.2 Methods of improving image quality

(1)   Use of a more suitable radiolabel

(2)   Use of tomoscintigraphy

(3)   Use of monoclonal antibody with greater preferential tumour uptake

(4)   Use of antibody fragments

(5)   Use of the 'second antibody' technique

reported gamma camera imaging using ^{111}In-labelled antibodies in a variety of tumours[71-73]. Rainsbury *et al.*[71] were able to demonstrate bony metastases from breast cancer which were not visualized using ^{131}I-labelled antibody. Using [^{111}In]791T/36 it was possible to interpret the images obtained without

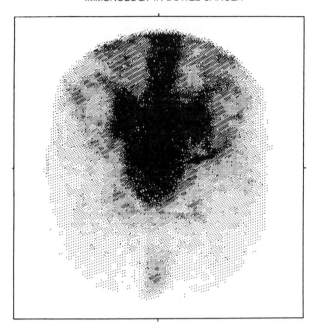

Figure 6.3 Posterior pelvic image of a patient with a large pelvic recurrence (→) using [^{111}In]C46

recourse to computer subtraction and obtain positive images in three of five primary and nine of 11 sites of secondary colorectal cancer. A T:NT of 2.8:1 was obtained from resected material indicating that the change of radiolabel had not altered the tumour localizing properties of the antibody[74]. However, the distribution of the ^{111}In-labelled antibody was different from that of ^{131}I-labelled antibody. Intense uptake was seen in liver and spleen and this may limit the detection of hepatic metastases. Uptake was also seen in the skeleton and testes which distribution has also been found by other workers and appears to be a characteristic of a radiolabel[73]. Emission tomography similar to X-ray CT involves taking images through an arc of 360° allowing the opportunity of visualization of antibody distribution through axial slices. Berche *et al.*[75] employed the technique and identified 16/17 sites of colorectal cancer compared with only 9/21 sites in the same patients using rectilinear scanning. They used ^{131}I as the radiolabel with its limitation and ^{111}In is a better radiolabel for this technique, as will be shown later. These first two methods refer only to methods of improving imaging while the next three methods rely on achieving a greater differential uptake of the antibody in the tumour compared with either blood or normal tissues. This may be potentially beneficial in targeting studies. Clearly a monoclonal antibody with a higher affinity will be an advantage in that the increased tumour uptake will give better images. We have recently reported a monoclonal antibody to CEA with such a high affinity. Using ^{111}In-labelled antibody we visualized 7/7 primary and 8/11 secondary tumours (Figure 6.3). Measurement of resected specimens gave[76] a T:NT of 5.8:1. Emission tomography was performed and

Table 6.3 Imaging of sites of recurrent colorectal cancer

Site of recurrence/ metastasis	Monoclonal antibody imaging	^{99m}Tc liver scan	Ultrasound scan	CT scan
Liver ^{131}I	12/18 (54%) +ve	14/24 (58%) +ve	9/14 (64%)+ve	12/14 (86%)+ve
^{111}In	1/6 (54%) +ve			
Abdomen	8/12 (67%) +ve	– – –	3/5 (60%) +ve	3/4 (75%) +ve
Pelvis	13/19 (68%) +ve	– – –	3/8 (38%) +ve	10/10 (100%) +ve
Other	4/7 (57%) +ve	– – –	– – –	2/2 (100%) +ve
All	38/62 (61%) +ve	– – –	16/27 (59%) +ve	27/30 (90%) +ve

MOAB imaging – Sensitivity: 62%

         – False positive: 4/10 patients who had no recurrence shown

although no further tumour deposits were identified several were identified with greater confidence.

The suggestion that fragments rather than intact antibodies may be useful rests on two factors. Firstly that removal of the Fc portion of the antibody will prevent non-specific uptake by Fc receptors in normal tissues, and secondly fragments are more rapidly cleared from the circulation giving improved tumour:non-tumour ratios. It has been shown that F(ab)'$_2$ fragments give superior tumour:blood ratios in animals studies[77]. Improved tumour imaging has been shown in patients by some workers[78]; our own experience using the Fab fragments of 791T/36 showed no localization. However, the affinity of 791T/36 is drastically reduced by cleavage of the Fc portion.

The second antibody technique depends upon the administration of radiolabelled antitumour antibody followed after a period by a second antibody to 'mop up' the first antibody. The resultant antibody/antibody complexes are cleared rapidly from the circulation. Begent et al.[79] showed improved imaging when a polyclonal anti-CEA was followed by liposomally entrapped second antibody, when images could be interpreted without subtraction.

Clinical potential of immunoscintigraphy

When considering the clinical usefulness of immunoscintigraphy it is unlikely that this technique will be of use in the diagnosis of primary colorectal cancers. The reason that in many studies primary tumours are imaged is that this gives the opportunity to study the distribution of the antibody and to measure uptake in resected specimens. However, immunoscintigraphy may have a place in the diagnosis of recurrent disease. We have recently reviewed 50 patients with suspected recurrent disease who had radioimmunoscintigraphy[80] (Table 6.3). The sensitivity was 62% at least as sensitive as ultrasound and although the resolution was less than that of CT scanning, gave valuable information in cases where differentiation between recurrence and fibrous/post-radiation change was not clear.

Begent et al.[81] reported a series of 31 patients in whom immunoscintigraphy was performed on the basis of a raised plasma CEA but no physical signs of recurrence. Eight patients were considered for surgery of whom three had tumour resections. In this series, four patients had tumours shown by immunoscintigraphy which were not detected by CT scanning.

Thus immunoscintigraphy may have a place in the follow-up of patients after resection of colorectal cancer either as an initial investigation or complementing other imaging modalities.

IMMUNOTHERAPY

In considering immunological treatment for colorectal cancer several aspects may be considered. These include stimulating a specific antitumour immune response and overcoming general immunosuppression due to tumour burden or to the effects of other treatment.

The stimulation of an antitumour response is a complex procedure and requires some understanding of the mechanisms involved. The cells involved in tumour cell killing include those designated as non-specific effector cells such as natural killer (NK) cells, lymphokine activated killer (LAK) cells and activated macrophages (AM) and more specific cytotoxic T-lymphocytes.

NK cells are thought to be in the first line defences for allograft rejection and viral surveillance[82] and have been shown to modulate tumour growth in vitro and in vivo in animal studies[83]. Clearance of radiolabelled lymphoma cells was markedly reduced in mice given anti-NK antisera[84] while mice treated with NK cells followed by melanoma B16 cells produced a 50–80% reduction in lung colonies compared with control mice[85].

In human studies it has been shown that peripheral blood NK cells are cytotoxic[86] and that NK activity in peripheral blood lymphocytes can be achieved by administration of interferons[87,88]. A phase 1 trial of interferon in patients with malignant melanoma and colorectal cancers has been reported which showed an initial fall of NK activity followed by a rise of activity for 7 days and a return to normal thereafter[89]. At the tumour level, however, although NK cells could be detected in axillary lymph nodes draining breast cancers[90] most tumours contain little or no NK activity due to both low frequency of NK cells and also the action of a suppressor cell[1].

Activated macrophages appear to act in a non-specific manner but have the ability to discriminate between malignant and non-malignant cells. They can be activated by many stimulating agents including bacterial vaccines and subcellular products such as muramyl dipeptide (MDP) especially when encapsulated in liposomes and Nocardia cell wall skeleton[91]. These activated macrophages can be shown to be cytotoxic to animal tumours and it has been shown that MDP can activate human peripheral blood monocytes and render them cytotoxic to tumour cell lines including colorectal cancer[92].

Various clinical trials have been reported of adjuvant therapy of colorectal cancer using a non-specific immune stimulator either alone or in combination with chemotherapy. However, the results of such trials have been dis-it is now possible to dissect the immunological aspects of colorectal cancer in greater detail than has been possible previously. The ability to understand the host response to colorectal cancer and to manipulate effector cells such as NK cells and macrophages may reverse immunosuppression and stimulate antitumour responses. Antigenic determinants may be important in helping to derive a prognostic index.

Labelling with radioisotopes allows tumour visualization by gamma camera and gives a potential for therapy, as does conjugation with other antitumour agents. These advances may in time bring about an improvement in survival for patients with colorectal cancer.

References

1. Vose, B. M. and Moore, M. (1985). Human tumour–infiltrating lymphocytes: a marker of lost response. *Semin. Hematol.*, **22**, 27–40
2. Riesco, A. (1970). 5 year cure: relation to total amount of peripheral lymphocytes and neutrophils. *Cancer*, **25**, 135
3. Kim, U. S. *et al.* (1976). Prognostic significance of peripheral blood lymphocyte counts and carcinoembryonic antigens in colorectal carcinoma. *J. Surg. Oncol.*, **8**, 257
4. Bone G. and Lauder, I. (1974). Cellular immunity, peripheral blood lymphocyte counts and pathological staging of tumours in the gastro intestinal tract. *Br. J. Cancer*, **30**, 215
5. Bolton, P. M., Mander, A. M., Davidson, J. M., James, S. N., Newcombe, R. G. and Hughes, L. E. (1976). Cellular immunity in cancer: comparison of delayed hyper-sensitivity skin tests in three common cancers. *Br. Med. J.*, **3**, 18–20
6. Wanebo, H. J. and Pinsky, C. M. (1978). A review of immunologic reactivity in patients with colorectal cancer. In Enker, W. (ed.) *Carcinoma of the Colon and Rectum*. (Chicago, London: Year Book Medical Publishers)
7. Manousos Economidao, J., Pathouli, C. H. and Merikas (1973). Disturbance of cell mediated immunity in patients with carcinoma of the colon and rectum. *Gut*, **14**, 739–42
8. Lauder, I. and Bone, G. (1973). Lymphocyte transformation in large bowel cancer. *Br. J. Cancer*, **28**, 78
9. Kaplan, M. S., Mino, F. O., Summerfield, K. B. and Lundak, R. L. (1975). Phytohaemag-glutin-stimulated immune reponse. *Arch. Surg.*, **110**, 1217
10. Hellstrom, I., Hellstrom, K. E., Pierce, G. E. and Yang, J. P. S. (1968). Cellular and humoral immunity to different types of human neoplasms. *Nature (London)*, **220**, 1352–4
11. Nind, A. P. P. *et al.* (1973). Lymphocyte anergy in patients with carcinoma. *Br. J. Cancer*, **28**, 108
12. Baldwin, R. W., Embleton, M. J. and Price, M. R. (1973). Inhibition of lymphocyte cytotoxicity for human colon carcinoma by treatment with solubilized tumour membrane fractions. *Int. J. Cancer*, **12**, 84
13. Umpleby, H. C., Heinemann, D., Symes, M. O. and Williamson, R. C. N. (1985). Expression of histocompatibility antigens and characterization of mono-nuclear cell infiltrates in normal and neoplastic colorectal tissues in humans. *J. Natl. Cancer Inst.*, **74**, 1161–8
14. Foley, E. J. (1953). Antigen properties of methyl cholanthrene-induced tumours in mice of strain of origin. *Cancer Res.*, **13**, 835
15. Baldwin, R. W., Embleton, M. J. and Price, M. J. (1979). Host response to spontaneous rat tumours. In Chandra, P. (ed.) *Antiviral Mechanisms in the Control of Neoplasia*. pp. 333–53.
16. Gold, P. and Freedman, S. O. (1965). Specific carcinoembryonic antigens of the human digestive system. *J. Exp. Med.*, **122**, 467
17. Primus, F. J., Newell, K. D., Blue, A. and Goldenberg, D. M. (1983). Immunological heterogeneity of carcinoembryonic antigen: antigenic determinants on carcinoembryonic antigen distinguished by monoclonal antibodies. *Cancer Res.*, **43**, 686–92
18. Herlyn, M., Steplewski, Z., Herlyn, D. and Koprowski, H. (1979). Colorectal carcinoma

specific antigen detection by means of monoclonal antibodies. *Proc. Natl. Acad. Sci. USA*, **76**, 5115-19

19. Olding, L. B., Thurin, J., Svalander, C. and Koprewski, H. (1984). Expression of gastrointestinal carcinoma associated antigen (GICA) detected in human foetal tissues by monoclonal antibody NS 19-9. *Int. J. Cancer*, **34**, 187-92

20. Finan, P. J., Grant, R. M., DeMattos, C., Takei, F., Berry, P. J., Lennox, E. S. and Bleehen, N. M. (1982). Immunohistochemical techniques in the early screening of monoclonal antibodies to human colonic epithelium. *Br. J. Cancer*, **46**, 9-17

21. Thompson, C. H., Jones, S. N., Pihl, E. and McKenzie, I. F. C. (1983). Monoclonal antibodies to human colon and colorectal carcinoma. *Br. J. Cancer*, **47**, 595-605

22. Brown, A., Ellis, I. O., Embleton, M. J., Baldwin, R. W., Turner, D. R. and Hardcastle, J. D. (1984). Immunohistochemical localization of Y Hapten and the structurally related H type 2 blood group antigen on large bowel tumours and normal adult tissues. *Int. J. Cancer*, **33(6)**, 727-36

23. Haggarty, A., Legler, C., Krantz, M. J. and Fuks, A. (1986). Epitopes of carcinoembryonic antigen defined by monoclonal antibodies prepared from mice immunized with purified carcinoembryonic antigen or HCT8R cells. *Cancer Res.*, **46**, 300-9

24. Embleton, M. J., Gunn, B., Byers, V. S. and Baldwin, R. W. (1981). Antitumour reactions of monoclonal antibody against a human osteogenic sarcoma cell line. *Br. J. Cancer*, **43**, 582-7

25. Campbell, D. G., Price, M. R. and Baldwin, R. W. (1984). Analysis of a human osteogenic sarcoma antigen and its expression on various human tumour cell lines. *Int. J. Cancer*, **34**, 31-7

26. Hansen, H. J., Synder, J. J., Miller, E., Vandervoorde, J. P., Muller, O. N., Hines, L. R. and Burns, J. J. (1974). Carcinoembryonic antigen. C.E.A. assay. A laboratory adjunct in the diagnosis and management of cancer. *Hum. Pathol.*, **5**, 139-47

27. Wanebo, J. H., Rao, B., Pinsky, C. M., Hoffman, R. G., Stearns, M., Schwartz, M. K. and Oettgen, H. F. (1978). Preoperative carcinoembryonic antigen level as a prognostic indicator in colorectal cancer. *N. Engl. J. Med.*, **229**, 448-51

28. Lewi, H., Blumgart, L. H., Carter, D. C., Gillis, C. R., Hole, D., Ratcliffe, J. G., Wood, C. B. and McArdle, C. S. (1984). Preoperative carcinoembryonic antigen and survival in patients with colorectal cancer. *Br. J. Surg.*, **71**, 206-8

29. Minto, J. P., Hoehn, J. L., Gerber, D. M., Horsley, J. S., Connolly, D. P., Salwan, F., Fletcher, W. S., Cruz, A. B., Gatchall, F. C., Oviedo, M., Meyer, K. K., Leffall, L. D., Bern, R. S., Stewart, P. A. and Kurucz, S. E. (1985). Results of a 400 patient carcinoembryonic antigen second look colorectal cancer study. *Cancer*, **55**, 1284-90

30. Koprowski, H., Herlyn, M., Steplewski, Z. and Sears, H. F. (1981). Specific antigen in the serum of patients with colon carcinoma. *Science*, **212**, 53-4

31. Del Villano, B. C., Brennan, S., Brock, P., Bucker, C., Liu, V., McClure, M., Rake B., Spale, S., Westrick, B., Schoemaker, H. and Zurawski, V. R. (1983). Radioimmunometric assay for a monoclonal antibody defined tumour marker CA 19-9. *Clin. Chem.*, **29**, 549-52

32. Kuusela, P., Jalanko, H., Roberts, P., Sipponen, P., Mecklin, J. P., Pitkanen, R. and Makela, O. (1984). Comparison of CA 19-9 and carcinoembryonic antigen (CEA) levels in the serum of patients with colorectal diseases. *Br. J. Cancer*, **49**, 135-9

33. Lindholm, L., Holmgren, J., Svennerholm, L., Fredman, P., Nilsson, O., Persson, B., Myrvold, H. and Lagergard, T. (1983). Monoclonal antibodies against gastro-intestinal tumour-associated antigens isolated as monosialoganlioside. *Int. Arch. Allergy Appl. Immunol.*, **77**, 178-81

34. Holmgren, J., Lindholm, C., Persson, B., Lagergard, T., Nilsson, O., Svennerholm, L., Rudenstaum, C. M., Unsgaard, B., Ingvason, F., Petterson, S. and Killander, A. F. (1984). Detection by monoclonal antibody of carbohydrate antigen CA 50 in serum of patients with carcinoma. *Br. Med. J.*, **288**, 1479-82

35. Vellacott, K. D. (1981). Colonic lavage and tumour related products. *DM thesis*, University of Nottingham.

36. Chester, K. A. and Begent, R. H. J. (1984). Circulating immune complexes (CIC) carcinoembryonic antigen (CEA) and CIC containing CEA as markers in colorectal cancer. *Clin. Exp. Immunol.*, **58**, 685-93

37. Vellacott, K. D., Baldwin, R. W. and Hardcastle, J. D. (1985). An immunofluorescent test for faecal occult blood. *Lancet*, **1**, 18-19

78. Moldofsky, P. J., Powe, J., Mulheen, C. B., Hammond N., Sears, H. F., Gattenby, R. A., Steplewski, Z. and Koprowski, H. (1983). Metastatic colon carcinoma detected with radiolabelled F(ab)₂ monoclonal antibody fragments. *Radiology*, **149**, 549–55

79. Begent, R. H., Keep, P. A., Green, A. J., Searle, F., Bagshawe, K. D., Jewkes, R. F., Jones, B. E., Barratt, G. M. and Ryman, B. E. (1982). Liposomally entrapped second antibody improved tumour imaging with radiolabelled (first) antitumour antibody. *Lancet*, **2**, 739–42

80. Ballantyne, K. C., Perkins, A. C., Armitage, N. C., Pimm, M. V., Wastie, M. L., Baldwin, R. W. and Hardcastle, J. D. (1986). Detection of metastatic and recurrent colorectal cancer by immunoscintigraphy. *Gut*, **27**, A600

81. Begent, R. H. J., Keep, P. A., Searle, F., Green, A. S., Mitchell, H. D. C., Jones, B. E., Dent, J., Pendower, J. E. H., Parkins, R. A., Reynolds, K. W., Cooke, T. G., Allen Mersh, T. and Bagshawe, K. D. (1986). Radioimmunolocalization and selection for surgery in recurrent colorectal cancer. *Br. J. Surg.*, **73**, 64–7

82. Herberman, R. B. (1982). Immunoregulation and natural killer cells. *Mol. Immunol.*, **19**, 313–21

83. Herberman, R. B. (1982). Natural killer cells and their possible relevance to transplantation biology. *Transplantation*, **34**, 1–7

84. Pollack, S. B. and Hallenbeck, L. A. (1982). *In vivo* reduction of NK activity with anti-NK1 serum: direct evaluation of NK cells in tumour diagnosis. *Int. J. Cancer*, **29**, 203

85. Warner, J. F. and Dennert, G. (1982). Effects of a cloned cell line with NK activity on bone marrow transplants, tumour development and metastases *in vivo*. *Nature (London)*, **300**, 31

86. Vose, B. M. and Moore, M. (1980). Natural cytotoxicity in humans susceptibility of freshly isolated tumour cells to lysis. *J. Natl. Cancer Inst.*, **65**, 257–63

87. Golub, S. H., Dorey, F., Hara, D., Morton, D. L. and Burk, M. W. (1982). Systemic administration of human leukocyte interferon to melanoma patients. 1. Effects on natural killer function and cell populations. *J. Natl. Cancer Inst.*, **68**, 703

88. Edwards, B. S., Hawkins, B. J. and Borden, E. C. (1984). Comparative *in vivo* and *in vitro* activation of human natural killer cells by two recombinant alpha interferon differing in antiviral activity. *Cancer Res.*, **44**, 3135

89. Fusi, S., Herbert, G. Z., Aritan, S., Ernstoff, M. and Kirkwood, J. M. (1982). Parameters of interferon action: T cell subjects and NK function during phase trial of recombinant human interferon alpha 2. *Clin. Res.*, **30**, 694

90. Kimber, I., Moore, M., Howell, A. *et al.* (1983). Nature and inducible levels of natural cytotoxicity in lymph nodes draining mammary carcinoma. *Cancer Immunol. Immunother.*, **15**, 32–8

91. Baldwin, R. W. (1985). Immunotherapy of cancer. In Pinedo, H. M. and Chabner, B. A. (eds.) *Cancer Chemotherapy*. Vol. 7, pp. 192–208. (Amsterdam: Elsevier Science)

92. Fidler, I. J., Jessup, J. M., Fogler, W. E., Staekel, R. and Mazumder, A. (1986). Activation of tumoricidal properties in peripheral blood monocytes of patients with colorectal carcinoma. *Cancer Res.*, **46**, 994–8

93. Mavligit, G. M., Gutterman, J. H., Burgess, M. A. *et al* (1978). Adjuvant immunotherapy and chemoimmunotherapy in colorectal cancer and Dukes C classification. *Cancer*, **36**, 2421

94. Higgins, G. A., Donaldson, R. C., Rogers, L. S., Juler, G. L. and Keehn, R. J. (1984). Efficacy of MER immunotherapy when added to a regimen of 5 fluorouracil and methyl CCNU following resection for carcinoma of the large bowel. 4. Veterans administration Surgical Oncology Group Report. *Cancer*, **54**, 193–8

95. Souter, R. G., Gill, P. G. and Morris, P. J. (1982). A trial of nonspecific immunotherapy using systemic *C. parvum* in treated patients with Dukes B and C colorectal cancer. *Br. J. Cancer*, **45**, 506–12

96. Enker, W. E. (1978). Adjuvant immunotherapy for large bowel cancer. Experimental studies in a relevant preclinical model. In Enker, W. (ed.) *Carcinoma of the Colon and Rectum*. pp. 259–82. (Chicago, London: Year Book Medical)

97. O'Dwyer, P., Dodson, T., Ravikumart, T. and Steele, G. (1986). The effect of alloimmunization on recurrence in an experimental colon cancer model. *Cancer*, **57**, 549–53

98. Hoover, H. C., Surdyke, M. G., Dangel, R. B., Peters, L. C. and Hanna, M. G. (1985). Prospectively randomized trial of adjuvant active-specific immunotherapy for human colorectal cancer. *Cancer*, **55**, 1236–43

99. Hollinshead, A., Elias, E. G., Arlen, M., Buda, B., Mosley, M. and Scherrer, J. (1985). Specific active immunotherapy in patients with adenomacarcinoma of the colon utilizing tumour-associated antigens (TAA). *Cancer*, **56**, 480–9

100. Rosenberg, S. A. (1985). Lymphokine-activated killer cells: a new approach to immunotherapy of cancer. *J. Natl. Cancer Inst.*, **75**, 595–603

101. Rayner, A. A., Grimm, E. A., Lotle, M. T., Chu, E. W. and Rosenberg, S. A. (1985). Lymphokine activated killer (LAK) cell phenomenon: iv. LAK cell clones lyse fresh tumour cells from autologous and multiple allogenic tumours. *Cancer*, **55**, 1327

102. Lafreniere, R. and Rosenberg, S. A. (1985). Successful immunotherapy of murine experimental hepatic metastasis with lymphokine activated killer cells and recombinant interleukin-2. *Cancer Res.*, **45**, 3735

103. Mazumder, A., Ebelein, T. J., Grimm, E. A., Wilson, D. J., Keenan, A. M., Aamodt, R. and Rosenberg, S. A. (1984). Phase 1 study of the adoptive immunity of human cancer with lectin activated autologous mononuclear cells. *Cancer*, **53**, 896

104. Lotze, M. R., Matory, Y. L., Ettinghausen, S. E., Rayner, A. A., Sharrow, S. O., Seipp, C. A. Y., Custer, M. C. and Rosenberg, S. A. (1985). *In vivo* administration of purified human interleukin-2. II. Halflife immunologic effects and expansion of peripheral lymphoid cells *in vivo* with recombinant IL2. *J. Immunol.*, **135**, 2865

105. Rosenberg, S. A., Lotze, M. T., Muul, L. M. *et al.* (1985). Observations on the systemic administration of autologous lymphokine-activated killer cells and recombinant interleukin-2 to patients with metastatic cancer. *N. Engl. J. Med.*, **313**, 1485–92

106. Herlyn, D. and Koprowski, H. (1982). IgG2a monoclonal antibodies inhibit human tumour growth through interaction with effector cells. *Proc. Natl. Acad. Sci. USA*, **79**, 4761–5

107. Sears, H. G., Herlyn, D., Steplewski, Z. and Koprowski, H. (1984). Effects of monoclonal antibody immunotherapy on patients with gastrointestinal adenocarcinoma. *J. Biol. Resp. Med.*, **3**, 138

108. Hammersmith Oncology Group and Imperial Cancer Research Fund (1984). Antibody guided irradiation of malignant lesions: three cases illustrating a new method of treatment. *Lancet*, **144**, 1–3

109. Rowland, G. F., Axton, C. A., Baldwin, R. W., Brown, J. P., Corvalan, J. R. F., Embleton, M. J., Gore, V. A., Hellstrom, I., Hellstrom, K. C., Jacobs, E., Marsden, C. H., Pimm, M. V., Simmonds, R. G. and Smith, W. (1985). Antitumour properties of vindesine–monoclonal antibody conjugates. *Cancer Immunol. Immunother.*, **19**, 1

110. Embleton, M. J., Rowland, G. F., Simmonds, R. G., Jacobs, E., Marsden, C. H. and Baldwin, R. W. (1983). Selective cytotoxicity against human tumour cells by a vindesine–monoclonal antibody conjugate. *Br. J. Cancer*, **47**, 43–9

111. Embleton, M. J. and Garnett, M. C. (1985). Antibody targetting of anti-cancer agents. In Baldwin, R. W. and Byers, V. (eds.) *Monoclonal Antibodies for Cancer Detection and Therapy*. (London: Academic Press)

112. Durrant, L. G., Armitage, N. C., Garnett, M. C., Baldwin, R. W. and Hardcastle, J. D. (1986). Sensitivity of methotrexate resistant colorectal cancer cells to monoclonal antibody targetted methotrexate. *Br. J. Cancer*, **54**, 186

113. Ballantyne, K. C., Perkins, A. C., Pimm, M., Garnett, M. C., Armitage, N. C., Baldwin, R. W. and Hardcastle, J. D. (1986). Localisation of monoclonal antibody drug conjugate 791T/36-methotrexate in colorectal cancer. *Br. J. Surg.*, **73**, 506

114. Canevari, S., Orlandi, R., Ripamonti, M., Tagliabue, E., Eguanno, S., Miotti, S., Menard, S. and Colnaghi, M. I. (1985). Ricin A chain conjugated with monoclonal antibodies selectively killing human carcinoma cells *in vitro*. *J. Natl. Cancer Inst.*, **75**, 831–9

115. Embleton, M. J., Byers, V. S., Garnett, M. C., Scannon, P. J. and Baldwin, R. W. (1986). *In vitro* comparison between monoclonal antibody targetted drug and toxin conjugates. *Br. J. Cancer*, In press

116. Bjorn, M. J., Ring, D. and Frankel, A. (1985). Evaluation of monoclonal antibodies for the development of breast cancer immunotoxins. *Cancer Res.*, **45**, 1214–21

117. Spitler, L. E., Del Rio, M., Khentigan, A. and Scannon, P. (1986). Therapy of patients with malignant melanoma with Xomazyme-MEL, a monoclonal antimelanoma antibody-ricin A chain immunotoxin: results of phase 1 Trial. In *Proceedings of International Conference on Monoclonal Antibody Immunoconjugates for Cancer,* San Diego, p. 30

118. Epenetos, A. A., Mather, S., Granowska, A. M., Nimmon, C. C., Hawkins, L. R., Britton, K. E., Shepherd, J., Taylor-Papadimitrou, J., Durbin, H., Malpas, J. S. and Bodmer, W. F. (1982) Targetting to iodine-123-labelled tumour-associated monoclonal antibodies to ovarian, breast and gastrointestinal tumours. *Lancet*, **2**, 999–1004

119. Smedley, H. M., Finan, P., Lennox, E. S., Ritson, A., Takei, F., Wraight, P. and Sikora, K. (1983). Localisation of metastatic carcinoma by a radiolabelled monoclonal antibody. *Br. J. Cancer*, **47**, 253–9

120. Mach, J. P., Chatal, J. F., Lumbruso, J. D., Buchegger, F., Forni, M., Ritschard, J., Berch, C., Douillard, J. Y., Carrel, S., Herlyn M., Steplewski, Z. and Koprowski, H. (1983). Tumour localisation in patients by radiolabelled monoclonal antibodies against colon cancer. *Cancer Res.*, **43**, 5593–600

121. Chatal, J. F., Saccavini, J. C., Fumolea, U. P., Douillard, J. Y., Curtet, C., Kremer, M., Lemevel, B. and Koprowski, H. (1984). Immunoscintigraphy of colon carcinoma. *J. Nucl. Med.*, **25**, 307–14

122. Allum, W. H., Anderson, P., MacDonald, F. and Fielding, J. W. L. (1985). Clinical evaluation of gastrointestinal cancer with a ^{131}I labelled monoclonal antibody to CEA. *Br. J. Cancer*, **53**, 203–10

123. Finan, P. J., Ritson, A., Ware, F., Parkin, A., Robinson, P. J., Sikora, K. and Giles, G. R. (1986). Monoclonal immunoscintigraphy for the detection of primary colorectal cancers: a prospective study. *Br. J. Surg.*, **73**, 177–9

124. Delaloye, B., Bishoff-Delaloye, A., Bucheger, F., Von Fliedner, V., Grob, J. P., Volant, J. C., Pettavel, J. and Mach, J. P. (1986). Detection of colorectal carcinoma by emission-computerized tomography after injection of ^{123}I-labelled F(ab) fragments from monoclonal anticarcinoembryonic antigen antibodies. *J. Clin. Inst.*, **77**, 301–11

125. Leyden, M. J., Thompson, C. H., Lichtensein, M., Andrews, J. T., Sullivan, J. R., Zalcberg, J. R. and McKenzie, I. F. C. (1986). Visualization of metastases from colon carcinoma using an iodine 131-radiolabelled monoclonal antibody. *Cancer*, **57**, 1135–9

126. Schlom, J. (1986). Basic principles and applications of monoclonal antibodies in the management of carcinoma: the Richard and Hinda Rosenthal Foundation Award Lecture. *Cancer Res.*, **46**, 3225–38

7
Recognition of Autologous Tumour Cells by Blood Lymphocytes in Patients with Lung Cancer

**F. VÁNKY, E. KLEIN, J. WILLEMS, K. BÖÖK,
T. IVERT AND A. PÉTERFFY**

AUTOLOGOUS TUMOUR STIMULATION (ATS)

On the basis of the knowledge which has emerged from experiments with well defined antigens it can be expected that if patients are sensitized against antigens present on their tumour cells, these can activate autologous blood lymphocytes *in vitro*. Indeed, blastogenesis and generation of cytotoxic lymphocytes have been induced in autologous mixed lymphocyte tumour cell cultures (MLTC). The frequency of positive results varied between 30 and 77% in the different reports (for review see ref. 1). The test conditions used in the different laboratories probably contributed to the variations. In our material of 359 patients, the frequencies varied between 29 and 72%, depending on the histological type of tumours (Table 7.1).

TECHNICAL ASPECTS OF THE TEST

Tumour cells

The main prerequisite of such experiments is the preparation of viable

Table 7.1 Frequency of autotumour stimulation

Tumours	Positive/No. tests	% positive tests
Adenocarcinoma of the lung	18/44	64
Squamous cell carcinoma of the lung	29/78	60
Malignant mesenchymal tumours	57/128	45
Small cell lung carcinoma	2/7	29
Adenocarcinoma of the kidney	13/18	72
Adenocarcinoma of the ovary	5/11	45
Malignant melanoma	7/10	70
Astrocytoma	24/60	40
Summary	155/359	43

*MLTC performed at the time of surgery; positive ATS = reactivity index 4.0 or higher

105

tumour cell suspensions without contaminating non-malignant cells. Among these, the imunologically active cells represent the most disturbing contaminants, since they may influence the outcome of the test. Some cell types such as B-cells and monocytes can stimulate T-lymphocytes[2,3], while others, such as activated T-cells and macrophages may suppress the immunological response[4,5].

We worked out a procedure based on velocity and density gradient sedimentations and exploitation of the adherence properties of certain cell types[6]. Changes of the initial procedure include the use of collagenase and DNase during the sedimentation steps, and monoclonal antibodies defining components in the cell suspensions. The bovine serum gradient used initially has been changed to Ficoll-Isopaque (FI) gradient[7] in order to avoid activation of the lymphocytes by the xeno-proteins adsorbed by tumour cells[8]. Recently, discontinuous Percoll gradients (in 10%, 15% and 20% concentrations) were introduced, that shortens the time required for processing and improves the quality of the tumour cell suspensions. The aim of producing single cell suspensions often led to impaired cell viability. Therefore, we accept the presence of clumps containing 3–10 tumour cells. Addition of collagenase and DNase counteracts cell aggregation.

The preparation of tumour cell suspensions is carried out as follows. Macroscopically distinguishable tumour tissue, without necrosis, is excised from the surgical specimens and minced with scissors in the presence of collagenase and DNase. The enzymes are added at 30 mg/ml and 2 mg/ml concentrations of stock solutions respectively, the amounts depending the appearance of the tissue. In general, the higher the proportion of dead cells, the larger amount of DNase added, and the more collagen material in the specimen the higher amount of collagenase added. The amount varies between 20 and 50 mg for collagenase between 2 and 5 mg for DNase.

The tumour material is then gently passed through a stainless steel mesh into collagenase (3 mg/ml), and DNase (0.2 mg/ml) containing BSS medium. If a tendency for cell aggregation is observed additional DNase is added. By sequential centrifugation, first at low speed (60 g, 5 min) followed by centrifugation of the supernatant at 500 g for 5 min, all debris are eliminated and a tumour cell-enriched (60 g sediment) and lymphoid cell-enriched (500 g sediment) suspensions are obtained. Each is further fractionated on Percoll discontinuous gradients[9]. 3 ml of 10%, 15% and 20% Percoll solutions are layered into 15 ml Falcon tubes (no. 2057). The cells (5×10^6–5×10^7) are placed on the top of the gradient in 1–2 ml volume, and the tube is centrifuged at 25 g for 5 min. The tumour cells usually collect at the lower part and at the bottom of the tube. Lymphocytes, erythrocytes and debris remain on the top and also pass into the intermediate layers.

If non-viable cells and erythrocytes are still present, the cell populations are further processed on FI gradients. The gradient is made up of 3 ml of 1.055 density FI solution (corresponding to 75% of the stock solution, diluted with balanced salt solution (BSS), layered on the stock solution (100% FI, density, 1.077). On this gradient, after centrifugation (900 g for 10 min at 4 °C) the viable cells are recovered at the interface between the 100% and 75% FI. A proportion of tumour cells from liposarcoma, melanoma and glioma may remain on the top of the 75% FI. Generally, the top fraction contains debris, macrophages and damaged (often unidentifiable) cells. Erythrocytes and non-viable cells sediment to the bottom. Following washes the viable cells are incubated into plastic tissue culture flasks in RPMI 1640 medium supplemented with 10% human serum for 30 min at 37 °C. The non-adherent cells containing the tumour cells are incubated overnight in culture conditions.

Culture conditions

Conventional synthetic media, supplemented with 5–10% serum, are suitable for the MLTC studies. Fetal calf serum (FCS) had to be avoided as supplement because it may activate the T-cells; therefore human serum for healthy male donors is provided. Blood group relationships do not influence the results. Serum samples with high lipoid content have to be avoided because they inhibit the reaction.

Evaluation of the results

Since lymphocyte stimulation is influenced by the cell concentration and the shape of the wells, the control samples, i.e. the lymphocytes without stimulators, are made up to concentrations identical with the MLTC. Therefore, though this does not represent a strict control, mitomycin-C (MMC)-treated cells from the responder lymphocyte population are added instead of tumour cells. The reactivity index (RI) is expressed as the ratio between [^{3}H]thymidine (^{3}H–TdR) uptake (cpm) in the test sample and in the control sample.

The results of autologous tumour stimulation (ATS) obtained by measurement of the isotope incorporation correlated well with the visually determined proportion of blasts[1]. Measurement of the thymidine incorporation may underestimate the degree of T-cell activation by tumour cells, due to the inhibitory effect of the tumour cells on the DNA synthesis of lymphocytes[10]. Furthermore, in order to proceed from the step of antigen recognition to cell division, production of monokines and lymphokines is required. A deficit in these activities may result in a lower proliferation response[11].

Reproducibility

The strategy of the experiments is mainly limited by the scarcity of tumour cells from tumour specimens. An important methodological improvement was the frozen storage of the tumour cells and lymphocytes[12,13]. This allows the performance of repeat experiments, and those types of experiments which require cultivation of the effector cells, e.g. in which autotumour cytotoxicity is generated. Frozen tumour cells were shown to maintain the stimulatory properties and can be used as targets in the cytotoxicity assay[1,14].

Kinetics and dose–response

The peak of thymidine incorporation in MLC is between the 6th and 7th days

107

of culture. With sensitized lymphocytes, the secondary response peaks on the 4th day[15]. In the MLTC the peak appears between the 3rd and 5th days. The response in MLTC is considerably weaker than in MLC and the peak values may appear on the 3rd, 4th or 5th days. Therefore measuring the ^{3}H-TdR incorporation at several time points is desirable. Due to the limited availability of the tumour cells, we usually measure the ^{3}H-TdR incorporation on the 5th day.

Stimulation of lymphocytes with allogeneic cells, bacteria and virus antigens shows a dose–response with an optimum beyond which the activity declines. The dose–response curve in the ATS system also is bell-shaped[1]. The peak values are usually obtained with lymphocyte:tumour cell ratios 5:1 and 10:1.

Specificity

The low frequency of stimulation with non-malignant cells and the dose dependency suggested that the ATS is a tumour-related antigen specific phenomenon. In our material stimulation of autologous lymphocytes by non-malignant cells was induced in three out of 51 tests[15]. These experiments were performed with connective tissue cells from soft tissue sarcoma, thyroid cells from patients with thyroid cancer, kidney cells from patients with kidney cancer, colon mucosa from patients with colorectal cancer, mesothelial cells from patients with ovarian carcinoma, and epidermal cells from malignant melanomas. For lung tumours, representative non-malignant cell preparation cannot be obtained. The cell population obtained from uninvolved lung tissue contains mainly macrophages and fibroblasts. The seemingly conflicting observation regarding the autologous stimulation with non-malignant tissue cell suspensions[17] may be attributed to the composition of cell suspensions used.

RESULTS WITH LUNG TUMOUR PATIENTS

Frequency of cases that react in ATS

The frequency of ATS obtained at the time of surgery was as follows: 64% of the patients with adenocarcinoma (44 cases), 60% with squamous cell carcinomas (78 patients) and 29% (7 cases) of small cell lung carcinomas (Table 7.1).

Specificity of ATS

Lymphocytes and tumour cells from the same individual were used in parallel as stimulators of allogeneic lymphocytes collected from tumour patients and healthy blood donors. The tumour cells were less efficient allogeneic stimulators than lymphocytes. There was a correlation between the two effects, showing that HLA antigen disparity determined the results. The cases with strong response to the allogeneic lymphocyte (MLC) were the ones that were stimulated also by the tumour cells (Figure 7.1). The autologous

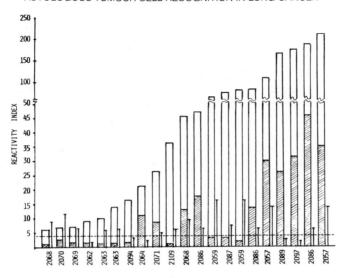

Figure 7.1 Stimulation of allogeneic lymphocytes by the patient's lymphocytes (□) and tumour cells (▨) related to the autotumour stimulation (⊤). Reactivity index 4.0 or higher is considered positive. Experiments are grouped according to the MLC reactivity. Tumours 2063, 2064, 2069, 2086, 2089, 2094 and 2109 are squamous cell carcinomas, 2057, 2062, 2070 and 2071 adenocarcinomas, 2059 and 2087 carcinoid tumours and 2086 large cell carcinomas.

Table 7.2   Lung tumour cell suspensions stimulating autologous and allogeneic lymphocytes in criss-cross assays

Lymphocytes from *	*Tumour cells from patient*†		
Exp. 1	SCC 1	AdC 1	AdC 2
SCC1	**30.6**⁺	1.7	1.8
AdC 1	2.4	**7.8**⁺	13.0⁺
AdC 2	1.0	0.5	**1.3**
Healthy	2.8	0.8	NT
Exp. 2	SCC 2	AdC3	AdC 4
SCC 2	**1.1**	1.1	1.7
AdC 3	1.8	**15.7**⁺	1.4
AdC 4	1.7	2.7	**8.5**⁺
Exp. 3	SCC 3	AdC 5	AdC 6
SCC 3	**7.2**⁺	2.3	NT
AdC 5	1.6	**8.6**⁺	1.7
AdC 6	1.5	3.7	**15.1**⁺
Healthy	2.2	1.2	NT
Exp. 4	SCC 4	SCC 5	
SCC 4	**6.2**⁺	1.7	
SCC 5	3.0	**0.5**	

* SCC = Squamous cell carcinoma; AdC = adenocarcinoma
† Results are expressed as reactivity index,
⁺ Positive ATS values, e.g. RI = 4.0 or higher. Autologous combinations in bold type

stimulatory capacity of tumour cells did not correlate with their ability to stimulate allogeneic lymphocytes. With ten of 21 tested tumours, the strength of ATS exceeded the values obtained when they were allogeneic stimulators.

In four experiments, with criss-cross combination using six adenocarcinoma, and five squamous cell carcinoma patients (Table 7.2), allogeneic stimulation occurred only in one of 23 combinations. Blood lymphocytes of one adenocarcinoma patient were stimulated both by the autologous and allogeneic adenocarcinoma cells (Exp. 1). The stimulating allogeneic tumour did not activate autologous lymphocytes. The five auto-stimulating adenocarcinomas did not stimulate the lymphocytes of three allogeneic adenocarcinoma donors, one squamous cell carcinoma donor, and two healthy

Table 7.3 ATS reactivity of lung carcinomas related to the expressed DR antigens on the tumour cells*

Patient No.	% Tumour cells†	Lymphocyte stimulation‡ Autologous	Allogeneic
*DR-negative squamous cell carcinomas***			
2059	98	**15**	2
2063	96	**4, 6**	1, 1, **9**
2069	98	**6**	2
2074	99	**6**	2
2097	93	2	**31**
2094	99	3	1
2093	95	**7**	1
2092	99	2	1
2091	98	1	2
2089	98	2	**27**
2175	98	1	2
DR-negative adenocarcinomas			
2061	97	**10, 9**	2, 1, 2, 1, 2, 1
2066	96	2	1, 1, 2
2096	100	3	**5**
2098	99	3	—
2183	96	**5**	3
DR-negative carcinoid tumours			
2087	97	**6**	2
2078	99	1	3
DR-positive adenocarcinomas			
2071	97	**5**	**8**
2182	92	3	**26**
DR-positive carcinoid tumour			
2127	98	2	12

* ³H-TdR incorporation during the last 16 hours of the 5 days MLTC. The results are expressed as reactivity indices. RI values 4.0 or higher are considered positive. The background values of cpm varied between 101 and 538

† The proportion of tumour cells was evaluated in Papanicolaou-stained cytopreparates: 400–800 cells were scored

‡ Autologous and allogeneic tumour stimulations were performed in the same conditions. In the allogeneic combinations each value represents different responders. Positive results are in bold type

** Expression of DR antigens was estimated by reactivity with anti-DR mAbs OKIa1 and LG-2-72 (LG-2-72 mAb was obtained from R. S. Accolla, Ludwig Inst. for Cancer Research, Lausanne Branch, Epalignes, Switzerland)

Table 7.4 Effect of anti-DR monoclonal antibody (mAb) LG-2-72 on the lymphocyte stimulation in various mixed cultures*

Group of tumours	Stimulators treated† with LG-2-72 mAb	Reactivity in‡ MLTC	AMLC	MLC
Squamous cell carcinoma of the lung	-	8/9	5/9	9/9
	+	8/8 (0)	1/5 (5)	7/9 (9)
Adenocarcinoma of the lung	-	2/4	0/4	4/4
	+	2/4 (1)	0/4	4/4 (4)
Large cell lung carcinoma	-	2/2	2/2	2/2
	+	2/2 (0)	0/2 (2)	2/2 (2)
Carcinoid	-	1/1	0/1	1/1
	+	1/1 (0)	0/1	0/1 (1)

* The experiments were performed in parallel using aliquots of the same responder lymphocytes in the three assays. MLTC = Mixed lymphocyte–tumour cell culture; AMLC = autologous mixed lymphocyte culture; MLC = mixed lymphocyte culture. Responder:stimulator ratios were 5:1 in the MLTC, and 1:1–2:1 in the AMLC and MLC. For mAb LG-2-72 see footnote **, Table 7.3.
† MMC-treated stimulators were incubated for 30 min with saturating (1 μg/10⁶ cells) concentration of mAb and washed three times prior to use in the tests.
‡ Positive/no. of tests. In parenthesis, number of tests in which the reduction exceeded 50%.

donors. The five squamous cell carcinomas stimulated only autologous lymphocytes (in three cases). Lymphocytes from two healthy donors were not activated.

The role of DR antigens in ATS

Malignant cells can express DR antigens even if the cell type of their origin does not carry them[18]. In 20 tumour cell suspensions of high purity (less than 5% contamination), DR-positive cells (detected with mAbs LG-2-72 and OKIal) were present in two adenocarcinoma preparations and in one carcinoid tumour (Table 7.3). Autologous lymphocytes responded often to the exposure of DR-negative tumours (5/11 squamous cell tumours, 2/5 adenocarcinomas and 1/2 carcinoid tumours). Among the three DR-positive tumours one stimulated. When these suspensions were used in allogeneic combinations (with lymphocytes of healthy donors or other patients) those which contained DR-positive tumour cells stimulated more often than the negative ones (3/3 and 4/26 respectively).

Aliquots of the tumour cell suspensions (nine squamous cell carcinomas, four adenocarcinomas, two large cell carcinomas and one carcinoid tumour) were used after pretreatment with anti-DR mAb LG-2-72 (Table 7.4). Untreated tumour cells induced a positive ATS response in 13/16 tests (8/9 with squamous cell carcinoma, 2/4 adenocarcinoma, 2/2 large cell carcinomas and 1/1 carcinoid tumour). Anti-DR mAb pretreatment of the tumour cells did not decrease their stimulatory capacity. When lymphocytes were the stimulators in AMLC and MLC, mAb pretreatment reduced their effect. These results together suggest that the DR antigens on the tumour cells are not essential in the induction of T-cell response in ATS.

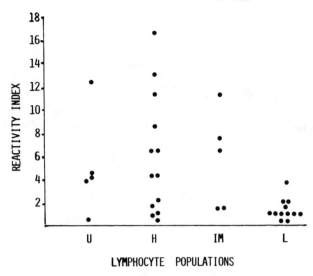

Figure 7.2 Reactivity of density fractionated lymphocyte subsets in the ATS. U, H, IM, and L are the unfractionated, high, intermediate, and low density lymphocyte populations

Lymphocyte subsets that react in ATS

Lymphocytes of 14 lung tumour patients were separated on discontinuous Percoll density gradients. The strongest proliferative response upon exposure to autologous tumour cells occurred in the high density T-cell fraction (Figure 7.2). This is the subset that reacts also in the MLC[19].

When sensitized lymphocytes are exposed to the relevant antigen, and when T-cells are co-cultured with allogeneic lymphocytes, both CD4+ (inducer/helper) and CD8+ (suppressor/cytotoxic) T-cells were shown to proliferate[20]. On the other hand, the AMLC reactive cells are in the CD4+ subset[21]. In three experiments (two squamous cell carcinomas and one large cell carcinoma) the nylon wool non-adherent blood lymphocytes were separated into CD8+ and CD4+ subsets, using negative selection. Aliquots of these were

Table 7.5 Reactivity of CD8+ and CD4+ T-cell subsets in MLTC and MLC*

Diagnosis†	cpm control‡			MLTC			MLC		
	NCp	CD8+	CD4+	NCp	CD8+	CD4+	NCp	CD8+	CD4+
SCC	455	679	327	6.3**	4.3	7.0	26.2	9.7	19.0
SCC	890	362	930	6.1	20.0	1.1	51.6	13.7	63.9
Carcinoid	223	735	335	4.3	1.2	7.3	74.6	26.6	23.7

* See also footnote *, Table 7.4. CD8+ and CD4+ subsets were separated from the NCp populations by negative selection in the paning method with OKT4 and OKT8 mAbs respectively.
† See footnote *, Table 7.2.
‡ Effectors cultured alone.
** See footnote †, Table 7.2.

Table 7.6 Reactivity of auto-erythrocyte rosetting T-lymphocytes in various types of mixed cultures*

Diagnosis†	cpm control‡			MLTC			AMLC			MLC		
	NCp	AR⁺	AR⁻**	NCp	AR⁺	AR⁻	NCp	AR⁺	AR⁻	NCp	AR⁺	AR⁻
AdC	385	302	230	**4.9**††	**9.3**	**6.8**	3.2	1.8	2.2	**118**	**120**	34
SCC	256	387	191	**5.6**	**7.3**	**8.5**	6.6	**12.4**	2.1	**81**	**73**	55
AdC	216	259	187	**7.8**	**8.6**	**12.2**	1.1	2.2	0.8	**60**	**44**	42
LCC	153	170	243	**21.0**	**14.4**	**9.0**	**5.5**	**5.7**	0.7	**90**	NT	51
SCC	571	269	339	**3.9**	**6.7**	**4.7**	**7.2**	**23.6**	**12.1**	**105**	**180**	**167**

* See footnote *, Table 7.4.
† See footnote *, Table 7.2. LCC = Large cell carcinoma of the lung.
‡ Effectors cultured alone.
** NCp = Unfractionated nylon column non-adherent cells. AR⁺ and AR⁻ are T-lymphocytes which form and do not form rosettes with autologous erythrocytes respectively.
†† Reactivity index 4 or higher in bold type.

tested in parallel for their ATS reactivity and in the MLC (Table 7.5). Both $CD8^+$ and $CD4^+$ cells were stimulated by the autologous tumours, each in two out of three tests and by allogenic lymphocytes in all three tests.

The responding T-cells in the AMLC were shown to form rosettes with autologous erythrocytes (AR^+)[22]. In five experiments comprising two adeno-carcinoma, two squamous cell carcinoma and one large cell carcinoma patients, using nylon wool non-adherent lymphocytes populations, the AR^+ and AR^- cells were compared for ATS reactivity. AMLC and MLC-s were initiated simultaneously with the same responder populations (Table 7.6). NCp populations were reactive in all five MLTC-s and MLC-s and in three of five AMLC-s. Both the AR^+ and AR^- subsets were stimulated in the MLTC and MLC. The AR^+ populations were reactive in three of five AMLC-s, while the AR^- only in one. These results indicate that different lymphocytes respond in the assays that reflect the recognition of the autologous malignant and non-malignant cells respectively, and also that the two phenomena are different.

ATS test results related to the clinical course

Among 31 patients with squamous cell carcinoma of the lung, 23 were ATS-positive (74%). After a mean observation time of 81 months (range 36–104) 15 patients in this group were tumour free. The negative tests predict a relatively unfavourable prognosis, because all non-reactive patients died with 36 months (mean 12) (Figure 7.3A). The survival time of the eight deceased ATS-positive patients did not differ significantly from that of the eight non-reactive individuals (mean 15 and 12 months respectively).

Among the 17 patients with adenocarcinoma 12 (71%) were ATS-positive at the time of surgery. Of these, nine were tumour free after a mean observation of 81 months (range 36–104). Four of the five ATS-negative individuals died within 36 months (mean 15) and one survived 62 months (Figure 7.3B).

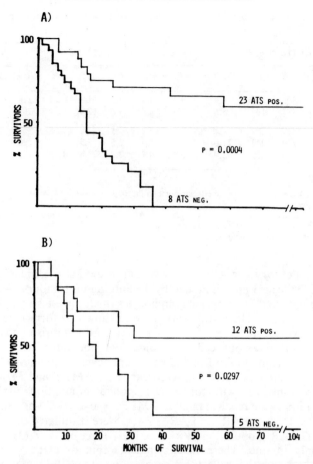

Figure 7.3 Life table analysis of the postsurgical clinical course of the patients with squamous cell carcinoma (A), and adenocarcinoma (B) of the lung, related to the ATS results obtained at the time of surgery

The results show that a negative ATS is a bad prognostic sign, while a proportion of patients with positive tests have a favourable clinical course.

AUTOLOGOUS LYMPHOCYTE-MEDIATED CYTOTOXICITY

Lymphocyte-mediated cytotoxicity is frequently used in studies of cellular immunology. Two important discoveries have led to new concepts. The first has established the participation of MHC gene products in the interaction of effectors and targets, even in those cases in which the response is directed against other than MHC gene products. The second has revealed that the cytotoxicity can occur in a seemingly indiscriminant fashion, i.e. when the

114

history of the lymphocyte donors does not indicate sensitization to the target cells used. It has been proposed that 'natural cytotoxicity', independent of priming, is an important antitumour mechanism. This should be based on the recognition of 'altered' membrane structures related to the malignant nature of the tumour cells. The basis of this assumption was the finding that the susceptible targets in such experiments were usually cultured tumour cells. In studies with human lymphocytes, K562 is the prototype of the sensitive target. Therefore, often the lysis of K562 cells is designated as natural killer (NK) function. With the demonstration that the active effector cell subset is mainly recovered in the low density population of the blood lymphocytes and that a proportion of these cells are distinguishable morphologically as large granular lymphocytes (LGL), this subset is usually referred to as NK cells. It has been debated whether these represent a separate cell lineage since increasing evidence places them into the T lineage.

The important distinction for the nature of the cytotoxic interaction is whether the function of the effector cell is related to a recognition involving a clonotypic antigen receptor (Ti).

When patients' lymphocytes lyse their own tumour cells the phenomenon does not correspond operationally to natural cytotoxicity, because sensitization may have occurred against the relevant antigens. In view of the lack of knowledge concerning the antigens, it is difficult to decide whether reactivity is the consequence of immunization. To approach this question, tests can be performed that exploit certain known characteristics that distinguish between antigen specific and non-discriminative cytotoxicities. Studies concerning the reactive subsets, the involvement of T-cell receptors and MHC antigens can lead to a closer definition of the nature of the cytotoxicity against autologous tumour cells.

RESULTS WITH LUNG TUMOUR PATIENTS

Frequency of cases that show ALC

With nylon wool non-adherent cell populations, that are enriched in T-lymphocytes, the proportion of positive ALC tests varied in the patient groups according to the histological type of the tumours. 20% of the patients with small cell lung carcinomas (20 tests) were positive. Among the 57 patients with adenocarcinoma 32%, and among the 119 squamous cell carcinoma 41% reacted (Table 7.7).

Table 7.7 Frequency of ALC

Histology	Cytotoxicity*	
Squamous cell carcinoma	49/119	(41%)
Adenocarcinoma	18/57	(32%)
Small cell lung carcinoma	4/20	(20%)

* Positive/no. test, 4 h ^{51}Cr release cytotoxicity assay. Criteria for the positivity: the difference between the cpm values of the test samples and control is significant and the increase (cpm) in the test is at least 10%.

Table 7.8 Specificity of ALC

	Source of		
Lymphocytes	*Target cells*	*Cytotoxicity**	
Lung cancer	Autologous tumour	69/196	(35%)
Lung cancer	Allogeneic lung tumour	3/53	(6%)
Lung cancer	Non-long tumour	3/45	(7%)
Non-lung tumour	Lung tumour	1/15	(7%)
Healthy donor	Lung tumour	1/26	(4%)

* See footnote Table 7.7

Specificity of ALC

Altogether 196 patients have been tested in the ALC assay. The test was positive in 69 (35%) (Table 7.8). Only a few reactions were detected against allogeneic lung tumour cells (6%) or allogeneic cells derived from other types of tumours (7%). Only in one test of 15 (7%) were lung tumour cells lysed by lymphocytes of patients with other types of malignancies and only in one test of 26 (4%) when the effectors were derived from healthy donors.

Table 7.9 Lymphocyte-mediated cytotoxicity against autologous and allogeneic tumours. Criss-cross assays

*Lymphocytes from**	*Tumour cells from patients†*			
Exp. 1	SCC 1	SCC 2	AdC 1	AdC 2
SCC 1	**27$^+$**	17	—	17
SCC 2	12	**36$^+$**	—	0
AdC 1	10	6	**51$^+$**	0
Healthy	10	0	7	—
Exp. 2	AdC 3	AdC 4	Caid 1	
AdC 3	**39$^+$**	10	8	
AdC 4	10	**22$^+$**	13	
Caid 1	9	—	**28$^+$**	
Healthy	2	5	—	
Exp. 3	SCC 3	SCC 4	SCLC 1	
SCC 3	**0**	0	11	
SCC 4	0	**23$^+$**	7	
SCLC 1	2		**31$^+$**	
Exp. 4	SCC 5	SCC 6	SCLC 1	
SCC 5	**15$^+$**	0	0	
SCC 6	3	**10**	—	
Exp. 5	SCC 7	SCC 8		
SCC 7	**22$^+$**	3		
SCC 8	13	**6**		

*SCC = Squamous cell carcinoma; AdC = adenocarcinoma; SCLC = small cell lung carcinoma; Caid = carcinoid tumour of the lung.
† Results are expressed as % specific ^{51}Cr release; + means significant. Autologous combinations in bold type. See also footnote Table 7.7.

Table 7.10 Frequency of ALC with low and high density lymphocyte subsets

Diagnosis*	n	Effector populations†		
		U	Ld	HD
SCC	32	7‡ (22) 3**	12 (38) 5**	12 (38) 5**
AdC	16	4 (25) 1**	4 (25) 1**	4 (25) 0**
SCLC	2	1	2	2

§ See footnote * Table 7.9.
† U, LD and HD = Unfractionated, low and high density lymphocyte populations.
‡ No. positive tests. In parenthesis their proportion.
** No. of positive cases obtained only with the indicated subset.

Tumour specificity of ALC could not be tested because non-malignant cells corresponding to the cell of origin cannot be obtained from the uninvolved lung tissue.

In criss-cross experiments, lysis of allogeneic cells was not detected even when ALC-positive cases were cross-tested and when the tests involved tumours of the same histological type (Table 7.9). The selectivity for the autologous tumour cells most likely reflects the MHC restriction of the cytotoxic interaction.

Lymphocyte subsets that react in ALC

In experiments performed with lymphocyte fractions of various densities, autotumour cytotoxic cells were detected both in the low (LD) and high density (HD) subsets (Table 7.10). In 50 experiments (32 squamous cell carcinomas, 16 adenocarcinomas of the lung and two small cell lung carcinomas), the frequencies of positive tests were 24% (12/50) with the unfractionated, 36% (18/50) with the LD fraction, and 36% (18/50) with the HD fraction. In 38 cases ALC was not detected by the unfractionated lymphocytes but in 11 of these the LD and in seven the HD subsets were positive. In five cases ALC occurred only in the LD and in another five only in the HD lymphocytes. These results suggest that the activities of the two populations may appear independently (Figure 7.4).

With 22 lung cancer patients (12 squamous cell carcinomas, eight adeno-carcinomas and two small cell lung carcinomas), density fractionated blood lymphocytes were also tested against allogeneic tumour biopsy cells (Table 7.11). Unmanipulated, unfractionated effectors were cytotoxic in 1/23 (4%) tests, LD cells in 7/25 (28%) and HD in none.

Cytotoxicity of blood lymphocytes from healthy blood donors showed a similar pattern of reactivity (Table 7.11). Unfractionated lymphocytes were cytotoxic against the allogeneic tumour targets in 1/27 (4%) cases, LD cells in 12/27 (44%) and HD in none.

K562 cells were included regularly in the cytotoxic assays for functional control of the effector subsets (Table 7.11). In 50 experiments with lung cancer patients (presented in Table 7.10), unfractionated lymphocytes lysed K562 in 30 (60%), LD in 47 (94%) and HD in none. In 30 cases unfractionated and LD lymphocytes from healthy donors lysed the K562 in all tests, and HD in one (data not presented). Thus the profile of ALC differed from that

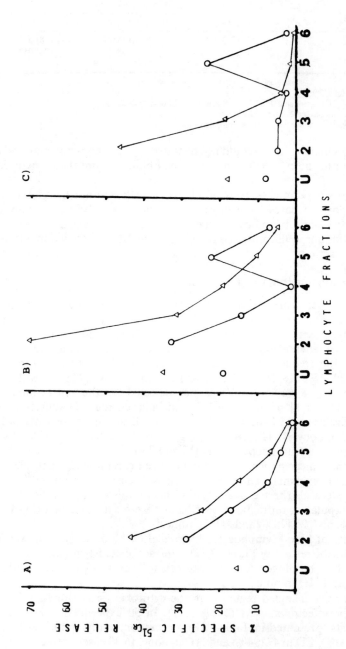

Figure 7.4 Lysis of autologous tumour cells (○) and K-562 (△) by density fractionated lymphocyte subsets. U = Unfractionated; 2–6 = fractions of the Percoll gradient from light to dense. A) Small cell lung carcinoma, ALC activity present in LD; B) adenocarcinoma of the lung, ALC present in U, LD and HD but absent in the intermediate fraction; C) adenocarcinoma of the lung, ALC in the HD but absent in LD and IM. Lysis of K-562 occured in the U and LD but not in the IM and HD fractions

Table 7.11 Cytotoxicity against allogeneic tumours

Lymphocytes from	Target cells	Lymphocytes*		
		U	LD	HD
Healthy donors	Fresh tumour	1/27 (4)†	12/27 (44)	0/27
Lung cancer patients	Fresh tumour	1/23 (4)	7/25 (28)	0/25
	K562	30/50 (60)	47/50 (94)	0/50

*See footnote † Table 7.10.
† See footnote *Table 7.7. In parenthesis percentage positive tests.

observed in allogeneic combinations and against K562. The function of HD cells was restricted to the autologous tumour cells.

The higher frequency of positive experiments with the density-separated subsets suggests that the active cells have to be enriched in order to detect activity.

For further characterization of the cytotoxic cells nylon wool passed populations were separated into OKT4 negative (CD8$^+$) and OKT8 negative (CD4$^+$) subsets (Table 7.12). Among the eight patients tested six had lung tumours. Unfractionated lymphocytes were cytotoxic in one, the CD8$^+$ fractions in five, and the CD4$^+$ in one of the eight tests each.

The HD subsets of three patients with adenocarcinoma of the lung were similarly separated into CD8$^+$ and CD4$^+$ populations. The former was ALC-positive in two cases and the latter subset in one. These results show that among the T-cells mainly the CD8$^+$ subset is responsible for ALC.

Participation of CD3 and CD2 receptors and the MHC class I antigens in the ALC

Monoclonal antibodies directed to the T-cell receptor complex CD3 inhibit

Table 7.12 ALC reactivity of CD8$^+$ and CD4$^+$ T-cell subsets*

Diagnosis†	Lymphocytes		
	Unfractionated	OKT4 depleted (CD8$^+$)	OKT8 depleted (CD4$^+$)
Nylon wool non-adherent lymphocytes			
Carcinoid	8	14$^+$	4
AdC	3	14	24$^+$
AdC	10	21$^+$	10
AdC	4	7	0
SCC	8	22$^+$	11
SCC	8	0	5
OSC	15$^+$	19$^+$	9
OSC	7	35$^+$	7
High density T-lymphocytes			
AdC	19$^+$	26$^+$	0
AdC	3	21$^+$	3
AdC	9	8	20$^+$

*See footnote *, Table 7.5.
† See footnote *, Table 7.9.

Table 7.15 Survival time and tumour-free period of the patients without known metastasis at the time of surgery, related to the ALC test results*

ALC test results	Number of tests	Status at the time of evaluation	n	Tumour-free period (months)	Survival/observation (months)	
Squamous cell carcinoma of the lung						
Positive	25	Alive	19			69.3±23
		Deceased	6	15.7±15.4	24.6±13.7	
Negative	11	Alive	0	6.1± 2.7	14.5±12.7	
Adenocarcinoma of the lung						
Positive	9	Alive	8			79.3±19.5
		Deceased	1		34.5	
Negative	8	Alive	0	11.0±4.7	23.6±9.5	

*ALC tests were performed at the time of surgery. Clinical relevance evaluated after a mean observation time of 80.2 months (range 36–108).

IN VITRO INDUCTION OF ALC

ALC induced in MLTC

20 MLTCs initiated with cells from lung tumour patients were tested for lysis of autologous and allogeneic lung tumour cells and K562 on the 7th day of the culture (Table 7.16). Autotumour lysis was generated in 12 (six

Table 7.16 Cytotoxicity generated in MLTC*

Lymphocyte donor† No. Diagnosis		Control culture‡	MLTC effectors Target cells			
		1°ALC	Autotumour	Autotumour	Allotumour**	K562
2063	SCC	4††	4	14	7	4
2089	SCC	—	17	22+	—	15+
2024	SCC	8	10	20+	3	25+
2028	SCC	—	0	74+	—	25+
2020	SCC	3	0	8	0	1
2014	SCC	14	4	11	0	12
2041	SCC	6	10	31+	14	0
2225	SCC	6	11	0	0	—
2240	SCC	—	9	72+	0	—
2244	SCC	18+	3	37+	0	—
2226	AdC	—	0	4	—	—
2096	AdC	10	20+	22+	—	3
2095	AdC	8	3	20+	4	55+
2091	AdC	—	13	61+	—	29+
2061	AdC	5	0	1	2	1
2057	AdC	39+	4	26+	8	3
2016	AdC	4	6	12	—	11
2019	AdC	17+	0	48+	—	22+
2293	AdC	0	12	19+	12	19+
2294	AdC	0	5	30+	0	24+

*Lymphocytes were cultured with autologous tumour cells for 6 days and then tested for cytotoxicity in 4 hours ^{51}Cr-release assay.
† See footnote *, Table 7.9.
‡ Lymphocytes cultured alone.
**All are lung tumours, except that tested with 2014 effectors. ††See footnote †, Table 7.9.

Table 7.17 Cytotoxicity generated in MLC*

Lymphocyte donor†			Targets		
No.	Diagnosis	1° ALC	Autotumour	Allotumour‡	K'562
2014	SCC	14**	22$^+$	24$^+$	55$^+$
2020	SCC	3	6	2	24$^+$
2055	SCC	25$^+$	37$^+$	11	—
2089	SCC	—	6	—	20$^+$
2293	AdC	0	9	9	56$^+$
2016	AdC	4	0	6	19$^+$
2057	AdC	39$^+$	31$^+$	36$^+$	—
2056	AdC	12	27$^+$	42$^+$	50$^+$
2065	AdC	9	7	4	—
2095	AdC	8	36$^+$	19$^+$	52$^+$

* Tumour patients' lymphocytes were cultured with MMC-treated allogeneic lymphocytes for 6 days and tested for cytotoxicity in 4 hours ^{51}Cr-release cytotoxicity assay. 1° ALC = direct cytotoxicity against autologous tumour cells.
† See footnote *, Table 7.9.
‡ The allogeneic tumours are 3rd party targets except in one case where lymphocytes 2056 were activated with lymphocytes 1143 and tested on tumour 1143.
** See footnote †, Table 7.9.

adenocarcinomas and six squamous cell carcinomas). Allogeneic tumour cells were not lysed. The majority of the active populations also lysed K562 cells. In 3/12 experiments only the autologous tumour cells were lysed. In 3/12 cases the freshly separated lymphocytes, and in one the control culture (not exposed to the autologous tumour) were also cytotoxic.

ALC induced in MLC

Cytotoxicity against the autologous tumour cells could be induced in MLC[28,29], when the patient's lymphocytes were cultured with MMC-treated allogeneic lymphocytes (Table 7.17). In MLC cultures initiated with lymphocytes from ten patients (four squamous cell carcinomas and six adeno-carcinomas), autologous tumour cells were lysed in five. In two of these the primary ALC was also positive. In all but one case third party allogeneic tumours were also lysed by those MLC populations which lysed autologous tumour cells.

Thus the lysis of autologous tumour cells can also be generated in MLC. These MLC-effector cells lysed third party tumour cells more frequently than the MLTC-s. The more efficient activation in the MLC-s compared to the MLTC-s is reflected in the difference in anti-K562 activity between these cultures. All MLC lysed K562 but only a proportion of MLTC-s did so.

Thus in the MLTC cytotoxic cells are generated against autologous, but rarely against allogeneic tumours. If the patient's lymphocytes are activated in MLC, autotumour cytotoxicity can be induced, but the effect is not selective for these cells.

Induction of ALC by interferon (IFN)

In a series of experiments with density fractionated lymphocytes from 14

Table 7.18 Interferon-induced ALC*

Lymphocyte donor†		Lymphocytes‡					
		U		LD		HD	
No. Diagnosis	IFN:	—	+	—	+	—	+++
2285 SCC		6**	22++	9	36++	0	1
2295 SCC		9	15++	3	0	0	2
2296 SCC		8	—	8	10	8	2
2297 SCC		19+	19+	15	32++	6	9
2004 SCC		26+	20+	22+	43++	3	8
2032 SCC		17+	20+	17+	27++	20+	20+
2036 SCC		12	27++	—	—	19+	17+
2041 SCC		6	3	6	32++	0	11
2042 SCC		6	11	6	32++	11	11
2045 SCC		12	14	32+	36+	23+	20+
2029 SCC		22+	14	5	15	2	5
2034 AdC		21+	52++	2	21++	11	0
2040 AdC		14	37++	0	14	0	8
2038 SCLC		15	17+	26+	30+	17+	17+
Summary††		5/14	9/13	4/13	9/13	4/14	4/14

* The effector populations were pretreated with human interferon alpha (1000 U/ml) for 16 h, and washed once prior to the test.
† See footnote *, Table 7.9.
‡ See footnote †, Table 7.10.
** See footnote †, Table 7.9; + the cytotoxicity is significant; ++ the potentiation is significant.
†† See footnote **, Table 7.13.

patients (11 squamous cell carcinomas, two adenocarcinomas, and one small cell lung carcinoma), the effect of IFN on their ALC function was compared (Table 7.18). Without IFN treatment ALC was obtained with unfractionated cells in 5/14 (36%), with LD in 4/13 (31%) and with HD in 4/14 (29%). Following IFN treatment, the frequencies of ALC with the unfractionated, LD and HD cells were 69% (9/13), 69% (9/13) and 29% (4/14) respectively. Thus IFN treatment induced ALC in the unfractionated and LD populations but not in the HD cells. IFN treatment induced cytotoxicity in the unfractionated and LD lymphocytes even against allogeneic tumours and K562, while HD effectors did not lyse these targets and interferon did not induce such function in this population[30].

Induction of ALC by OK-432

OK-432 is an immunopotentiator preparation derived from *Streptococcus pyogenes*[31]. It has been shown to elevate the natural killer function both *in vitro* and *in vivo*[32]. The effects of OK-432 on the cytotoxic potential of the unfractionated, LD, and HD lymphocytes were compared in 14 lung cancer patients (five adenocarcinomas, six squamous cell carcinomas, two small cell lung carcinomas and one carcinoid tumour). Unfractionated lymphocytes lysed the autologous tumour cells in three experiments (21%), LD and HD each in six (43%) (Table 7.19). Pretreatment of the effectors with OK-432 induced lysis in the unfractionated population in five additional cases, in the LD subsets in four and in HD in two and potentiated the existing effect of HD cells in one. The experiments confirmed that OK-432 induced or

Table 7.19 OK-432-induced autotumour lysis*

Lymphocyte† donor			Lymphocytes‡				
			U		LD		HD	
No. Diagnosis	OK-432:	−	+	−	+	−	+
2117 AdC		8**	22++	30+	32+	19+	50++
2118		11	14++	3	18++	3	14++
2119		9	17++	9	15++	9	18++
2111		4	4	10	10	13+	21+
2113		0	14+	0	0	0	0
2116 SCC		9	5	12	41++	17+	24+
2122		0	25++	24+	22+	16+	25+
2142		30+	21+	10	61++	20+	26+
2133		0	—	9	6	7	7
2143		7	10	5	10	10	2
2109		10	11	15+	19+	0	1
2144 SCLC		15+	15+	18+	15+	8	0
2110		15+	24+	30+	24+	54+	44+
Mean:		9.1	16.0	13.4	21.2	13.6	17.9
Summary††		3/13	7/12	5/13	9/13	6/13	8/13

* Lymphocytes were exposed to OK-432 (50 μg/ml) for 16 h and washed prior to the test.
† See footnote *, Table 7.9.
‡ See footnote †, Table 7.10.
** See footnote †, Table 7.9.
†† See footnote **, Table 7.13.

potentiated the lysis of K562 exerted by the unfractionated and LD effectors. HD cells did not lyse K562 even after pretreatment with OK-432.

CONCLUSIONS

The concept that patients with solid tumours may develop an immunological response against their own tumour is supported by several types of immunological assays. The results of available tests must be interpreted with caution, however, and the issue is far from being decisively proven. The lack of correlation between the outcome of various assays and the clinical course of the disease together with the usually disappointing results of immunotherapy are obvious reasons for doubting the relevance of seemingly tumour-specific *in vitro* tests. However, even in experimental tumour grafting-rejection tests, where a host response can be unequivocally demonstrated *in vivo, in vitro* parameters do not necessarily reflect the *in vivo* events (see Chapter 1). Moreover, it is hardly possible to influence an established tumour by immunological means even in experimental tumour systems with proven antigenicity. Our knowledge concerning the regulation and the mechanisms of immune reactions against autologous tumours is clearly deficient.

In the search for immunological reactivities against freshly isolated tumour cells we have employed two assay systems:

(1) Induction of DNA synthesis in blood lymphocytes of patients by *in vitro* exposure to the freshly isolated tumour cells,

(2)   Lymphocyte-mediated lysis of these tumour cells (MLTC and ALC).

Cellular recognition of the autologous tumour cells has been demonstrated in both assay systems. The frequency of positive cases was considerably higher in the former assay. The correlation between the postsurgical clinical course and the test results of ALC and ATS suggest that these *in vitro* activities may reflect an immune control of tumour growth *in vivo*. The correlations were only partial, however.

The weakness of these studies is the undefined nature of the antigens responsible for these reactivities. Nevertheless, by application of the knowledge that has emerged from the classical cellular immunology, tentative conclusions can be reached. Thus antigenic recognition in the ALC is indicated by the existing analogies between the effectors involved in the autotumour reactivities in comparison with the primed T-lymphocytes[33]. In both systems the major population of the cytotoxic effectors belonged to the CD8[+] subset and pretreatment of the effectors with mAb to the CD3 complex or the target cells with mAb to the MHC class I antigens inhibited the ALC functions.

On the other hand, recognition of the autologous tumour cells in the MLTC was not inhibited by the mAbs directed against the MHC class II antigens, known to be involved in T-cell activation. ATS reactivities obtained with tumour cells that do not express DR antigens further proved the notion that these structures are not essential in the induction of proliferative response by the autologous tumour cells[34,35].

ACKNOWLEDGEMENTS

This work was supported by The Swedish Cancer Society; by PHS grant No. 5R01 CA25184-05 awarded by the National Cancer Institute DHHS.

We thank Mrs Eva Oldmark and Mrs Birgitta Wester for skilful technical assistance.

References

1.   Vánky, F. and Stjernswärd, J. (1979). Lymphocyte stimulation. In Herberman, R. B. and McIntire, K. R. (eds.) *Immunodiagnosis of Cancer*. pp. 998–1032. (New York: Marcel Decker)

2.   Opelz, G., Kiuchi, M., Takasugi, M. and Terasaki, P. I. (1975). Autologous stimulation of human lymphocyte subpopulations. *J. Exp. Med.*, **142**, 1327–33

3.   Weksler, M. E. and Kozak, R. (1977). Lymphocyte transformation induced by autologous cells. Generation of immunological memory and specificity during the autologous mixed lymphocyte reaction. *J. Exp. Med.*, **146**, 1833–8

4.   Vose, B. M., Ferguson, R. and Moore, M. (1982). Mitogen responsiveness and inhibitory activity of mesenteric lymph node cells. Conditionated medium containing T cell growth factor reverses suppressor function. *Cancer Immunol. Immunother.*, **13**, 105–11

5.   Akiyama, M., Bean, M. A., Sadamoto, K., Takahashi, Y. and Brankovan, V. (1983). Suppression of the responsiveness of lymphocytes from cancer patients triggered by co-culture with autologous tumor-derived cells. *J. Immunol.*, **131**, 3085–90

6.   Klein, E., Vánky, F., Galili, U., Vose, B. M. and Fopp, M. (1980). Separation and characteristics of tumor-infiltrating lymphocytes in man. In Witz, I. P. and Hanna, M. G. Jr.

(eds.) *Contemporary Topics in Immunobiology*. Vol 10, pp. 79–107. (New York: Plenum)

7. Bøyum, A. (1974). Separation of blood leukocytes, granulocytes and lymphocytes. *Tissue Antigens*, **4**, 269–74

8. Kagan, J. and Choi, Y. S. (1983). Failure of the human autologous mixed lymphocyte reaction in the absence of foreign antigens. *Eur. J. Immunol.*, **13**, 1031–6

9. Timonen, T., Saksela, E., Ranki, A. and Hayry, P. (1979). Fractionation, morphological and functional characterization of effector cells responsible for human natural killer activity against cell line targets. *Cell. Immunol.*, **48**, 133–48

10. Taramelli, D., Fossati, G., Balsari, A., Marolda, R. and Parmiani, G. (1984). The inhibition of lymphocyte stimulation by autologous human metastatic melanoma cells correlates with the expression of HLA-DR antigens on the tumor cells. *Int. J. Cancer*, **34**, 797–806

11. Herman, J., Kew, M. C. and Rabson, A. R. (1984). Defective interleukin-1 production of monocytes from patients with malignant disease. Interferon increases IL-1 production. *Cancer Immunol. Immunother.*, **16**, 182–5

12. Wood, N., Baskir, H., Greally, J., Amos, D. B. and Yunis, E. J. (1972). Simple method of freezing and storing live lymphocytes. *Tissue Antigens*, **2**, 27–31

13. Oldham, R. K., Dean, J. H., Cannon, J. B., Ortaldo, J. R., Dunston, G., Applebaum, I., McCoy, L., Djeu, J. and Herberman, R. B. (1976). Cryopreservation of human lymphocyte function as measured by *in vitro* assays. *Int. J. Cancer*, **18**, 145–55

14. Vánky, F., Klein, E. and Stjernswärd, J. (1976). Lymphocyte stimulation test for detection of tumour specific reactivity in humans. In Wybran, J. and Staquet, M. (eds.) *Clinical Tumor Immunology*. pp. 55–8. (Oxford: Pergamon Press)

15. Fradelizi, D. and Dausset, J. (1975). Mixed lymphocyte reactivity of human lymphocytes primed *in vitro*. I. Secondary response to allogeneic lymphocytes. *Eur. J. Immunol.*, **5**, 295–301

16. Vánky, F., Klein, E., Stjernswärd, J., Rodriguez, L., Péterffy, Á., Steiner, L. and Nilsonne, U. (1978). Human tumor–lymphocyte interaction *in vitro*. III. T lymphocytes in autologous tumor stimulation (ATS). *Int. J. Cancer*, **22**, 679–86

17. Grimm, E. A., Vose, B. M., Chu, E. W., Wilson, D. J., Lotze, M. T., Rayner, A. A. and Rosenberg, S. A. (1984). The human mixed lymphocyte–tumor cell interaction test. I. Positive autologous lymphocyte proliferative responses can be stimulated by tumor cells as well as by cells from normal tissues. *Cancer Immunol. Immunother.*, **17**, 83–9

18. Natali, P. G., De Martino, C., Quaranta, V., Bigotti, A., Pellegrino, M. A. and Ferrone, S. (1981). Changes in Ia-like antigen expression on malignant human cells. *Immunogenetics*, **12**, 409–13

19. Ortaldo, J. R., Seeley, J. M., Mori, N. and Bolhuis, R. L. H. (1984). Responses of human large granular lymphocytes and classical T cells in culture to allogeneic cells, lectins and soluble antigen. *J. Leukocyte Biol.*, **35**, 537–48

20. Meuer, S. C., Schlossman, S. F. and Reinherz, E. L. (1982). Clonal analysis of cytotoxic T lymphocytes: $T4^+$ and $T8^+$ effector T cells recognize products of different major histocompatibility complex regions. *Proc. Natl. Acad. Sci. USA*, **79**, 4395–9

21. Damle, N. K., Hansen, E. A., Good, R. A. and Gupta, S. (1981). Monoclonal antibody analysis of human T lymphocyte subpopulations exhibiting autologous mixed lymphocyte reaction. *Proc. Natl. Acad. Sci. USA*, **78**, 5096–8

22. Palacios, R., Llorente, L., Alarcon-Segovia, D., Ruiz-Arguelles, A. and Diaz-Jouanen, E. (1980). Autologous rosette-forming T cells as the responding cells in human autologous mixed lymphocyte reaction. *J. Clin. Invest.*, **65**, 1527–30

23. Landgren, U., Ramstedt, U., Axberg I., Ullberg, M., Jondal, M. and Wigzell, H. (1982). Selective inhibition of human T cell cytotoxicity at levels of target recognition or initiation of lysis by monoclonal OKT3 and Leu2a antibodies. *J. Exp. Med.*, **155**, 1579–84

24. Meuer, S. C., Hussey, R. E., Hogdgon, J. C., Hercend, T., Schlossman, S. F. and Reinherz, E. L. (1982). Structures involved in target recognition by human cytotoxic T lymphocytes. *Science (Wash. DC)*, **218**, 471–3

25. Moretta, A., Pantaleo, G., Lopez-Botet, M., Mingari, M-C., Carrel, S. and Moretta, L. (1985). Involvement of T11 molecules antigen receptor-mediated T lymphocyte functions: effect of anti-T11 monoclonal antibody on functional capabilities of alloreactive T cell clones. *Eur. J. Immunol.*, **15**, 841–4

26. Schlossman, S. F. (1972). Antigen recognition: the specificity of T cells involved in the cellular immune response. *Transplant. Rev.*, **10**, 97–134

27. Zinkernagel, R. M. and Doherty, P. G. (1976). Major transplantation antigens, virus and specificity of surveillance T cells: The 'altered self' hypothesis. *Contemp. Top. Immunobiol.*, **7**, 179–220

28. Vánky, F., Klein, E., Willems, J., Böök, K., Ivert, T., Péterffy, A., Nilsonne, U., Kreicbergs, A. and Aparisi, T. (1986). Lysis of autologous tumor cells by blood lymphocytes tested at the time of surgery. Correlation with the postsurgical clinical course. *Cancer Immunol. Immunother.*, *21*, 69–76

29. Vánky, F., Argov, S. and Klein, E. (1981). Tumor biopsy cells participating in systems in which cytotoxicity of lymphocytes is generated. Autologous and allogeneic studies. *Int. J. Cancer*, **27**, 273–80

30. Strausser, J. L., Mazumder, A., Grimm, E. A., Lotze, M. T. and Rosenberg, S. A. (1981). Lysis of human solid tumors by autologous cells sensitized *in vitro* to alloantigens. *J. Immunol.*, **127**, 266–71

31. Vánky, F., Masucci, M. G., Bejarano, M. T. and Klein, E. (1984). Lysis of tumour biopsy cells by blood lymphocytes of various densities. *Int. J. Cancer*, **33**, 185–92

32. Hoshino, T. and Uchida, A. (1984). OK-432 (Picibanil): property, action and clinical effectiveness. In Hoshino, T. and Uchida, A. (eds.) *Clinical and Experimental Studies in Immunotherapy.* pp. 3–19. (Tokyo: Excerpta Medica)

33. Uchida, A. and Micksche, M. (1982). Augmentation of human natural killing activity by OK-432. In Herberman, R. B. (ed.) *NK Cells and Other Natural Effector Cells.* pp. 431–6. (London: Academic Press)

34. Reinherz, E. L., Acuto, O., Fabbi, M., Bensussan, A., Milanese, C., Royer, H. D., Meuer, S. C. and Schlossman, S. F. (1984). Clonotypic surface structure on human T lymphocytes: functional and biochemical analysis of the antigen receptor complex. *Immunol. Rev.*, **81**, 95–129

35. Vánky, F., Klein, E. and Willems, J. (1985). DR antigens expressed on tumor cells do not contribute to the blastogenic response of autologous T cells. *Cancer Immunol. Immunother.*, **19**, 219–25

8
Melanoma

Ph. RÜMKE and J. E. DE VRIES

Melanoma is one of the malignancies in which immunologists have a special interest. The reasons are that particularly in melanoma, spontaneous disappearance of the primary tumour and of metastases has been witnessed, that micrometastases may remain for a long time in a dormant state before they grow out and that histologically primary tumours may often show regression together with infiltration of mononuclear cells, whereas regional lymph nodes also may bear the histological characteristics of immune reactivity. It seems therefore that melanoma may induce an immune response in its host.

CLINICAL EVIDENCE OF SPONTANEOUS REGRESSION

Primary tumours

Occasionally, patients will present with lymph node or other metastases, while there is no evidence of a primary tumour. Patients with such occult primaries may constitute 4–12% of patients with metastatic melanoma[1]. Although the majority of these patients have no history of a possible disappearance of a primary, some of them may have noticed that in the previous 1–3 years, a mole or wart had disappeared after it had changed in colour or appearance, or had bled. In these cases often a small depigmented area of the skin has been left.

Metastases

It has been estimated that 0.25% of all melanoma patients show spontaneous regression of metastases[2]. Compared to other malignancies, this is a high frequency, illustrated by the observation that, although melanomas represent not more than 1% of all human malignancies, they account for 11% of the reported cases of spontaneous regression[3]. It has also been estimated that about 40% of the melanoma patients with spontaneous regression were cured, since at more than 5 years follow-up or at autopsy performed after death from other causes, no recurrence had occurred[4].

OTHER CLINICAL INDICATIONS OF DEFENCE MECHANISMS

Extremely long time intervals (up to 20 years) occasionally observed before metastases appear after removal of a primary tumour, seem to suggest host responsiveness against the tumour which keeps tumour cell growth under control. Another argument why particularly in melanoma, host defence factors may play a role, is that relatively often at early stages of metastatic disease, isotope scanning shows an enlarged spleen or a spleen–liver uptake ratio of >1, which is rarely observed in other malignancies[5]. Yet another argument is that immune suppressed patients, such as those with kidney transplants, are at risk to develop skin cancers, including melanomas, suggesting that immunosurveillance is an active mechanism in the natural prevention of developing a melanoma[6,7]. Melanoma may even occur five times more frequently than expected in the age-matched general population[8].

HISTOLOGICAL SIGNS OF SPONTANEOUS REGRESSION IN PRIMARIES

Histologically confined partial regression in primary melanoma is not a rare phenomenon. For instance, McGovern[9] observed it in 54 of 437 (12%) cases. The incidence in thin melanomas may even be much higher[10]. It is characterized by dense lymphocyte infiltration around the melanoma cells that undergo degeneration and disintegration. In a recent prospective study for the presence of histologic regression within the primary melanoma of 844 patients, regression was found in 173 cases (20.5%). However, no statistically significant effect of regression on survival was found in any of the three thickness strata[11]. These observations suggest that the regression is confined to one or more clones of cells that evoke an immune response while other clones that grow out into metastases are much less immunogenic or not at all.

IMMUNE HISTOLOGICAL CHARACTERISTICS OF REGIONAL LYMPH NODES

Cochran et al.[12] observed that lymph nodes adjacent to nodes partly or completely replaced by melanoma often contained single melanoma cells, a rare finding in tumour-free node groups draining the site of a melanoma. This suggested that nodes affected in this way might have some functional abnormality which permitted the survival of melanoma cells which they harboured. Therefore, orientated lymph nodes from melanoma patients who had undergone lymphadenectomy for suspected metastasis were carefully examined, seeking evidence for immune dysfunction. Histological and immunohistological examination indicated that these nodes had significantly less paracortical hyperplasia than nodes further removed from the melanoma-infiltrated lymph nodes. This was supported by quantitative studies of antigen-presenting interdigitating dendritic cells in the paracortices of the lymph nodes[13]. Functional studies of the orientated lymph nodes involving spontaneous incorporation of [³H]thymidine and incorporation induced by exposure to PHA, ConA, alloantigens and IL-2, supported the histological observations[13]. Significant immune suppression of tumour proximal nodes was demonstrated in most patients. Studies in progress demonstrated an excess of ConA-inducible suppressor cells in the tumour proximal nodes and the possible complicity of tumour-derived gangliosides as immune suppressing agents[13].

The coexistence of occult minimal tumour penetration in the lymph nodes which are immune suppressed suggests a cause and effect relationship, with tumour modifying lymph node function to a degree that permits tumour growth in an area where this would not previously have been possible. Local immune suppression may thus be an important factor of permitting local tumour extension and eventual metastases.

AUTOIMMUNITY TO MELANOMA ANTIGENS - CASE REPORTS

Occasionally patients have been transfused with blood from other melanoma patients in order to see whether rejection mechanisms could be transferred. Sumner and Foraker[14] described a 28-years-old man in whom skin metastases disappeared 6 months after transfusion of 250 ml blood from a 30-years-old woman in whom metastases had disappeared spontaneously. Teimourian and McCune[15] observed a nearly complete disappearance of lung metastases 4 months after transfusion of blood from a patient who had had a surgical resection of a melanoma with lymph node metastases 10 years earlier.

Although these case reports are remarkable and show that immune mechanisms may have been the cause of the regression in these patients, no further reports have appeared on the issue of transferring rejection mechanisms from one patient to the other.

IN VITRO TESTING

Expression of MHC antigens on human melanoma

Human melanoma cells were found to express both class I and class II HLA antigens. Analysis of frozen melanoma sections derived from primary tumours and metastases indicated that class I and class II HLA antigens are heterogeneously expressed[16-18]. Since a decrease in class I HLA antigen expression was observed during tumour progression[16,19,20] and the expression of HLA-DR antigens on primary melanomas and metastasis seemed to be associated with high risk of metastases and poor prognoses, it has been suggested that tumour progression correlates with reduced expression of class I and an increased expression of class II HLA antigens[20]. However, contrasting results were obtained in a recent study by Taramelli *et al.*[21]. Although these authors also demonstrated considerable heterogeneity in class I and class II HLA expression within single tumours and among different metastases, no differences in class I and class II HLA antigen expression were observed. Fresh melanoma cell suspensions obtained from primary tumours or metastases contained similar percentages of class I and II HLA antigen positive cells. Whether these discrepancies are related to the different techniques used or to limits arbitrarily set to define positive cells remains to be elucidated.

HLA-DR antigens are not expressed on normal melanocytes[22] that are considered to represent the normal counterparts of malignant melanoma cells. Therefore, it may be concluded that HLA-DR antigens appear on melanoma cells as a consequence of a malignant transformation process.

Class II HLA antigens expressed on monocytes/macrophages and B-lymphocytes have been shown to be required for antigen presentation[23,24] and are associated with the activation of autologous and allogeneic lymphocytes. Recently, it has been demonstrated that HLA-DR antigens expressed on human melanoma cells are also involved in the activation of autologous lymphocytes[25]. Melanoma cells, strongly expressing HLA-DR antigens selected from a melanoma cell line which was heterogeneous for HLA-DR, were more effective in inducing autologous lymphocyte activation than melanoma cells lacking HLA-DR expression. In addition, this lymphocyte activation was shown to be inhibited by an allospecific anti-HLA-DR antiserum. Fossati et al.[26] demonstrated that lymphocytes from melanoma patients could be activated by stimulation with autologous HLA-DR$^+$ melanoma cells derived from primary tumours, whereas HLA-DR$^-$ cells from primary tumours failed to do so. In some cases these activated lymphocytes were also found to be cytotoxic for autologous melanoma cells. In contrast, metastatic melanoma cells were unable to induce proliferative or cytotoxic autologous lymphocytes, irrespective of the presence or absence of HLA-DR antigens on these melanoma cells. However, in 60% of the cases HLA-DR$^+$ metastatic melanoma cells were able to stimulate allogeneic lymphocytes of normal individuals, indicating that the HLA-DR antigens on metastatic melanoma were functionally active.

Gamma interferon has been shown to enhance the expression of class II HLA antigens on human melanoma[26,27]. This enhanced class II HLA expression resulted in an increased proliferation of allogeneic lymphocytes, whereas no effects were observed with autologous lymphocytes[26]. Although in the studies mentioned above autostimulation with melanoma cells was only induced by cells from primary tumours[26,28–30], others have shown that successful induction of cytotoxic lymphocytes by autologous melanoma cells was also obtained with cells from pleural effusions[31] or melanoma cell lines[32]. On the other hand, a recent study in which the role of HLA-DR antigens in stimulating autologous lymphocytes was investigated, showed that both HLA-DR$^-$ and HLA-DR$^+$ tumour cells were able to stimulate autologous T-cells. Since monoclonal anti-HLA-DR antibodies did not inhibit the proliferation-inducing effect, these authors concluded that HLA-DR antigens did not significantly contribute to T-cell activation induced by autologous tumour cells[33].

Thus, although some of the studies suggested a potential role of HLA-DR antigens in regulating tumour–host interactions, others led to opposite conclusions. Therefore the exact role of class II HLA antigens on melanoma cells in lymphocyte activation remains to be established.

Melanoma-associated antigens

Several test systems such as mixed haemadsorption, immunoadsorption, cytotoxicity and immunofluorescence have been used in the search for melanoma-associated antibodies in sera of patients. In this review we will only refer to a study where autologous typing was performed with sera and cells from the same patient using several techniques in parallel and carried out in combination with absorption analysis to determine the occurrence and quantity of antigen on cells from various sources[34]. Antibodies to three different classes of surface antigens were described. Class 1 antigens are restricted to the autologous tumour and cannot be detected on autologous normal cells or on any other normal or malignant cell type. Class 2 antigens are shared tumour antigens found on autologous as well as on allogeneic tumours of similar and in some cases dissimilar origins. Recent information indicates that some class 2 antigens are autoantigenic differentiation antigens since they are also detected on a restricted range of normal tissues[35]. Class 3 antigens are widely distributed and not restricted to tumour cells.

Autologous typing of sera from 75 melanoma patients showed that in 75% of the patients IgG or IgM anti-melanoma antibody could be detected. Of the 30 patients in whom the antibody analysis was complete, four patients had antibody identifying class 1 antigens, five patients class 2 antigens and 21 patients class 3 antigens[34]. The low frequencies of class 1 and class 2 reactivity may have several explanations, ranging from lack of class 1 antigens on the majority of melanomas to lack of antibody to melanoma class 1 and class 2 antigens in the majority of melanoma patients. It is also possible that the serological tests used are of insufficient sensitivity to detect antibodies of low titre or low avidity. In addition, it has been shown that class 1 reactivity with cultured melanoma cells could only be detected in one out of six different metastases obtained from the same patient[36], suggesting that class I reactivity may be more common than the studies carried out with one single cell culture from each melanoma patient would indicate. However, these class 1 antigens are of the greatest interest as they show absolute restriction to the autologous melanoma cells and they can be considered as tumour specific antigens that are able to induce the immune response (although infrequently) in the tumour-bearing host. Class 2 antigens have a high degree of specificity for melanoma cells but are also detected on human melanocytes[37], on tumours from neurectodermal origin and on fetal as well as on adult brain. Class 2 antigens are not only recognized by melanoma patients, since antibodies with anti-class 2 reactivity have been detected in 5% of the sera from normal non-transfused individuals[38] and in the serum of a patient with astrocytoma[39]. Despite relatively high antibody titres it has not been possible to characterize class 1 antigens biochemically. Class 2 antigens should be considered as autoantigenic differentiation antigens. The clinical significance of antibodies to class 1 and class 2 antigens on human melanoma cells is unclear. In one melanoma patient it was demonstrated that the presence of antibody appeared to be associated with the presence of tumour, since tumour recurrence was associated with a rising antibody titre, whereas removal of the tumour resulted in a decreasing titre[34]. Irie et al.[40] demonstrated a correlation between survival of postoperative stage 2 and 3 melanoma patients and their serum levels of antibodies to one particular type of class 2 antigen, the oncofetal antigen 1 (OFA-1). This OFA-1 antigen is expressed on 50% of the melanoma cells, on human tumours of various histological types and on human fetal brain[41]. Antibodies to OFA-1 could be detected in 60% of the melanoma patients and were shown to be cytotoxic for melanoma cells *in vitro* in the presence of complement. This OFA-1 antigenic system has recently been shown to contain two specificities, OFA-1-1 and OFA-1-2, which are both present on melanoma cells. Like the original OFA-1, OFA-1-1 is also found on various histological types of human cancer cells and fetal brain, whereas OFA-1-2 is only detected on tumour cells of neuroectodermal origin[40]. The OFA-1-1 is related to the AH class 2 antigen[42] and both antigens are found to be comparable to the GD2 ganglioside[35,43]. An immunotherapeutic trial with a vaccine prepared from melanoma cells expressing OFA-1 indicated that anti-OFA-1 antibodies could be enhanced in 19 out of 23 melanoma patients treated[44]. In contrast, a recent immunotherapeutic trial carried out with a whole cell vaccine prepared from the melanoma cell line SK-MEL-13 expressing the AH class 2 antigen appeared to be very ineffective in inducing anti-AH antibody responses[45]. Only in 1 of 20 patients were anti-AH antibodies generated, whereas all 20 patients developed antibodies against surface HLA alloantigens of the immunizing SK-MEL-13 cells. These latter results may explain why antibodies against these types of antigens are so rare in melanoma patients despite the presence of these antigens on over 50% or more of melanomas. Comparable data were obtained in a trial in which 13 melanoma patients were treated with autologous melanoma cell vaccines. Humoral immune responses could only be detected in two patients[45] and were found to be directed against class 2 melanoma antigens. The reason for the general lack of responsiveness to class 1 and class 2 melanoma antigens remains to be determined, but may be attributed to unfavourable presentation of the antigen, antigen modulation, inhibition of the antibody response by suppressor mechanisms or restriction of the response to cellular rather than humoral immune reactivity.

CELLULAR IMMUNE REACTIVITY

In the mid-1970s several investigators attempted to establish that melanoma patients had circulating lymphocytes with specificity for the autologous melanoma cells. Lymphocyte stimulation, leukocyte migration inhibition or direct cytotoxicity techniques were used. Only when proper control experiments for specificity were carried out, was it recognized that much of the reactivity was non-specific and could also be found in healthy individuals. This reactivity, called natural killer (NK) cell activity of lymphocytes, is one of the important activities believed to play a role in the natural immune resistance. Whether this activity is important in the tumour–host relationship is still a matter of debate.

Melanoma-NK cell interaction

NK cells belong to a subset of lymphocytes that without any presensitization of the host are able to kill a large variety of tumour cells *in vitro*. They comprise 1–2.5% of the total peripheral lymphocyte population[46]. Most NK cell activity resides in a distinct subpopulation of lymphocytes bearing a receptor for the Fc portion of human IgG and designated as large granular lymphocytes. Anatomically, NK cell activity is easily detectable in the peripheral blood, lymph nodes and spleen and to a lesser degree in the bone marrow and peritoneal cavity. NK cells are absent from the thymus[47]. The cytotoxic activity of NK cells from all anatomical sites can be enhanced by exposure to tumour cells[48], viruses[49], bacterial products like BCG[50] and *Corynebacterium parvum*[51], and chemical agents[52] like poly I:C. These NK-enhancing effects were shown to be mediated by biological response modifiers such as interferon and interleukin-2[53,54]. Many studies in recent years have demonstrated that NK cells may play a role in the host control of nascent tumours[46,47,52,55]. However, the majority of these early experimental studies were carried out with lymphoma cell lines that were selected for their suscept-ibility for NK cell activity. Recent evidence suggests that NK cells are predominantly effective in early tumour cell elimination but have no effect on later tumour progression[56]. Furthermore, it has been shown that NK cells may play a role in the control of tumour metastasis. Adoptive transfer of cloned NK cells[57] resulted in a 50–85% reduction in the development of melanoma B16 lung metastases following intravenous inoculation of tumour cells in mice rendered NK deficient by cyclophosphamide treatment[57]. NK cells that are able to kill fresh autologous and allogeneic melanoma cells *in vitro* have been demonstrated in the peripheral blood of melanoma patients[58]. However, for these NK cells to exert antitumour effects, they have to traffic to and become localized within the tumours. Since low numbers of NK cells are detected in lymphocytic infiltration of melanoma[59] and very low levels of NK cell activity were found in lymphocytes isolated from these tumours[60], it seems fair to conclude that NK cells play an insignificant role in the host defence against already existing melanoma tumours. Although advanced tumour growth in humans is associated with reduced NK activity[61] and advanced tumour patients have significantly lower numbers of circulating NK cells[62], NK cell activity had no clear prognostic significance in melanoma patients. The notion that NK cells have no significant effects on the growth of existing melanomas is supported by the disappointing results of many immunotherapeutic trials carried out with biological response modifiers. Systemic administration of BCG, *C. parvum* and interferon resulted in enhanced NK activity, but had no effect on tumour growth and progression of the disease[53,54].

Melanoma-T-lymphocyte interaction

The close association observed between T-lymphocytes and melanoma cells in lymphocytic infiltrates in melanomas suggested that T-lymphocyte–melanoma cell interaction may play a role in tumour–host interactions[9,22,59,63–65]. It has been demonstrated that purified T-lymphocytes from melanoma patients were able to lyse autologous cultured melanoma cells in 18 of 32 patients tested[66]. The presence of this cytotoxic reactivity seemed to be correlated with tumour volume but not with tumour stage. However, like most of these types of studies carried out to demonstrate specific cell-mediated immunity, the cytotoxic reactivity was insufficiently controlled and on many occasions the results may have been obscured by natural killer cell activity present in these bulk effector cell populations. On the other hand, it is well established that peripheral blood lymphocytes from melanoma patients can be induced to proliferate by co-cultivation with autologous irradiated melanoma cells[26,28]. Stimulation of peripheral blood lymphocytes from melanoma patients by co-cultivation with autologous melanoma cells resulted in the generation of lymphocytes that were cytotoxic for autologous T-lymphoblasts[29-31]. Furthermore, cytotoxic T-lymphocytes that were able to lyse autologous melanoma cells were also generated, when peripheral blood lymphocytes from melanoma patients were activated by co-cultivation with pooled allogeneic peripheral blood lymphocytes or allogeneic EBV-transformed B-lymphoblastoid cell line cells[29-31]. However, these lymphocytes had a much broader specificity and were often found to be cytotoxic for a variety of other tumour cells[29].

These data imply that activation of peripheral blood lymphocytes from melanoma patients can result in the generation of cytotoxic T-lymphocyte (CTL) clones that recognize and interact with determinants expressed on autologous melanoma cells, but which are absent on autologous normal cells. This notion prompted us to investigate whether such CTL clones with auto-melanoma reactivity could be isolated from bulk cultures in which lymphocytes from a melanoma patient were either activated by co-cultivation with autologous melanoma cells from a pleural effusion, or by stimulation with cells of an allogeneic EBV-transformed B-cell line[31]. Limiting dilutions of these bulk cultures carried out in the presence of feeder cells resulted in the isolation of CTL clones that lysed autologous melanoma cells. Both T4[+] and T8[+] CTL clones were obtained. Analysis of the specificity of the clones showed that they were cytotoxic for autologous melanoma cells but not for autologous fibroblasts or autologous T-lymphoblasts. Furthermore, these CTL clones lysed approximately 60% of the allogeneic melanoma cells tested, whereas in a panel containing 25 normal and other non-melanoma tumour target cells (including many that are very susceptible for natural killer cell activity) less than 10% of the cells were lysed. Inhibition studies with monoclonal antibodies directed against class I and class II MHC antigens excluded the possibility that the anti-melanoma reactivity of the CTL clones was directed against HLA antigens. This notion was confirmed by the finding that monoclonal antibodies directed against T3, which inhibits the cytotoxic reactivity of CTL clones specific for HLA antigens, did not affect the cytotoxic reaction of the anti-melanoma CTL clones[31]. Taken together, these data indicate that CTL clones can be obtained which recognize determinants preferentially expressed on melanoma cells. This anti-melanoma reactivity was not MHC-restricted. In order to characterize the antigenic structures recognized by these CTL, monoclonal antibodies were produced against melanoma cells and selected on their capacity to block the cytotoxic reactivity of the autologous CTL clones. Two monoclonal antibodies were found to inhibit the cytotoxic reactivity of an anti-melanoma CTL clone. Biochemical analysis revealed that one antibody (AMF-6) reacted with a melanoma-associated high molecular weight proteoglycan (MW>450–250 kD). The other monoclonal antibody (AMF-7) reacted with a melanoma-associated antigen with a molecular weight of 150–95 kD (J. E. de Vries *et al.*, submitted for publication). The antigens detected by AMF-6 and AMF-7 were selectively expressed on human melanoma. Significant cross-reactivity of AMF-6 was only observed with most naevi, perineurium and astrocytomas. AMF-7 cross-reacted with some naevi and endothelial cells of very small vessels, but not with those of the large vessels. Both monoclonal antibodies did not react with normal skin melanocytes or B16 murine melanoma. Both melanoma-associated antigens were shown to be involved in the adhesion to endothelium and in the fibronectin-induced motility of human melanoma cells *in vitro*, suggesting that the high molecular weight proteoglycan and the 150–95 kD molecule may play a role in metastasis of human melanoma. This notion was supported by the finding that AMF-7 stained primary melanoma tumours heterogeneously and that many AMF-7 negative cells were present. In contrast, metastases showed a strong and homogeneous staining with AMF-7[67]. Interestingly, the finding that these antigens are also recognized *in vitro* by the T-cell clones with anti-melanoma reactivity, suggests that these cells have receptors for these molecules and that interaction of the receptors and the melanoma-associated antigens results in lysis of the melanoma cells.

IMMUNOTHERAPEUTIC APPROACHES

Based on the assumption that melanoma cells may carry surface antigens to which the host is naturally not able to develop effective rejection mechanisms, several immunotherapeutic approaches have been clinically applied in the hope of improving the prognosis in all stages of the disease.

Non-specific stimulation

Mainly in the adjuvant setting, immunostimulators such as BCG, *C. parvum,* levamisole, transfer factor, and many other agents have been administered in the hope that outgrowth of micrometastases could be postponed or even that tumour cells could be killed. However, extensive randomized studies have not shown that non-specific stimulation of the immune response results in a better prognosis[68,69].

Notwithstanding the negative results in many of the trials, new immuno-stimulating drugs continue to be tested in randomized adjuvant trials. For instance, in a randomized study on patients surgically treated for regional lymph node metastases, the WHO Melanoma Cooperative Group is testing the effect of polyadenylic-polyuridylic acid (poly A-poly U). This non-toxic double-stranded complex of synthetic polyribonucleotides is an inducer of interferon and a modulator of humoral and cellular immune responses, which may have improved the prognosis of breast cancer patients[70]. In mouse tumour models it has been shown that it retards tumour growth.

Non-specific stimulation as an adjuvant to chemotherapy in advanced disease has not shown that it improves the response rate to chemotherapy. For instance, in the WHO-sponsored trial no. 8, in which BCG or *C. parvum* was added to dacarbazine in a randomized trial of 196 evaluable patients, no improvement of the response rate of dacarbazine was observed[71].

Interferons

Recently, non-specific immunotherapy has focussed on the use of interferons in patients with metastatic disease. Generally, when patients with visceral metastases are involved, no effects are seen. However, in patients with soft tissue metastases and occasionally also with lung metastases, remissions have been observed[72-75]. Carter[76] analysed six abstracts of the 1984 ASCO–AACR meeting and concluded that a cumulative response rate in 159 evaluable patients was nearly 10%, and 18%, if mixed responses and stable disease are included. No obvious differences are seen between recombinant IFN-γ, human leukocyte or lymphoblastoid IFN. It has been claimed that, by treating patients simultaneously with cimetidine orally, T-suppressor cell activation is inhibited and, as a consequence, leukocyte interferon may become more effective[77]. It does not appear that the interferon effect is highly dependent on the dose. 12 mega units recombinant IFN-γ three times a week[74] seemed as effective as the more toxic dose of 50 mega units, three times a week[73,74]. Complete responses of more than 2.5 years' duration have been obtained in two out of 23 patients[78].

As yet, interferons have not been employed in adjuvant trials, nor have they been tested in combination with chemotherapy

Topical and intralesional 'immuno'therapy for primaries and skin metastases

A number of drugs and immunomodulating organisms or fractions thereof have been applied to primary melanomas, in-transit metastases, and other skin metastases. One of the substances that have been used to eradicate primary melanomas of the superficial type, is the hapten dinitrochloro-benzene (DNCB). About 2 weeks after skin sensitization, repeated applications of DNCB in acetone or Vaseline on normal skin as well as on primary tumours or metastases provoke a delayed type of skin reaction with, in the more severe forms, an eczematous component. This reaction, if locally induced in primary superficial spreading melanoma, may lead to complete regression. After the first report on three cases by Malek-Mansour[79], several investigators have tried the method. We refer here to the recent publication of Illig *et al.*[80] who have reported induction of 46 complete responses in 50 patients. The complete regression was histologically proven in the first 16 cases, after which no further patients were therefore submitted to excision of the skin where the melanoma had completely regressed. With a 5-year disease-free survival of 88%, the results seem excellent, but the lack of histological proof and thickness measurements makes it impossible to definitely evaluate the value of this approach. It still remains to be investigated whether this method has the notable advantage over surgery that it may promote an immune response to the tumour.

Another agent that has been used intralesionally in primary melanomas is vaccinia virus[81,82]. In a non-randomized study in 48 patients who received vaccinia virus before surgical removal, the ultimate prognosis seemed better than could be expected[82].

Topical DNCB treatment of cutaneous metastases may result in disappearance of these metastases, but in most patients new metastases will continue to appear[79].

Intralesional BCG injections in superficial metastases are probably the most frequently applied way of topical or intralesional treatment of metastases. Mastrangelo et al.[83] have reviewed 14 publications and concluded that regression of injected nodules was seen in 95 out of 127 (66%) nodules, while regression of uninjected nodules was seen in 21 out of 120 (21%) metastases. In 26 out of 98 (27%) of the patients a complete response was achieved.

It can be concluded that topical or intralesional immunotherapy may occasionally be appropriate as a therapy for primary melanomas that cannot be surgically removed, or for skin metastases, in particular when in-transit metastases are involved.

Topical treatment combined with chemotherapy

Topical or intralesional immunotherapy has, until now, not been employed as an adjuvant to chemotherapy in haematogenous metastases. This is remarkable since, on the one hand, systemic immunostimulation has been tested in many trials and on the other, intralesional application of BCG has already proved more effective in the eradication of metastases than systemic BCG[84]. Rümke and Israels[85] pretreated 39 patients with skin metastases with DNCB before DTIC was given. 19 patients had skin metastases only. Remarkably, nine patients (23%) achieved a complete response and five of them (13%) were still in complete remission 3–8.5 years after the start of the therapy. Because of these time intervals, and also because two of these patients had lung metastases as well, it seems likely that the DNCB treatment, presumably by enhancing an immune response, had potentiated the DTIC effect. Synergistic activity of a specific antitumour immune response and chemotherapy has been shown to occur in some experimental systems[86,87].

Specific immunization

With the aim of inducing or reinforcing a melanoma-specific immune response, irradiated or neuraminidase-treated autologous or allogeneic melanoma cells or fractions of these cells have been employed as vaccines. Viral lysates have also been used to prepare fractions containing melanoma-associated antigens. So far it has not been shown that vaccination results in the formation of antibodies against melanoma-associated antigens. Some clinical observations suggest, however, that vaccination may improve the prognosis. For instance Seigler et al.[88] used neuraminidase-treated melanoma cells with BCG to inject 719 patients as an adjuvant to surgery of primary

antigens has recently been reviewed by several authors[105-107].

Although none of the antigens identified so far are specific for melanoma, some of them are so much more concentrated on or in melanoma cells than in other cells, that the antibodies against these antigens can potentially be used in the diagnosis and treatment of melanoma. Some of them are directed against antigens whose functions are largely known. These mabs are important tools for fundamental research in the pathogenesis, immuno-genicity, metabolism, metastasis formation and progression of melanoma.

The clinical research, carried out *in vitro* and *in vivo*, with various mabs will be discussed with reference to the molecules identified by these antibodies. The emphasis will be on those antigens and antibodies that are potentially of interest for immunotherapy.

p97

p97 is a glycoprotein with a molecular weight of 97000 expressed on the surface of over 80% of melanoma cell lines and in melanoma extracts[108]. Later studies showed that the antigen also occurred on normal and fetal cells, but the concentration was still 10–100-fold higher on melanoma cells, naevi and fetal intestine. Structurally and functionally it is related to transferrin[109].

Imaging studies with ^{111}In-labelled antibodies against p97 showed that half of 100 metastases could be imaged dependent on the amount of antibody administered and site of the metastases. With the higher dosage skin metastases could all be detected, while 89% of lymph node, 75% of bone, 67% of lung and 33% of brain metastases could be imaged. Considerable back-ground uptake was observed in blood pool and other organs with gradual acquisition of label in tumour sites by 48–72 h[110]. It was also shown that the antibodies were cleared slowly from the circulation and that early rapid distribution of labelled antibody to the liver can be reduced by increasing the dose of unlabelled antibody[111].

High molecular weight proteoglycans

A high molecular weight antigen consisting of chondroitin sulphate moiety with a molecular weight of >450 kD and a core glycoprotein with a molecular weight of 250 kD is present in high concentration on 90% of melanomas, but also on some astrocytomas and skin cancer[112,113]. Selective localization of an antibody (coded 9.2.27) against this antigen was demonstrated in nude mice xenografted with human melanoma[114]. In one study the antibody was administered intravenously to eight metastatic patients. Biopsies of nodules demonstrated the selective localization of the antibody on the cell surface of the melanoma cells with dose response to the quantity administered. 4 days after 200 mg antibody had been injected nearly all viable melanoma cells appeared to be coated, albeit not saturated, by the antibody[115]. The patients experienced few side-effects from the administration of the monoclonal antibody. Only three of the eight patients developed antibodies against the mouse immunoglobulin; moreover, the antiglobulin response seemed to be transient and seemingly regulated by higher doses of antibody. Although in this study no clinical responses were seen, it paved the way for further studies to explore the use of higher doses of monoclonal antibody and conjugates thereof. In a preliminary communication it was stated that 500 mg antibody was also well tolerated[116]. Interestingly, when combined with mononuclear cells of mouse spleens, the antibody could completely destroy human melanoma xenografted in nude mice[117].

Recently it was shown that the antibody labelled with ^{125}I could selectively inhibit the colony-forming ability of a melanoma cell line carrying the antigen[118]. Clinical trials with the isotope labelled antibodies are therefore warranted.

Ganglioside GD3

GD3 ganglioside has mainly been studied by the mab R24, developed by Dippold et al.[119]. GD3 is a prominent ganglioside on the surface of melanoma cells and other cells of neurectodermal origin such as melanocytes and astrocytes. The antibody R24 mediates a variety of biological functions, including detachment of melanoma cultures, and tumour cell aggregation. In addition, complement-mediated cytotoxicity and antibody-dependent cell-mediated cytotoxicity with human effector cells were observed[120]. The antibody binds to all primary melanomas and metastases, also with most benign naevi, but not with normal and fetal tissues. Within a tumour there can be quantitative differences of the cells in the binding of the antibody[121]. Biopsies of metastases of patients infused with the antibody show binding of the antibody, and of complement factors, as well as infiltration of mono-nuclears[121]. In another study 12 patients were injected intravenously with 8, 80 and 240 mg antibody/m^2 in a period of 2 weeks. Biopsies showed lymphocyte and mast cell infiltration, mast cell degranulation and complement deposition. Side-effects were mild and readily controlled by antihistamines. Clinically, partial responses were observed in five patients, with major tumour regression in three patients. In all patients antibodies to mouse immunoglobulin developed within 15–40 days. It was considered that for further studies higher doses can be employed[120].

Future aspects of immunotherapy with monoclonal antibodies

Although in the studies described above a few impressive responses were observed, it is clear that passive immunotherapy with a single monoclonal antibody as such, does not have much future. Since the expression of tumour-associated antigens may vary considerably even among the cells of the same tumour, it is likely that single mab immunotherapy will lead to selective outgrowth of tumour cell clones expressing other antigens. Therefore, if passive immunotherapy as such should be given a chance, at least mab cocktails should be employed in order not to leave a number of cells unsensitized. Obviously, a prerequisite of such an approach should be that the biological capacities of all antibodies are such that effector mechanisms of the host can be switched on. Since only some classes of murine mabs have the capacity of activating human complement and of mediating cellular cyto-toxicity, selection for these biological characteristics is a necessity. If the effectiveness of mab immunotherapy is dependent on humoral and cellular mechanisms of the host, it is clear also that these mechanisms may have to be enforced in conjunction with the administration of the mabs. Particular antibody-dependent killer cell systems would have to be activated and amplified with the appropriate lymphokines.

Therapy with conjugates of mabs with radioactive isotopes, toxins, biological response modifiers and cytostatic drugs is another possibility. Results of the first clinical trials can be expected to appear soon. However, the main obstacle will still be the formation of anti-mouse immunoglobulin antibodies. Particularly if they are directed to the idiotypes of the mabs, i.e. against those epitopes that are part of the binding sites, these anti-antibodies will prevent the binding of the mabs to the target cells even if the mabs are of human origin.

There may well be a reason to exploit the possibility of synergistic actions between mabs and chemotherapy. Some mabs, such as those of the IgG2a and IgG3 isotypes, are able to activate human complement by which they may kill the cell. However, nucleated cells will seldom all be killed by complement and some clones are resistant to lysis in spite of the appropriate binding of the antibodies. Destruction of active complement factors by membrane enzymes and repair mechanisms that heal complement-induced lesions are responsible for the resistance. Adriamycin was found to render resistant cells sensitive to complement lysis by inhibiting these mechanisms[122,123]. Moreover, adriamycin increases cellular-induced cytotoxicity by different mechanisms[124].

If indeed a synergistic action of monoclonal antibody therapy (with antibodies of the appropriate isotypes) and chemotherapy can be definitely proven in animal models, there is every reason to embark on combination therapy trials in patients whose tumours are found to be resistant to the respective single agents, including the antibody.

References

1. Balch, C. M. and Milton, G. W. (1985). Diagnosis of metastatic melanoma at distant sites. In Balch, C. M. and Milton, G. W. (eds.) *Cutaneous Melanoma*. pp. 221–50. (Philadelphia: J. B. Lippincott)
2. Everson, T. C. and Cole, W. H. (1966). *Spontaneous Regression of Cancer*. (Philadelphia: W. B. Saunders)
3. Bodurtha, A. J., Berkelhammer, J., Kim, Y. H. *et al.* (1976). A clinical histologic and immunologic study of a case of malignant melanoma undergoing spontaneous remission. *Cancer*, **37**, 735
4. Nathanson, L. (1976). Spontaneous regression of malignant melanoma: a review of the literature on incidence, clinical features and possible mechanisms. *Natl. Cancer Inst. Monogr.*, **44**, 67
5. Ikonopisov, R. L. and Oreshkov, V. I. (1974). Possible immunological significance of hepatomegaly and splenomegaly as recorded by hepatic gamma scanning in patients with malignant melanoma. *Tumori*, **60**, 99–104
6. Penn, I. (1984). Cancer in immunosuppressed patients. *Transpl. Proc.*, **16**, 492–4
7. Greene, M. H., Young, T. I. and Clark, W. H. Jr. (1981). Malignant melanoma in renal-transplant recipients. *Lancet*, **1**, 1196
8. Sheil, A. G. R., Flavel, S., Disney, A. P. S. and Mathew, T. H. (1985). Cancer development in patients progressing to dialysis and renal transplantation. *Transplant. Proc.*, **17**, 1685–8

9. McGovern, V. J. (1975). Spontaneous regression of melanoma. *Pathology*, 7, 91
10. McGovern, V. J. and Murad, T. M. (1983). Pathology of melanoma: an overview. In Balch, C. M. and Milton, G. W. (eds.) *Cutaneous Melanoma*. pp. 29–53. (Philadelphia: J. B. Lippincott)
11. Kelly, J. W., Sagebiel, R. W. and Blois, M. S. (1985). Regression in malignant melanoma. A histologic feature without independent prognostic significance. *Cancer*, 56, 2287–91
12. Cochran, A. J., Wen, D.-R. and Herschman, H. R. (1984). Occult melanoma in lymph nodes detected by antiserum to S-100 protein. *Int. J. Cancer*, 34, 159–63
13. Cochran, A. J. and Hoon, D. B. (1986). Immunological aspects of malignant melanoma. In Veronesi, U., Cascinelli, N. and Santinami, M. (eds.) *Cutaneous Melanoma. Status of Knowledge and Future Perspective*. (Academic Press) In press
14. Sumner, W. C. and Foraker, A. G. (1960). Spontaneous regression of human melanoma. *Cancer*, 13, 79
15. Teimourian, B. and McCune, W. S. (1963). Surgical management of malignant melanoma. *Am. Surg.*, 29, 515
16. Ruiter, D. J., Berman, W., Welvaart, K., Scheffer, E., Van Vloten, W. A., Russo, C. and Ferrone, S. (1984). Immunohistochemical analysis of malignant melanomas and nevocellular nevi with monoclonal antibodies to distinct monomorphic determinants of HLA antigens. *Cancer Res.*, 44, 3930–5
17. Natali, P. G., Bigotti, A., Cavaliere, R., Lia, S. K., Taniguchi, M., Matsui, M. and Ferrone, S. (1985). Heterogeneous expression of melanoma-associated antigens and HLA antigens by primary and multiple metastatic lesions removed from patients with melanoma. *Cancer Res.*, 45, 2883–9
18. Burshiell, S. W., Martin, J. C., Imai, K., Ferrone, S. and Warner, N. L. (1982). Heterogeneity of HLA-A, HLA-B, DR-like and melanoma-associated antigen expression by human melanoma cell lines analyzed with monoclonal antibodies and flow cytometry. *Cancer Res.*, 42, 4110–15
19. Bröcker, E.-B., Suter, L., Brüggen, J., Ruiter, D. J., Macher, E. and Sorg, C. (1985). Phenotypic dynamics of tumour progression in human malignant melanoma. *Int. J. Cancer*, 36, 29–35
20. Van Duinen, S. G., Ruiter, D. J., Bröcker, E.-B., Sorg, C., Welvaart, K. and Ferrone, S. (1984). Association of low level of HLA-ABC antigens or high level of Ia antigens in metastatic melanoma with a high grade of malignancy. *J. Invest. Dermatol.*, 82, 558
21. Taramelli, D., Fossati, G., Mazzocchi, A., Delia, D., Ferrone, S. and Parmiani, G. (1986). Classes I and II HLA and melanoma-associated antigen expression and modulation on melanoma cells isolated from primary and metastatic lesions. *Cancer Res.*, 46, 433–9
22. Ruiter, D. J., Bhan, A. K., Harrist, J. *et al.* (1982). Major histocompatibility antigens and mononuclear inflammatory infiltrate in benign nevomelanocytic proliferations and malignant melanoma. *J. Immunol.*, 129, 2808
23. Spits, H., De Vries, J. E. and Terhorst, C. (1981). The cell mediated lympholysis inducing capacity of highly purified human monocytes and T lymphocytes in primary and secondary leukocyte cultures. *J. Immunol.*, 126, 2275
24. Winchester, R. and Kunkel, H. (1979). The human Ia system. *Adv. Immunol.*, 126, 222
25. Guerry, D. IV, Alexander, M. A., Herlyn, M. F., Zehngebot, L. M., Mitchell, K. F., Zmijewski, C. M. and Lusk, E. J. (1984). HLA-DR histocompatibility leukocyte antigens permit cultured human melanoma cells from early but not advanced disease to stimulate autologous lymphocytes. *J. Clin. Invest.*, 73, 267–71
26. Fossati, G., Taramelli, D., Balsari, A., Bogdanovich, S., Andreola, A. and Parmiani, G. (1984). Primary but not metastatic human melanomas expressing DR antigens stimulate autologous lymphocytes. *Int. J. Cancer*, 33, 591–7
27. Basham, J. Y. and Merigan, T. C. (1983). Recombinant interferon-gamma increases HLA-DR synthesis and expression. *J. Immunol.*, 130, 1492
28. Vose, B. M. and Bonnard, G. D. (1982). Human tumour antigens defined by cytolytic and proliferative responses of cultured lymphoid cells. *Nature (London)*, 296, 359
29. Vanky, F., Gorsky, T., Gorsky, Y. *et al.* (1982). Lysis of tumour biopsy cells by autologous T lymphocytes activated in mixed cultures and propagated with T cell growth factor. *J. Exp. Med.*, 155, 83
30. Murkerdji, B. and MacAlister, T. J. (1983). Clonal analysis of cytotoxic T cell response against human melanoma. *J. Exp. Med.*, 158, 240

31. De Vries, J. E. and Spits, H. (1984). Cloned human cytotoxic T lymphocyte (CTL) lines reactive with autologous melanoma cells. I. *In vitro* generation, isolation and analysis to phenotype and specificity. *J. Immunol.*, **132**, 510

32. Knuth, A., Dippold, W. and Meyer zum Buschenfelde K. H. (1984). Target level blocking of T-cell cytotoxicity for human malignant melanoma by monoclonal antibodies. *Cell. Immunol.*, **83**, 398

33. Vanky, F., Klein, E. and Willems, J. (1985). DR antigens expressed on tumour cells do not contribute to the blastogenetic response of autologous T cells. *Cancer Immunol. Immunother.*, **19**, 219–55

34. Old, L. J. (1981). Cancer immunology: the search for specificity. *Cancer Res.*, **41**, 361

35. Watanabe, T., Pukel, C. S., Takeyama, H. *et al.* (1982). Human melanoma antigen AH is an autoantigenic ganglioside related to GD2. *J. Exp. Med.*, **156**, 1884

36. Albino, A. P., Lloyd, K. O., Houghton, A. N. *et al.* (1982). Heterogeneity in surface antigens and glycoprotein expression of cell lines derived from different melanoma metastases of the same patient. *J. Exp. Med.*, **154**, 1764

37. Mattes, M. J., Thomson, T. and Old, J. L. (1983). A pigmentation associated different-iation antigen of human melanoma defined by a precipitating antibody in human serum. *Int. J. Cancer*, **32**, 717

38. Houghton, A., Taormina, M., Ikeda, H. *et al.* (1980). Serological survey of humans for natural antibody to cell surface antigens of melanoma. *Proc. Natl. Acad. Sci. USA*, **77**, 4260

39. Pfreundschuh, M., Shiku, H., Takahashi, T. *et al.* (1980). Serological analysis of cell surface antigens of malignant human brain tumours. *Proc. Natl. Acad. Sci. USA*, **75**, 5122

40. Irie, R. F., Sze, L. and Saxton, R. E. (1982). Human antibody to OFA-1, a tumour antigen, produced *in vitro* by EBV transformed human B lymphoid cell lines. *Proc. Natl. Acad. Sci. USA*, **79**, 5666–70

41. Sidell, N., Irie, R. and Morton, D. (1979). Oncofoetal antigen 1: a target for immune cytolysis of human cancer. *Br. J. Cancer*, **40**, 950

42. Shiku, H., Takahashi, T., Oettgen, H. F. and Old, L. J. (1976). Cell surface antigens on human malignant melanoma. II. Serological typing with immune adherence assays and definition of two new surface antigens. *J. Exp. Med.*, **144**, 873–81

43. Cahan, L. D., Irie, R. F., Singh, R., Cassidenti, A. and Paulson, J. C. (1982). Identification of human neuroectodermal tumour antigen (OFA-1-2) as ganglioside GD2. *Proc. Natl. Acad. Sci. USA*, **79**, 7629–33

44. Irie, R., Giuliano, A. and Morton, D. (1979). Oncofetal antigen, a tumour associated fetal antigen immunogenic in man. *J. Natl. Cancer Inst.*, **63**, 367–73

45. Livingston, P., Takeyama, H., Pollack, M. *et al.* (1983). Serological responses of melanoma patients to vaccines derived from allogeneic cultured melanoma cells. *Int. J. Cancer*, **31**, 567

46. Roder, J. and Haliotes, T. (1980). Do NK cells play a role in antitumour surveillance? *Immunol. Today*, **1**, 96

47. Herberman, R. B. and Holden, H. (1978). Natural cell mediated immunity. *Adv. Cancer Res.*, **27**, 305

48. Herberman, R. B., Nunn, M. E., Holden, H. T. *et al.* (1977). Augmentation of natural cytotoxic reactivity of mouse lymphoid cells against syngeneic and allogeneic target cells. *Int. J. Cancer*, **19**, 555

49. Welsh, R. M., Zinkernagel, R. M. and Hallenbeck, L. A. (1979). Cytotoxic cells induced during LCM virus infection in mice. II. Specificities of the natural killer cells. *J. Immunol.*, **122**, 475

50. Wolfe, S. A., Tracey, D. and Henney, C.-S. (1976). Induction of natural killer cells by BCG. *Nature (London)*, **262**, 584

51. Milas, L. and Scott, M. T. (1977). Antitumor activity of *Corynebacterium parvum*. *Adv. Cancer Res.*, **26**, 257

52. Herberman, R. B. (1980). *Natural Cell Mediated Immunity against Tumors*. (New York: Academic Press)

53. Baldwin, R. W. (1982). Manipulation of host resistance in cancer therapy. *Springer Sem. Immunopathol,*, **5**, 113

54. Baldwin, R. W. (1983). Immunotherapy. In Pinedo, H. M. and Chabner, B. (eds.) *Cancer*

Chemotherapy. The EORTC Cancer Chemotherapy Annual 5. pp. 193–216. (Amsterdam: Elsevier)

55. Herberman, R. B. (1983). Immunoregulation and natural killer cells. *Mol. Immunol.*, **19**, 1313

56. Hanna, N. (1982). Role of natural killer cells in control of cancer metastases. *Cancer Metastasis Rev.*, **1**, 45

57. Warner, J. F. and Dennert, G. (1982). Effects of a cloned line with NK activity on bone marrow transplants, tumour development and metastasis *in vivo. Nature (London)*, **300**, 31

58. Serrate, S., Vose, B., Timonen, T. *et al.* (1982). Natural killer activity against human primary solid tumours. *Fed. Proc.*, **41**, 601

59. Poppema, S., Bröcker, E. M., De Ley, L. *et al.* (1983). *In situ* analysis of mononuclear cell infiltrate in primary malignant melanoma of the skin. *Clin. Exp. Immunol.*, **51**, 77

60. Vose, B., Vanky, F. and Klein, E. (1977). Human tumour lymphocyte interaction *in vitro.* V. Comparison of the reactivity of tumour infiltrating blood and lymphnode lymphocytes with autologous tumour cells. *Int. J. Cancer*, **20**, 512–19

61. Takasugi, M., Ramsyer, A. and Takasugi, J. (1977). Decline of natural non selective cell-mediated cytotoxicity in patients' tumour progression. *Cancer Res.*, **37**, 431

62. Balch, C. M., Tilden, A. B., Dougherty, P. *et al.* (1983). Depressed level of granular lymphocytes with natural killer cell function in 247 cancer patients. *Ann. Surg.*, **198**, 192

63. Dvorak, A. M., Mihm, M. C., Osage, J. F. *et al.* (1980). Melanoma, an ultrastructural study of the host inflammatory and vascular responses. *J. Invest. Dermatol.*, **75**, 388

64. Szekeres, L. and Daraczy, J. (1981). Electron microscopic investigation on the local cellular reaction to primary malignant melanoma. *Dermatologica*, **163**, 137

65. Kornstein, M. H., Brooks, J. S. and Elder, D. E. (1983). Immunoperoxidase localization of lymphocyte subsets in the host response to melanoma and nevi. *Cancer Res.*, **43**, 2749

66. Livingston, P., Shiku, H., Bean, M. A. *et al.* (1979). Cell mediated cytotoxicity for cultured autologous melanoma cells. *Int. J. Cancer*, **24**, 34

67. De Vries, J. E., Keizer, G. D., Te Velde, A. A., Voordouw, A., Ruiter, D., Rümke, P., Spits, H. and Figdor, C. G. (1986). Characterization of melanoma-associated surface antigens involved in the adhesion and motility of human melanoma cells. *Int. J. Cancer*, **38**, 465–73

68. Mulder, J. H. (1984). Immunotherapy in melanoma. In MacKie, R. M. (ed.) *Clinics in Oncology.* Vol 3, p. 587. (London: W. B. Saunders)

69. Cascinelli, N., Bajetta, E., Vaglini, M. *et al.* (1983). Present status and future perspectives of adjuvant treatment of cutaneous malignant melanoma. In Mackie, R. M. (ed.) *Malignant Melanoma.* Vol. 6, p. 187. (Basel: Karger)

70. Lacour, J., Lacour, F., Spira, A. *et al.* (1984). Adjuvant treatment with polyadenylic-polyuridylic acid in operable breast cancer: updated results of a randomised trial. *Br. Med. J.*, **288**, 589

71. Veronesi, U., Aubert, C., Bajetta, E. *et al.* (1984). Controlled study with imidazole carboxamide (DTIC), DTIC + Bacillus Calmette-Guérin (BCG) and DTIC + *Corynebacterium parvum* in advanced malignant melanoma. *Tumori*, **70**, 41

72. Retsas, S., Priestman, T. J., Newton, K. A. *et al.* (1983). Evaluation of human lymphoblastoid interferon in advanced malignant melanoma. *Cancer*, **51**, 273

73. Creagan, E. T., Ahmann, D. L., Green, S. J. *et al.* (1984). Phase II study of recombinant leukocyte A interferon (rIFN-αA) in disseminated malignant melanoma. *Cancer*, **54**, 2844

74. Creagan, E. T., Ahmann, D. L., Green, S. J. *et al.* (1984). Phase II study of low-dose recombinant leukocyte A interferon in disseminated malignant melanoma. *J. Clin. Oncol.*, **2**, 1002

75. Krown, S. E., Burk, M. W., Kirkwood, J. M. *et al.* (1984). Human leukocyte (alpha) interferon in metastatic malignant melanoma: The American Cancer Society phase II trial. *Cancer Treat. Rep.*, **68**, 723

76. Carter, S. K. (1984). Perusing the ASCO abstracts with a focus on interferon in malignant melanoma and renal cell carcinoma. *Cancer Chemother. Pharmacol.*, **13**, 153

77. Flodgren, P., Borgstrom, S., Jonsson, P. E. *et al.* (1983). Metastatic malignant melanoma: regression induced by combined treatment with interferon (HuIFN-α(Le)) and cimetidine. *Int. J. Cancer*, **32**, 657

78. Kirkwood, J. M., Ernstoff, M. S., Davis, C. A. *et al.* (1985). Comparison of intramuscular

and intravenous recombinant alpha-2 interferon in melanoma and other cancers. *Ann. Int. Med.*, **103**, 32

79. Malek-Mansour, S. (1973). Remission of melanoma with DNCB treatment. *Lancet*, **2**, 503

80. Illig, L., Paul, E. and Bodeker, R.-H. (1984). Epifocal dinitrochlorobenzene therapy in malignant melanoma (experience during the last eight years). *Anticancer Res.*, **4**, 293

81. Hunter-Craig, I., Newton, K. A., Westbury, G. and Lacey, B. W. (1970). Use of vaccinia virus in the treatment of metastatic malignant melanoma. *Br. Med. J.*, **2**, 512–15

82. Everall, J. D., Ward, J., O'Doherty, C. J. and Dowd, P. M. (1975). Treatment of primary melanoma by intralesional vaccinia before excision. *Lancet*, **2**, 583–6

83. Mastrangelo, M. J., Rosenberg, S. A., Baker, A. R. *et al.* (1982). Cutaneous melanoma. In De vita, V. T. Jr., Hellman, S. and Rosenberg, S. A. (eds.) *Cancer. Principles and Practice of Oncology.* Ch. 31, p. 1124. (Philadelphia: J. B. Lippincott)

84. Nathanson, L., Schoenfeld, D., Regelson, W. *et al.* (1979). Prospective comparison of intralesional and multipuncture BCG in recurrent intradermal melanoma. *Cancer*, **43**, 1630

85. Rümke, P. and Israels, S. P. (1985). Continuous complete remissions of long duration after topical DNCB and subsequent DTIC treatment in patients with skin and other metastases. *Proceedings First International Conference on Skin Melanoma*, Venice, Italy, May 6–9, p. 10 (abstract)

86. Hanna, M. G. Jr. and Key, E. (1982). Immunotherapy of metastases enhances subsequent chemotherapy. *Science*, **271**, 367

87. Currie, G. A. and Bagshawe, K. D. (1970). Active immunotherapy with *Corynebacterium parvum* and chemotherapy in murine fibrosarcomas. *Br. Med. J.* **1**, 541

88. Seigler, H. F., Cox, E., Mutzner, F. *et al.* (1979). Specific active immunotherapy for melanoma. *Ann. Surg.*, **190**, 366

89. Balch, C. M. and Hersey, P. (1985). Current status of adjuvant immunotherapy. In Balch, C. M. and Milton, G. W. (eds.) *Cutaneous Melanoma. Clinical Management and Treatment Results Worldwide.* p. 197 (Philadelphia: J. P. Lippincott)

90. Cassel, W. A., Murray, D. R. and Phillips, H. S. (1983). A phase II study on the postsurgical management of stage II malignant melanoma with a Newcastle disease virus oncolysate. *Cancer*, **52**, 856

91. Weisenburger, T. H., Jones, P. C., Ahn, S. S. *et al.* (1982). Active specific intralymphatic immunotherapy in metastatic melanoma: evidence of clinical response. *J. Biol. Response Modifiers*, **1**, 57

92. Hollinshead, A., Arlen, M., Yonemoto, R. *et al.* (1982). Pilot studies using melanoma tumour-associated antigens (TAA) in specific-active immuno-chemotherapy of malignant melanoma. *Cancer*, **49**, 1387

93. Werkmeister, J., Zaunders, J., McCarthy, W. H. *et al.* (1980). Characterization of an inhibitor of cell division in tumour cell cultures. *Clin. Exp. Immunol.*, **41**, 487

94. Thornes, R. D., Lynch, G. and Sheelan, M. V. (1982) Cimetidine and coumarin therapy of melanoma. *Lancet*, **2**, 328

95. Asherson, G. L., Zembala, M., Thomas, W. R. *et al.* (1980). Suppressor cells and the handling of antigen. *Immunol. Rev.*, **50**, 3

96. Russell, P. S., Chase, C. M. and Burton, R. C. (1983). Studies of allogeneic tumour transplants: induced rejection of advanced tumours by immune alterations of recipients. *J. Immunol.*, **130**, 951

97. Cheema, A. R. and Hersh, E. M. (1972). Local tumour immunotherapy with *in vitro* activated autochthonous lymphocytes. *Cancer*, **29**, 982–6

98. Frenster, J. H. and Rogoway, W. M. (1970). Immunotherapy of human neoplasma with autologous lymphocytes activated *in vitro*. In Harris, J. E. (ed.) *Proceedings of the 5th Leucocyte Culture Conference.* pp. 359–73

99. Slankard-Chahinian, M., Holland, J. F., Gordon, R. E., Becker, J. and Ohnuma, T. (1984). Adoptive autoimmunotherapy: cytotoxic effect of an autologous long-term T-cell line on malignant melanoma. *Cancer*, **53**, 1066–72

100. Rosenberg, S. A., Lotze, M. T., Muul, L. M. *et al.* (1985). Observations on the systemic administration of autologous lymphokine-activated killer cells and recombinant interleukin-2 to patients with metastatic cancer. *N. Engl. J. Med.*, **313**, 1485–92

101. Parmiani, G., Fossati, G., Taramelli, D., Anichini, A., Balsari, A., Gambacorti-Passerini,

C., Sciorelli, G. and Cascinelli, N. (1985). Autologous cellular immune response to primary and metastatic human melanomas and its regulation by DR antigens expressed on tumour cells. *Cancer Metastasis Rev.*, **4**, 7–26

102. Natali, P. G., Cavaliere, R., Bigotti, A., Nicotra, M. R., Russo, C., Ng, A. K., Giacomini, P. and Ferrone, S. (1983). Antigenic heterogeneity of surgically removed primary and autologous metastatic human melanoma lesions. *J. Immunol.*, **130**, 1462–6

103. Yeh, M. Y., Hellström, I. and Hellström, K. E. (1981). Clonal variation in expression of a human melanoma antigen defined by a monoclonal antibody. *J. Immunol.*, **126**, 1312–17

104. Anichini, A., Fossati, G. and Parmiani, G. (1986). Heterogeneity of clones from a human metastatic melanoma defected by autologous cytotoxic T lymphocyte clones. *J. Exp. Med.*, **163**, 215–20

105. Johnson, J. P. and Riethmüller, G. (1985). The search for transformation related antigens in human tumours: the experience with monoclonal antibodies to melanoma. In Ferrone, S. and Dierich, M. P. (eds.) *Handbook on Monoclonal Antibodies: Application in Biology and Medicine*. pp. 347–59 (Parkridge, NJ: Noyes)

106. Natali, P. G., Cavaliere, R., Matsui, M., Buraggi, G., Callegaro, L. and Ferrone, S. (1984). Human melanoma associated antigens identified with monoclonal antibodies: characterization and potential clinical application. In Ruiter, D. J., Welvaart, K. and Ferrone, S. (eds.) *Cutaneous Melanoma and Precursor Lesions*. pp. 19–37. (Boston: Martinus Nijhoff)

107. Hersey, P. (1985). Review of melanoma antigens recognized by monoclonal antibodies (MAbs). Their functional significance and applications in diagnosis and treatment of melanoma. *Pathology*, **17**, 346–54

108. Woodbury, R. G., Brown, J. P., Yeh, M. Y., Hellström, I. and Hellström, K. E. (1980). Identification of a cell surface protein, P97, in human melanomas and certain other neoplasms. *Proc. Natl. Acad. Sci. USA*, **77**, 2183–6

109. Brown, J. P., Hewick, R. M., Hellström, I., Hellström, K. E., Doolittle, R. F. and Dreyer, W. J. (1982). Human melanoma-associated antigen p97 is structurally and functionally related to transferrin. *Nature (London)*, **296**, 171–3

110. Murray, J. L., Rosenblum, M. G., Sobol, R. E. *et al.* (1985). Radioimmunoimaging in malignant melanoma with In-111 labeled monoclonal antibody 96.5. *Cancer Res.*, **45**, 2376–81

111. Rosenblum, M. G., Murray, J. L., Haynie, T. P. *et al.* (1985). Pharmacokinetics of In-111 labeled anti-p97 monoclonal antibody in patients with metastatic malignant melanoma. *Cancer Res.*, **45**, 2382–6

112. Morgan, A. C., Galloway, D. R. and Reisfeld, R. A. (1981). Production and characterization of monoclonal antibody to a melanoma-specific glycoprotein. *Hybridoma*, **1**, 27

113. Bumol, T. F. and Reisfeld, R. A. (1982). Unique glycoprotein–proteoglycan complex defined by monoclonal antibody on human melanoma cells. *Proc. Natl. Acad. Sci. USA*, **79**, 1245–9

114. Hwang, K. M., Fodstadt, O., Oldham, R. K. *et al.* (1985). Radiolocalization of xenografted human malignant melanoma by a monoclonal antibody (9.2.27) to a melanoma-associated antigen in nude mice. *Cancer Res.*, **45**, 4150

115. Oldham, R. K., Foon, K. A., Morgan, A. C. *et al.* (1984). Monoclonal antibody therapy of malignant melanoma: *in vivo* localization in cutaneous metastasis after intravenous administration. *J. Clin. Oncol.*, **2**, 1235

116. Woodhouse, C. S., Schroff, R., Morgan, A. *et al.* (1984). Immunohistological assessment of localization of monoclonal antibody administered for therapy of malignant melanoma. *Fed. Proc.*, **43**, 1514

117. Schulz, G., Staffileno, L. K., Reisfeld, R. A. *et al.* (1985). Eradication of established human melanoma tumours in nude mice by antibody-directed effector cells. *J. Exp. Med.*, **161**, 1315

118. Lindmo, T., Boven, E., Mitchell, J. B., Morstyn, G. and Bunn, P. A. Jr. (1985). Specific killing of human melanoma cells by I-125 labeled 9.2.27 monoclonal antibody. *Cancer Res.*, **45**, 5080–7

119. Dippold, W. G., Lloyd, K. O., Li, L. T. C., Ikeda, H., Oettgen, H. F. and Old, L. J. (1980). Cell surface antigens of human malignant melanoma. Definition six antigenic systems with monoclonal antibodies. *Proc. Natl. Acad. Aci. USA*, **77**, 6114–18

120. Houghton, A. N., Mintzer, D., Cordon-Cardo, S. *et al.* (1985). Mouse monoclonal IgG3

antibody detecting GD3 ganglioside: a phase I trial in patients with malignant melanoma. *Proc. Natl. Acad. Sci, U.S.A,* **82**, 1242

121. Dippold, W. G., Dienes, H. P., Knuth, A. and Meyer zum Buschenfelde, K.-H. (1985). Immunohistochemical localization of ganglioside GD3 in human malignant melanoma, epithelial tumors, and normal tissues. *Cancer Res.,* **45**, 3699–705

122. Panneerselvam, M., Welt, S., Old, L. J. *et al.* (1985). Studies of C3 binding to complement resistant and complement sensitive human melanoma cells. *Fed. Proc.,* **44**, 1976 (abstract)

123. Panneerselvam, M., Welt, S., Old, L.J. *et al.* (1986). A molecular mechanism of complement resistance of human melanoma cells. *J. Immunol.,* **136**, 2534

124. Ehrke, M. J., Maccubbin, D., Ryoyama, K. *et al.* (1986). Correlation between adriamycin-induced augmentation of interleukin-2 production and of cell-mediated cytotoxicity in mice. *Cancer Res.,* **46**, 54

9
Immunological Features of Human Bladder Cancer

S. PAULIE AND P. PERLMANN

INTRODUCTION

Bladder carcinoma is globally one of the ten most common types of malignant diseases, being more than twice as frequent in men as in women. In contrast to some other carcinomas such as colon carcinoma, the frequency of bladder cancer is showing a world-wide increase, in several areas being as high as 100% over the last 20 years. The exact aetiology is unknown but a relationship to cigarette smoking and to the exposure to certain chemical substances (e.g. β-naphthylamine, benzidine) has been demonstrated[1,2]. In the great majority of cases (>95%) tumours arise in the transitional epithelium of the bladder wall, ureter or renal pelvis and the disease is often referred to as transitional cell carcinoma (TCC). Treatment has generally been performed by transurethral resection or irradiation but successful therapy of superficial tumours has also been achieved with intravesical instillations of chemo-therapeutic agents[3]. Regardless of the type of treatment, prognosis is closely dependent on the stage and malignancy of the individual tumours stressing the importance of early and accurate diagnosis.

Bladder cancer is also one of the tumours for which immune defence mechanisms have been assigned a role in affecting the course of the disease. This presumption originates from the frequent observations that patients with leukocyte infiltrated tumours generally show a better prognosis than patients without such infiltration. Moveover, spontaneous regressions of established bladder tumours have occasionally been reported[4] and an activation of the immune response is also believed to be the reason behind the therapeutic effects of BCG, especially in preventing tumour recurrence[5,6]. In the present report we will discuss some of the studies performed to analyse the specificity and the mechanisms of this immune response, especially emphasizing the recent identification of a number of TCC-associated antigens.

IMMUNE RESPONSE IN TCC PATIENTS

Bladder carcinoma has, together with malignant melanoma, become one of

151

the most extensively studied human tumours with regard to the host's antitumour response. A brief recollection of these studies shows that TCC patients can respond immunologically to the development of their tumours. From *in vitro* experiments assessing lymphocyte cytotoxicity several investigators have found that lymphocytes from TCC patients are more prone to kill bladder tumour cells than a variety of control cells[7-10]. Such TCC-related killing was not observed if lymphocytes were obtained from patients with other malignant diseases or from healthy donors. The TCC-related cytotoxicity was seen to be superimposed upon a normal NK activity and was most pronounced in untreated patients with localized non-invasive tumours[10,11]. Reactivity was lower in patients with a heavy tumour burden and was often seen to disappear after removal of the tumour[7]. Interestingly, a similar TCC-related cytotoxicity as demonstrated in patients has also been observed with lymphocytes from clinically tumour-free industrial workers having been exposed to chemical carcinogens known to induce tumours of the urinary tract[12]. Although cytotoxicity *in vitro* is an artificial system, the *in vivo* relevance of these studies has been supported by prospective follow-up studies where a significantly lower rate of survival was seen in patients displaying low specific cytotoxicity than in a comparable group of patients with high specific cytotoxicity[13].

Considerable effort has also been made to determine the effector lymphocyte population active in these reactions. Although confounded by the simultaneous presence of non-specific cytolysis (NK, natural antibodies) these studies have clearly demonstrated the participation of antibodies as a substantial part of the specific cytotoxicity against allogeneic TCC cells[14]. Consistent with this finding, it has also been established that serum antibodies from TCC patients exert a similar disease-related cytotoxicity when tested in ADCC (antibody dependent cellular cytotoxicity)[15,16]. A minor but significant part of the specific cytolytic activity seen with patients' lymphocytes could, however, not be assigned to humoral factors, suggesting the simultaneous operation of other effector mechanisms.

BLADDER CANCER ANTIGENS

Although most of the investigations referred to above were performed with limited panels of target cells these studies indirectly support the existence of TCC-associated antigens acting both as stimulators and targets for the immune response of TCC patients. A better knowledge of the characteristics and cellular distribution of these putative antigens is of prime importance for the further elucidation of this immune response. The definition of such neoplastic markers should also contribute to the development of improved methods for diagnosis and, in a longer perspective, possibly also serve as the basis for immunotherapeutic approaches. Moreover, the recent recognition of cellular oncogenes and some of the physiological functions of their products has also stimulated the search for corresponding properties of tumour-associated antigens (TAA). Although the formal evidence proving that antibody-defined TAAs are directly involved in cellular transformation is lacking at present, it seems likely that some TAAs will turn out to be products of activated oncogenes.

With our own findings as a basis we will in the following describe what is presently known about TAAs in the bladder cancer system. In doing so we have deliberately excluded earlier work performed with hyperimmune sera. Due to the inherent difficulties in using extensively absorbed antisera these studies have rarely if ever been conclusive. For discussion of these earlier results and of the use of enzymatic and other markers in diagnosis of bladder cancer see Wahren and Perlmann[17].

Derivation of monoclonal antibodies

As repeatedly affirmed, the hybridoma technique has dramaticlly improved the possibilities of defining individual characteristics of tumour and normal cells. With the use of monoclonal antibodies one can dissect the tumour cell into its constituents enabling a detailed comparison with normal cells. In our studies of bladder cancer we have raised a large number of hybridomas with the expectations that some of them may produce antibodies directed towards antigens expressed only by malignant cells. The approach that we have used has been outlined in Figure 9.1 and is similar to that of other investigators. The use of cultured cells for immunization and for the primary selection of hybridomas was based solely on practical considerations. However, the relevance of using cell lines has been widely demonstrated in other tumour systems. While the hybridoma technique does not require purified antigen for immunization it is, however, dependent on easily performed screening methods to single out the hybridomas of interest. For this purpose we have used an ELISA assay where antibodies from hybridoma supernatants were assessed for binding to glutaraldehyde-fixed target cells[18]. In the primary selection this included the cells used for immunization, normal urothelial cells and a few non-TCC tumour targets. Hybridomas showing production of TCC-associated antibodies were selected and subcloned. Monoclonal antibodies from such cultures were then tested against a large panel of *in vitro* grown cells (as exemplified in Figure 9.1 with mab S2C6) and finally with fresh tumour and normal tissue sections.

TCC-associated antigens

By the procedure described above we have obtained monoclonal antibodies to five distinct antigens being preferentially expressed by bladder carcinoma cells. This TCC-associated distribution was first revealed as tested against a large panel of *in vitro* cultured cells[18,19] and was further confirmed and extended with freshly isolated tissues of normal and malignant origin (Table 9.1)[20]. As seen from Table 9.1, all of the antigens were expressed on a majority or all of the TCC specimens tested but could not be demonstrated on normal uroepithelium. Moreover, three of the antigens (4E8, SK4H-12 and 8F4) have so far not been seen on any other types of tissues, while the remaining two were also found to be expressed by a few other distinct cell types. One of these, S2C6, was found to also be a highly specific marker for B-lymphocytes expressed by normal as well as by malignant cells of the B-lineage[21]. It was

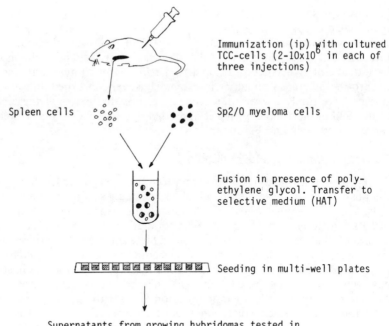

Immunization (ip) with cultured TCC-cells (2-10x10⁶ in each of three injections)

Spleen cells

Sp2/0 myeloma cells

Fusion in presence of poly-ethylene glycol. Transfer to selective medium (HAT)

Seeding in multi-well plates

Supernatants from growing hybridomas tested in cell-ELISA against TCC and non-TCC targets.

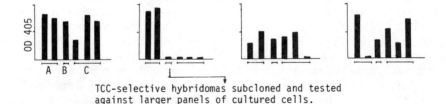

TCC-selective hybridomas subcloned and tested against larger panels of cultured cells.

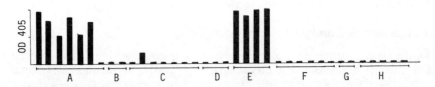

Figure 9.1 General procedure for derivation and selection of monoclonal anti-TCC antibodies. Cultured target cells used in ELISA screening were A) TCC cells; B) normal urothelial cells; C) non-TCC carcinomas; D) malignant melanoma; E) B-cell lymphoma; F) T-cell lymphoma; G) fibroblasts; H) normal blood cells

not found on any other type of blood cells and is likely to represent a hitherto undetected B-cell marker. This antigenic relationship between two so disparate cell types is intriguing and may also provide clues as to the functional properties of this molecule.

Table 9.1 Reactivity of anti-TCC antibodies with frozen sections of tumours and normal tissues*

| Tissue/cells | No. | Monoclonal antibodies | | | | |
		4E8 IgG2a	SK4H-12 IgG2a	S2C6 IgG1	7E9 IgG3	8F4 IgG2a
Tumour						
Bladder ca.	14	8/14	10/14	10/14	10/14	12/12
Breast ca.	3	—	—	—	—	—
Pancreas ca.	1	—	—	—	—	—
Lung ca.	2	—	—	—	—	—
Hypernephroma	1	—	—	—	—	—
Colon ca.	1	—	—	—	—	—
Melanoma	5	—	—	—	—	—
B-CLL†	13	—	—	13/13	—	—
IC‡	6	—	—	6/6	—	—
HCL**	4	—	—	4/4	—	—
Myeloma	2	—	—	—	—	—
CML††	3	—	—	—	—	—
T-CLL‡‡	4	—	—	—	—	—
Normal						
Bladder	3	—	—	—	—	—
Liver	1	—	—	—	—	—
Salivary gland	2	—	—	—	—	—
Skin	2	—	—	—	—	—
Colon	1	—	—	—	—	—
Ileum	1	—	—	—	—	—
Tonsil	2	—	—	2/2	—	—
Spleen	1	—	—	1/1	—	—
Lymph node	1	—	—	1/1	—	—
Thymus	3	—	—	3/3	—	—
Placenta	2	—	—	—	—	—
Prostatic hyperplasia	5	—	—	—	4/5	—
Granulocytes	2	—	—	—	—	—
Monocytes	2	—	—	—	—	—
Lymphocytes	2	—	—	—	—	—
RBC A,B,O		—	—	—	—	—

*Tissues were stained by indirect methods for immunoperoxidase and immunofluorescence;† B-cell chronic lymphocytic leukaemia; ‡immunocytoma; **hairy cell leukaemia; ††chronic myeloid leukaemia; ‡‡T-cell chronic lymphocytic leukaemia

As revealed by immunoprecipitation studies (for procedure see Figure 9.2) all five antibodies recognized distinct cell surface antigens of varying molecular size (Figure 9.2)[19,22]. Three of the antibodies were seen to precipitate more than a single component. All antigens were of glycoprotein nature showing affinity for the lectin concanavalin A.

Using similar approaches, other groups have recently reported on the production of monoclonal antibodies with TCC-associated specificity. Some of these are listed in Table 9.2. In the most comprehensive of these reports, Fradet and co-workers have obtained monoclonal antibodies to a number of

poorly differentiated cells showing a rapid and invasive growth pattern. An interesting question is whether or not these marked differences in biological behaviour are also reflected in the expression of cell surface antigens. That this may in fact be the case has been shown for at least some of the now defined antigens. Thus, the Om5 antigen has been seen to be almost solely confined to low grade papillary tumours and cancer *in situ*[23] (C. Cordon-Cardo, personal communication) while a corresponding association to high grade tumours has been seen with the G4 antigen of Chopin *et al.*[28] and with a 90 kD antigen defined by Young *et al.*[26]. These findings are of considerable interest as the antibodies may detect qualitative characters of the tumour cells and could provide the means for a differential diagnosis of aggressive and non-aggressive tumours.

However, the majority of TCC antigens, including those studied by our own group, seem to be expressed without any apparent correlation to the grading and staging of the disease.

Urothelial antigens

In addition to the antibodies directed to malignancy-associated antigens, antibodies to urothelial tissue type specific antigens have also been obtained. With reactivities being more or less restricted to the uroepithelium these antibodies can be further divided into those recognizing all urothelial cells and those detecting distinct subpopulations of cells[31-33]. In most cases a corresponding distribution was observed for the neoplastic cells. Although this type of antibodies may prove most useful in studies concerning embryo-genesis and differentiation of this tissue type, they should also be explored for possible correlations between the antigenic phenotype and the biological characteristics of tumour cells. Such a relationship has previously been observed for blood group antigens of the A, B, H type where deletions of these antigens appear to be associated with a more aggressive clinical behaviour[34].

Nature of TCC-associated antigens – possible role in oncogenesis

From the above it is now clear that malignant urothelial cells can be distinguished from their normal counterpart as well as from most other tumour or normal cells by virtue of their cell surface phenotype. As discussed in a later section, this may have several clinical implications for the diagnosis and management of this disease but also raises questions as to the nature and physiological functions of these antigens. Extensive studies of TAAs in the melanoma system[35] have shown that many of these represent differentiation antigens expressed during distinct stages of melanocyte maturation[36]. As malignant transformation is known to include the arrest of cells at a certain stage preventing further differentiation, the tumour clone may become antigenically distinct from the majority of cells forming the normal tissue. Although most of the TCC-related antigens have not been seen on urothelium, discrete stages comprising a minority of cells may have escaped detection. Furthermore, TAAs in other tumour systems have been claimed to represent fetal differentiation antigens which are re-expressed as a consequence of transformation. The most well known examples of such oncofetal antigens are CEA (carcinoembryonic antigen) and AFP (alphafetoprotein). These are abundantly found in gastrointestinal tumours (CEA) and hepatomas (AFP) as well as in the corresponding fetal tissues. The possibility of such a relationship between the TCC antigens and fetal tissue antigens has not been extensively elucidated. However, studies by Fradet et al. and by ourselves have been unable to demonstrate any reactivity of the anti-TCC antibodies with fetal urothelium of the bladder or ureter[20,23]. Although most or all of the TCC-related antigens may ultimately be classified as belonging to the group of differentiation-related molecules, the possibility that some of the most restricted ones (e.g. Om5 and 4E8) represent tumour-specific products should not be excluded.

Another group of molecules expressed in a differentiation-associated manner are those coded for by cellular oncogenes (proto-oncogenes). Fulfilling fundamental roles in normal cells, activation of these genes either by critical mutational changes or by deregulation at the transcriptional level may have profound physiological effects on the cells where this occurs. Isolation and incorporation of such DNA into certain susceptible premalignant cell cultures (transfection) have been shown to confer malignant features, like growth in nude mice, upon the transfected cells. Other studies have shown that the activation of at least two different oncogenes is required to fully transform normal cells (oncogene co-operation)[37]. To date more than 30 different cellular oncogenes have been identified as constituents of the normal cell genome[38,39]. For one of these, c-ras, coding for a 21 kD polypeptide, the transforming capacity is induced by a single amino acid substitution[40,41]. As this was first revealed in transfection studies using DNA from two TCC cell lines (T24 and EJ)[40,41] the ras gene has been implicated in the genesis of this tumour type, a conclusion which was further supported by the demonstration that the specific type of mutation required could be induced by several chemical carcinogens[42]. Other studies have, however, disproved ras activation as a common feature of all bladder cancers in that the transforming gene could only be traced in a proportion of TCC tumours investigated[43,44].

Although oncogene products and TAAs are usually looked upon as two distinct groups of molecules, this is more a reflection of the different ways by which they were first detected (at the DNA and protein level, respectively) than of established differences in their properties. Whether the expression of some TAAs will also show a causal relationship to the transformation process is something that can be finally settled only with the isolation and transfection of the corresponding DNA. Recent developments in penetrating the physiological activities of certain oncogene-coded molecules have, however, yielded important guide lines as to the probable functions of some transforming proteins. Thus, in scrutinizing the properties of oncogene products displaying a similar cell surface location as the now defined TCC antigens, several have been shown to be structurally and functionally homologous to growth factor receptors[45,46]. A characteristic and assayable feature of these molecules is their phosphoprotein nature and their capability to phosphorylate themselves or other suitable substrate molecules primarily using tyrosine as the site for phosphorylation[47]. Such protein kinase activity has been assigned an important role in which cells can respond to and propagate external growth signals.

In a first attempt to indirectly relate our TCC antigens with a possible receptor function, we have recently examined them for this particular type of enzymatic activity using the *in vitro* protein kinase test described by Collett and Erikson[48]. The results indicate that the 8F4 antigen, but not any of the others, constitute a protein kinase capable of autophosphorylation (unpublished results). Whether or not this indeed indicates that the 8F4 antigen is a receptor site for an active growth factor remains to be elucidated but is intriguing especially in the light of recent findings where some TCC cell lines have been shown to produce their own growth promoting factors[49]. Such mutual expression of growth factors and the corresponding receptor has been suggested to be an important way by which tumour cells can make themselves independent of normal growth signals (autocrine stimulation)[50].

CLINICAL APPLICATIONS

Anti-TCC antibodies in diagnosis

As is the situation with many types of tumours, successful treatment of bladder cancer is closely dependent upon an early and accurate diagnosis. Hopes of improving the present methods for tumour detection have been centred on the use of specific tumour markers combined with sensitive immunological test systems. In its most attractive form tumour detection may be achieved by analysing serum or urine for presence of TAAs. This requires that the antigens are released from the tumour into the body fluids where their demonstration would be indicative of a progressing tumour. Due to the short history of the now defined TCC-associated antigen/antibody systems their practical use in this type of assay has not yet been evaluated. Great efforts are, however, being made to develop such test systems. A certain amount of cross-reactivity with normal tissues or other tumours should not *a priori* exclude antibodies from being used in this kind of assay. Although such antibodies can be expected to give some false positives this is difficult to foresee and should be tried empirically.

More direct applications of the anti-TCC antibodies would be as a diagnostic adjunct to conventional histopathology and to cytologic examination of cell sediments from urine or bladder washings. These methods which both rely on the identification of characteristic morphological features are by definition most efficient in detecting tumours of higher malignancy grading while tumours of lower grades may often be difficult to clearly differentiate from normal cells. As several of the anti-TCC antibodies discussed above appear to be detecting early (possibly premalignant) changes in the urothelium, they should be particularly useful for the determination of these low grade tumours. While the efficiency in immunostaining of tissue isolates has already been proven for most TCC-related antibodies, the corresponding staining of exfoliated cells in urine or bladder washings has not been extensively studied. Chopin and co-workers have, however, recently reported on the use of two of the antibodies (G4 and E7)[51] for immuno-peroxidase staining of bladder washings from TCC patients and control groups. The sensitivity of these antibody tests appeared to be similar to conventional Papanicolaou staining in that the same numbers of TCC patients appeared positive (14/18). The four negative samples were all low grade tumours which is in accordance with the previously reported selectivity of these antibodies for high grade tumours[28]. Positive staining of the normal and tumour control groups was limited to one out of 51 with both methods.

Immunolocalization and approaches to therapy

The idea of using tumour-specific antibodies for *in vivo* localization of tumours dates back more than 20 years. Labelled with short-lived radio-isotopes such antibodies, administered systemically, may trace the tumour and the accumulated radioactivity revealed by whole body gamma scinti-graphy. Without doubt, also here, monoclonal antibodies have added a new dimension to this type of approach, not only due to their proven potential in selecting suitable target antigens but also for providing an inexhaustible source of stable and monospecific reagents. By using carefully selected antibodies, often in a fragmented form (Fab or F(ab')₂) and under well defined conditions immunolocalization has become a powerful tool in the detection of certain types of tumours[52]. While immunoimaging is primarily intended as a way of early detection and guidance for conventional therapy the same principle may, however, also be applied for targeting therapeutic doses of radiation or chemotherapeutic agents to the tumour site. Moreover, recent results have shown that administration of tumour-specific mouse antibodies by themselves, probably mainly through the arming of host effector cells, may exert therapeutic effects[53].

Although immunolocalization, *per se*, can be assumed to be of limited additional value for the detection of localized bladder tumours it should provide meaningful help in cases where one has reason to suspect lymph node involvement or metastasis to other body locations. This and the prospect of immunotherapy has led us to make preliminary investigations of the suitability of some of our antibodies for localization *in vivo*. Using the nude mouse as a carrier of transplanted human TCC and control tumours we have so far been able to demonstrate the specific localization of three of the antibodies (7E9, 4E8 and 8F4)[54] (unpublished results). With a tumour/normal tissue radioactive ratio between 2 and 10 these results were similar to those obtained by others employing different monoclonal antibodies and tumour types. As expected, blood and blood-rich organs contained the major background radioactivity while antigen negative control tumours and most normal tissues showed no specific uptake.

HUMAN ANTIBODIES

The surface location and cellular distribution of the now defined TCC antigens make them compatible with being targets for the patient's immune response. Although information to this effect is presently lacking, purification of these antigens will in time provide the means for assessing their possible *in vitro* and *in vivo* relevance. Despite this apparent efficiency in using xenogeneic antibodies for the identification of antigens there also exist several reasons for more direct approaches exploiting the antibodies produced in tumour patients. Thus, it can be assumed that patients' antibodies are more liable to recognize relevant antigens and epitopes than are xenogeneic antibodies. Moreover, human antibodies, as such, represent a more suitable reagent for applications *in vivo* in that they do not normally give rise to neutralizing anti-Ig antibodies as is often the case after repeated injections of murine immunoglobulin. In spite of these advantages, reports on the characterization of tumour antigens defined by human antibodies are scarce and none have so far been described in association with bladder tumours.

However, this is primarily a reflection of the difficulties connected with obtaining suitable antibody reagents. Thus, the generally low titres and plurispecificity of patients' sera have in most cases disqualified their use in immunoprecipitation or related methods for antigen analysis. Although several techniques for enriching the specific antibodies have been described it is first with the introduction of methods for *in vitro* growth and cloning of human B-lymphocytes that this question could be properly addressed. In addition to the formation of human hybridomas, human B-cell cultures may also be obtained by immortalization with Epstein–Bar virus[55]. Unfortunately none of the methods have so far proved to perform as efficiently as the mouse hybridoma technique but improvements are constantly being made and the derivation of human monoclonal antibodies to a variety of antigens, including some of tumour-related nature, have recently been reported with both methods (for review see refs. 55, 56). In line with this and hoping to find antibody reactivities reflecting the humoral antitumour response of TCC patients we have established a series of B-cell cultures and clones after transformation with EBV. Using similar assays as for the mouse monoclonal antibodies, i.e. cell-ELISA and immunofluorescence, we have to date examined antibodies from more than 35 patients for target cell specificity and for antigenic location[57] (unpublished results). Clones producing antibodies to cellular antigens were in this way obtained from a majority (>70%) of the patients tested. The antibodies reacted with antigens in all cellular compartments including nucleus, cytoskeleton, cytoplasma as well as plasma membrane. These results are similar to those of others employing lymphocytes from patients with other malignant diseases[58]. While most of the antibodies were directed to common antigens more selectively reacting antibodies were also occasionally encountered. As these have so far only been tested against cultured cell lines further assessment with fresh and also with autologous tissue sections should be awaited before concluding on their specificity. Whatever the outcome of these tests, this study has clearly demonstrated the potential of the approach in dissecting the antitumour response of patients. Further improvements in methodology including the definition of growth requirements of B-cells and in techniques for *in vitro* activation will no doubt stimulate this line of research.

Although not covered in this report, corresponding developments in the culturing and cloning of human T-cells have also provided new means for elucidating the involvement of T-cells as cytolytic effector cells and regulators of the immune reponse in tumour patients. No such studies with relevance to bladder, carcinoma have, however, been reported as yet.

References

1. Wynder, E. L. and Stellman, S. D. (1977). Comparative epidemiology of tobacco-related cancers. *Cancer Res.*, **37**, 4608–22
2. Meigs, J. W., Marrett, L. D., Ulrich, F. U. and Flannery, J. T. (1985). Bladder tumor incidence among workers exposed to benzidine: a thirty-year follow up. *J. Natl. Cancer Inst.*, **76**, 1–8
3. Connolly, J. G. (ed.) (1981). Carcinoma of the bladder. In *Progress in Cancer Research and Therapy*. Vol. 18, pp. 165–75. (New York: Raven Press)
4. Smith, J. A. and Herr, H. W. (1980). Spontaneous regression of pulmonary metastases from transitional cell carcinoma. *Cancer*, **46**, 1499–502
5. Morales, A., Eidinger, D. and Bruce, A. W. (1978). Adjuvant BCG immunotherapy in recurrent superficial bladder cancer. *Prog. Cancer Res. Ther.*, **6**, 225–32
6. Lamm, D. L., Thor, D. E., Harris, S. C., Reyna, J. A., Stogdill, V. D. and Radwin, H. W. (1979). BCG immunotherapy of superficial bladder cancer. *J. Urol.*, **124**, 38–42
7. O'Toole, C., Perlmann, P., Unsgaard, B., Almgård, L. E., Johansson, B., Moberger, G. and Edsmyr, F. (1972). Cellular immunity to human urinary bladder carcinoma. II. Effect of surgery and preoperative irradiation. *Int. J. Cancer*, **10**, 92–8
8. Bean, M. W., Pees, H., Fogh, J. E., Grabstald, H. and Oettgen, H. F. (1974). Cytotoxicity of lymphocytes from patients with cancer of the urinary bladder: detection by a ^{3}H-proline microcytotoxicity test. *Int. J. Cancer*, **14**, 186–95
9. Vilien, M. and Wolf, H. (1978). The specificity of the microcytotoxicity assay for cell-mediated immunity in human bladder cancer. *J. Urol.*, **119**, 338–42
10. Troye, M., Pape, G. R., Larsson, Å., Paulie, S., Karlsson, M., Perlmann, P., Blomgren, H. and Johansson, B. (1980). Disease-related lymphocyte cytotoxicity *in vitro* in patients with transitional cell carcinoma of the urinary bladder. Comparisons with other malignancies, acute cystitis, and healthy controls. *Cancer Immunol. Immunother.*, **8**, 13–26
11. O'Toole, C., Perlmann, P., Unsgaard, B., Moberger, G. and Edsmyr, F. (1972). Cellular immunity to human urinary bladder carcinoma. I. Correlation to clinical stage and radiotherapy. *Int. J. Cancer*, **10**, 77–91
12. Kumar, S., Taylor, G., Wilson, P. and Hurst, W. (1980). Prognostic significance of specific immunoreactivity in occupational bladder cancer. *Br. Med. J.*, **280**, 512–13
13. Vilien, M., Wolf, H. and Rasmussen, F. (1981). Follow-up investigations of bladder cancer patients by titration of natural and specific lymphocyte mediated cytotoxicity. Prognostic significance of specific activity. *Cancer Immunol. Immunother.*, **10**, 171–80
14. Troye, M., Perlmann, P., Pape, G. R., Spiegelberg, H. L., Näslund, I. and Gidlöf, A. (1977). The use of Fab-fragments of rabbit anti-human immunoglobulins as analytic tools for establishing the involvement of immunoglobulins in the spontaneous cytotoxicity of lymphocytes from patients with bladder carcinoma and from healthy donors. *J. Immunol.*, **119**, 1061–7
15. Troye, M., Hansson, Y., Paulie, S., Perlmann, P., Blomgren, H. and Johansson, B. (1980). Lymphocyte mediated lysis of tumor cells *in vitro* (ADCC) induced by serum from patients with urinary bladder carcinoma or controls. *Int. J. Cancer*, **25**, 45–51
16. Hansson, Y., Paulie, S., Larsson, Å., Lundblad, M.-L., Perlmann, P. and Näslund, I. (1983). Humoral and cellular immune reactions against tumour cells in patients with urinary bladder carcinoma. Correlation between direct cell mediated cytotoxicity and antibody-dependent cell mediated cytotoxicity. *Cancer Immunol. Immunother.*, **16**, 23–9
17. Wahren, B. and Perlmann, P. (1982). Bladder and renal tumor markers. In Sell, S. and Wahren, B. (eds.) *Human Cancer Markers*. pp. 303–19. (New Jersey: The Humana Press)

18. Koho, H., Paulie, S., Ben-Aissa, H., Jonsdottir, I., Hansson, Y., Lundblad, M. L. and Perlmann, P. (1984). Monoclonal antibodies to antigens associated with transitional cell carcinoma of the human urinary bladder. I. Determination of the selectivity of six antibodies by cell-ELISA and immunofluorescence. *Cancer Immunol. Immunother.*, **17**, 165–72

19. Ben-Aissa, H., Paulie, S., Koho, H., Biberfeld, P., Hansson, Y., Lundblad, M. L., Gustafson, H., Jonsdottir, I. and Perlmann, P. (1985). Specificities and binding properties of 2 monoclonal antibodies against carcinoma cells of the human urinary bladder. *Br. J. Cancer*, **52**, 65–72

20. Ben-Aissa, H., Paulie, S., Koho, H., Biberfeld, P., Hansson, Y., Braesch-Anderson, S., Lagerkvist, M., Lundblad, M. L., Gustafson, H. and Perlmann, P. (1986). Monoclonal antibodies against carcinoma cells of the human urinary bladder: immunohistochemical staining of tissues. *Anticancer Res.*, **6**, 165–70

21. Paulie, S., Ehlin-Henriksson, B., Mellstedt, H., Koho, H., Ben-Aissa, H. and Perlmann, P. (1985). A p50 surface antigen restricted to human urinary bladder carcinomas and B lymphocytes. *Cancer Immunol. Immunother.*, **20**, 23–8

22. Paulie, S., Koho, H., Ben-Aissa, H., Hansson, Y., Lundblad, M. L. and Perlmann, P. (1984). Monoclonal antibodies to antigens associated with transitional cell carcinoma of the human urinary bladder. II. Identification of the cellular target structures by immuno-precipitation and SDS-PAGE analysis. *Cancer Immunol. Immunother.*, **17**, 173–9

23. Fradet, Y., Cordon-Cardo, C., Thomson, T., Daly, M. E., Whitmore, W. F. Jr., Lloyd, K. O., Melamed, M. R. and Old, L. J. (1984). Cell surface antigens of human bladder cancer defined by mouse monoclonal antibodies. *Proc. Natl. Acad. Sci. USA*, **81**, 224–8

24. Messing, E. M., Bubbers, J. E., Whitmore, K. E., deKernion, J. B., Nestor, M. S. and Fahey, J. L. (1984). Murine hybridoma antibodies against human transitional carcinoma-associated antigens. *J. Urol.*, **132**, 167–72

25. Mazuko, T., Yagita, H. and Hashimoto, H. (1984). Monoclonal antibodies against cell surface antigens on human urinary bladder cancer cells. *J. Natl. Cancer Inst.*, **72**, 523–30

26. Young, D. A., Prout, G. R. and Lin, C. W. (1985). Production and characterization of mouse monoclonal antibodies to human bladder tumor-associated antigens. *Cancer Res.*, **45**, 4439–46

27. Starling, J. J., Sieg, S. M., Beckett, M. L., Schelhammer, P. F., Ladga, L. E. and Wright, Jr. G. L. (1982). Monoclonal antibodies to human prostate and bladder tumor-associated antigens. *Cancer Res.*, **42**, 3084–9

28. Chopin, D. K., Bubbers, J. E., deKernion, J. B. and Fahey, J. L. (1984). Monoclonal antibodies against tumor-associated antigens (TAA) on human transitional cell carcinoma (TCC) of human bladder. *Annual Meeting of American Urological Association*, May 6–10, New Orleans

29. Baricordi, O. R., Sensi, A., De Vinci, C., Melchiorri, L., Fabris, G., Marcetti, E., Corrado, F., Mattiuz, P. L. and Pizza, G. (1985). A monoclonal antibody to human transitional-cell carcinoma of the bladder cross-reacting with a differentiation antigen of neutrophilic lineage. *Int. J. Cancer*, **35**, 781–6

30. Grossmann, B. H. (1983). Hybridoma antibodies reactive with human bladder carcinoma cell surface antigens. *J. Urol.*, **130**, 610–14

31. Sommerhayes, I. C., McIlhinney, R. A. J., Ponder, B. A. J., Shearer, R. J. and Pocock, R. D. (1985). Monoclonal antibodies raised against cell membrane components of human bladder tumor tissue recognizing subpopulations in normal urothelium. *J. Natl. Cancer Inst.*, **75**, 1025–38

32. Rearden, A., Nachtsheim, D. A., Frisman, D. M., Chiun, P., Elmajian, D. A. and Baird, S. M. (1983). Altered cell surface antigen expression in bladder carcinoma detected by a new hemagglutinating monoclonal antibody. *J. Immunol.*, **131**, 3073–7

33. Cordon-Cardo, C., Bander, N. H., Fradet, Y., Finstad, C. L., Whitmore, W. F., Lloyd, K. O., Oettgen, H. F., Melamed, M. R. and Old, L. J. (1984). Immunoanatomic dissection of the human urinary tract by monoclonal antibodies. *J. Histochem. Cytochem.*, **32**, 1035–40

34. Johnson, J. D. and Lamm, D. L. (1980). Prediction of bladder tumor invasion with the mixed cell agglutination test. *J. Urol.*, **123**, 25–8

35. Real, F. X., Houghton, A. N., Albino, A. P., Cordon-Cardo, C., Melamed, M. R., Oettgen, H. F. and Old, L. J. (1985). Surface antigens of melanomas and melanocytes

defined by mouse monoclonal antibodies: specificity analysis and comparison of antigen expression in cultured cells and tissues. *Cancer Res.*, **45**, 4401–11

36. Houghton, A. N., Eisinger, M., Albino, A. P., Cairncross, J. G. and Old, L. J. (1982). Surface antigens of melanocytes and melanomas. Markers of melanocyte differentiation and melanoma subsets. *J. Exp. Med.*, **156**, 1755–66

37. Land, H., Parada, L. F. and Weinberg, R. A. (1983). Tumorigenic conversion of primary embryo fibroblasts require at least two cooperating oncogenes. *Nature (London)*, **304**, 596–602

38. Bishop, J. M. (1983). Cellular oncogenes and retroviruses. *Ann. Rev. Biochem.*, **52**, 301–54

39. Hunter, T. (1984). Oncogenes and proto-oncogenes: how do they differ. *J. Natl. Cancer Inst.*, **73**, 773–86

40. Tabin, C. J., Bradley, S. M., Bargmann, C. I., Weinberg, R. A., Papageorge, A. G., Scolnick, E. M., Dhar, R., Lowy, D. R. and Chang, E. (1982). Mechanism of activation of a human oncogene. *Nature (London)*, **300**, 143–9

41. Reddy, E. P., Reynolds, R. K., Santos, E. and Barbacid, M. (1982). A point mutation is responsible for the acquisition of transforming properties by the T24 human bladder carcinoma oncogene. *Nature (London)*, **300**, 149–52

42. Zarbl, H., Sukumar, S., Arthur, A. V., Martin-Zanca, D. and Barbacid, M. (1985). Direct mutagenesis of Ha-ras-1 oncogenes by N-nitroso-N-methylurea during initiation of mammary carcinogenesis in rats. *Nature (London)*, **315**, 382–5

43. Fujita, J., Yoshida, O., Yuasa, Y., Rhim, J. S., Hatanaka, M. and Aaronson, S. A. (1984). Ha-ras oncogenes are activated by somatic alteration in human urinary tract tumors. *Nature (London)*, **309**, 464–6

44. Feinberg, A. P., Vogelstein, B., Droller, M. J., Baylin, S. B. and Nelkin, B. D. (1983). Mutation affecting the 12th amino acid of the c-Ha-ras oncogene product occurs infrequently in human cancer. *Science*, **220**, 1175–7

45. Downward, J., Yarden, Y., Mayes, E., Scrace, G., Totty, N., Stockwell, P., Ullrich, A., Schlessinger, J. and Waterfield, M. D. (1984). Close similarity of epidermal growth factor receptor and v-erbB oncogene protein sequences. *Nature (London)*, **307**, 521–7

46. Sherr, C. J., Rettenmier, C. W., Sacca, R., Roussel, M. F., Look, A. T. and Stanley, E. R. (1985). The c-fms proto-oncogene product is related to the receptor for the mononuclear phagocyte growth factor, CSF-1. *Cell*, **41**, 665–76

47. Hunter, T. and Cooper, J. A. (1985). Protein tyrosine kinases. *Ann. Rev. Biochem.*, **54**, 897–930

48. Collett, M. S. and Erikson, R. L. (1978). Protein kinase activity associated with the avian sarcoma virus src gene product. *Proc. Natl. Acad. Sci. USA*, **75**, 2021–4

49. Messing, E. M., Bubbers, J. E., deKernion, J. B. and Fahey, J. L. (1984). Growth stimulating activity produced by human bladder cancer cells. *J. Urol.*, **132**, 1230–4

50. Sporn, M. B. and Roberts, A. B. (1985). Autocrine growth factors and cancer. *Nature (London)*, **313**, 745–7

51. Chopin, D. K., deKernion, J. B., Rosenthal, D. L. and Fahey, J. L. (1985). Monoclonal antibodies against transitional cell carcinoma for detection of malignant urothelial cells in bladder washing. *J. Urol.*, **134**, 260–5

52. Burchiel, S. W. and Rhodes, B. A. (1983). *Radioimmunoimaging and Radioimmuno-therapy.* (Amsterdam: Elsevier/North Holland Biomedical Press)

53. Sears, F. G., Herlyn, D., Steplewski, Z. and Koprowski, H. (1984). Effects of monoclonal antibody immunotherapy on patients with gastrointestinal adenocarcinoma. *J. Biol. Response Mod.*, **3**, 138–47

54. Bubenik, J., Kieler, J., Perlmann, P., Paulie, S., Koho, H., Christensen, B., Dienstbier, Z., Koprivova, H., Pospisil, J., Pouckova, P., Novak, F., Dvorak, P., Lauerova, L., Kovarik, J., Iversen, H. G., Hou-Jensen, C., Rasmussen, F., Bubenikova, D., Jandlova, T. and Simova, J. (1985). Monoclonal antibodies against human urinary bladder carcinomas: selectivity and utilization for gamma scintigraphy. *Eur. J. Cancer Clin. Oncol.*, **21**, 701–10

55. Engleman, E. G., Foung, S. K. H., Larrick, J. and Raubitschek, A. (eds.) (1985). *Human Hybridomas and Monoclonal Antibodies.* (New York, London: Plenum Press)

56. Olsson, L. (1985). Human monoclonal antibodies in experimental cancer research. *J. Natl. Cancer Inst.*, **75**, 397–403

57. Paulie, S., Lundblad, M. L., Hansson, Y., Koho, H., Ben-Aissa, H. and Perlmann, P. (1984). Production of antibodies to cellular antigens by EBV-transformed lymphocytes from patients with urinary bladder cancer. *Scand. J. Immunol.*, **20**, 461–70
58. Cote, R. J., Morrissey, D. M., Houghton, A. N., Beattie, E. J. Jr., Oettgen, H. F. and Old, L. J. (1983). Generation of human monoclonal antibodies reactive with cellular antigens. *Proc. Natl. Acad. Sci. USA*, **80**, 2026–30

10
Immunobiology of Human Breast Cancer

A. E. FRANKEL, C. M. BOYER and R. C. BAST

BREAST CANCER-ASSOCIATED ANTIGENS

The analysis of surface membrane and intracellular antigens in breast carcinoma cells has been greatly accelerated by the discovery of monoclonal antibodies produced by somatic cell hybridization[1]. Such antibodies provide a large supply of a reagent which reproducibly recognizes a single antigenic epitope. This allows analysis of epitope and antigen expession as well as purification and characterization of the antigen.

Monoclonal antibodies to breast cancer have been of rodent or human origin. The rodent monoclonals have been derived by immunizing mice or rats with live breast tumour cell lines[2], breast cancer membrane, cytosolic extracts[3] and human milk fat globule preparations[4]. The immunized rodent splenocytes are then isolated and fused to appropriate HGPRT-negative myeloma partners and grown in HAT media. Hybridomas are selected which produce rodent antibodies capable of binding to breast cancer antigens. Human monoclonals are derived from breast cancer patients' draining axillary node lymphocytes which are fused to either rodent or human myeloma cells[5]. Hybridomas secreting human immunoglobulin reactive with breast tumour antigens are selected and cloned.

Monoclonal antibodies have been used to characterize the physical and chemical properties of breast cancer-associated antigens as well as the tissue distribution and cellular location of these antigens. For many of the monoclonal antibodies to breast cancer there is very little information concerning the relevant antigen. From a review of the literature we can, however, recognize several immunodominant antigens and speculate on both structure–function relationships and clinical applications. Immunodominant antigens include high molecular weight mucins and receptors for transferrin, epidermal growth factor (EGF), oestrogen, and progesterone, as well as a number of proteins which are shed from tumour cells or internalized rapidly by tumour cells (see Table 10.1).

167

well as physical trauma. The antigen appears identical to the previously described breast mucins EMA (epithelial membrane antigen) and PAS-O[19,27].

Breast mucin is present on the apical borders and secretions of normal and lactating breast epithelium. Well differentiated breast tumours, benign lesions and normal ducts show a delicate staining of the apical luminal surface. In contrast, poorly differentiated tumours demonstrate cytoplasmic localization of the antigen[28]. When breast cancer cell lines are exposed to sodium butyrate (a potent inducer of differentiation in haematopoietic cell lines), there is a ten-fold increase in surface membrane expression of breast mucin[29]. These observations can be understood by considering the mucin as a breast differentiation protein which must be normally extensively glycosylated and transported both to the apical cell surface and into the lumen. Defects in proper differentiation signals affecting either glycosylation or protein transport can lead to the malignant phenotype.

Unusual glycosylation and modification of intracellular transport of mucins may be important components in the embryonic and neoplastic process. When breast cancer cell lines are grown in conditions which promote three-dimensional growth and cell-to-cell contact there is from a ten- to 100-fold increase in the expression of the Tn epitope on the cell surface[30]. Tn is also expressed on cell surfaces in a discrete phase of fetal development[31]. Thus, a normal role for the T and/or Tn determinant on mucins may involve adhesion to other cells or their substratum. Breast cancer cells express far more T/Tn intracellularly and on their cell surface than do their normal adult counterparts. This is probably due to the efficient glycosylation and transport of mucins to the apical membrane and lumen in normal breast tissue which is disrupted in cancer cells. The diffuse surface T/Tn expression of breast mucins in breast cancer cells may increase their metastatic potential. This hypothesis is supported by the dependence of a T or Tn–lectin interaction for adherence of lymphoma cells to hepatocytes *in vitro* and for metastatic growth *in vivo*[32]. There has been minimal study of the nature or function of most of the oligosaccharide side-chains recognized by monoclonal antibodies to breast cancer mucins.

There are several recognized clinical applications of monoclonal antibodies to breast mucins. The antigen is shed into the serum of breast cancer patients and elevated serum levels are found in 80–85% of patients with distant metastases and 40–50% of patients with only axillary node metastases[33–38]. Unfortunately, 2% of healthy individuals and 20–50% of smokers and patients with renal insufficiency also have elevated levels. However, as in the case of CA125 for ovarian cancer[39,40], there is an excellent correlation between the course of the disease and the serum mucin levels.

Most of the monoclonal antibodies to the breast mucins do not react with normal mesothelial or endothelial cells and can aid in immunohistochemical diagnoses of carcinoma on smears of cells from serous effusions[41,42]. This is useful in approximately 15% of samples in which the similarity of well differentiated adenocarcinoma cells and reactive mesothelial cells prevents routine cytologic diagnosis. Similarly, monoclonal antibodies to the breast mucin have been applied to detect micrometastatic involvement of bone marrow in patients with primary breast cancer[43,44]. Patients with microscopic mucin positive cells have been demonstrated to relapse more frequently and earlier than their cohorts without positive marrow cells. Cases of carcinomatous meningitis can be differentiated from lymphoma, neural tumours and reactive pleocytosis in the CSF using immunocytology with panels of monoclonal antibodies[45]. Since anti-breast cancer mucin monoclonals react with a broad range of carcinomas they may be useful in future panels for this application. Lymphoid tissues and tumours do not express epitopes of breast mucins. Consequently, the monoclonal antibodies to the mucin have also shown value in confirming the epithelial origin of neoplasms in formalin-fixed paraffin-embedded tissues[46,47]. At least one monoclonal antibody to the breast mucin (NCRC11) has been used in an immunoperoxidase assay on paraffin sections of primary breast cancer to predict clinical course[48]. With NCRC11 the intensity of staining was directly related to survival and was independent of other prognostic factors. Such an assay when used in combination with the other known prognostic factors may permit more accurate prediction of clinical course.

Radioimmunoimaging of breast carcinoma metastases has been accomplished[49-51] with the anti-mucin antibodies DF3, 115D8, L1CR-LON-M8, HMFG1, and HMFG2. Metastases in bone only were visualized with ^{111}In-labelled M8. Factors which may have contributed to this result were the high epitope density on bone metastases, the excellent medullary blood supply and the variable epitope expression and poor vascular access of extraskeletal metastases. The high non-specific reticuloendothelial uptake may also have limited the ability to detect non-skeletal metastases. Radioiodinated HMFG1 and HMFG2 were used successfully to image non-skeletal metastases in the chest, abdomen and pelvis. Both the use of single photon emission computerized tomography (SPECT) and ^{123}I-labelling may have facilitated the detection of extraskeletal metastases. DF3 has been radioiodinated and injected intralymphatically to detect axillary nodal metastases prior to axillary dissection. The results are too preliminary to judge. Excellent specific lymphatic imaging has, however, been obtained with the anti-breast cancer monoclonal antibody 3E1-2 for which the antigen is unknown[52].

Transferrin receptor

An ubiquitous antigen on breast cancer cell lines is the transferrin receptor. Monoclonal antibodies which have been made to breast cancer cell lines and which react with the transferrin receptor[8,53] include 24-17.1 and 454A12. The transferrin receptor is a 180 000 molecular weight glycoprotein composed of two equal subunits of 94 000 daltons[54-58]. The glycoprotein antigen contains 5% carbohydrate by weight and a small amount of fatty acid. The transferrin binding site has an affinity of about 10^9 L/mol for transferrin with a higher affinity for iron-saturated, diferric transferrin than non-ferric or apotransferrin. Each subunit of the transferrin receptor binds one molecule of transferrin.

The complete sequence of the transferrin receptor is known and deductions can be made about its structure[59,60]. There is a cytoplasmic N-terminal tail of 61 amino acids. This region has four serine residues which can act as

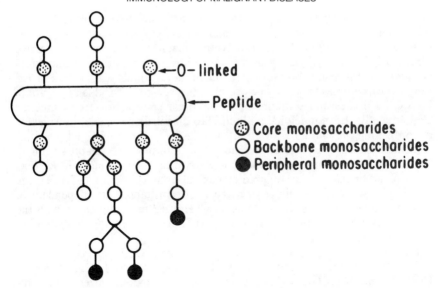

Figure 10.2 Structure of the transferrin receptor

acceptors for phosphate modification. Immediately preceding the transmembrane segment is a very basic sequence lys-pro-lys-arg which is a
cytoplasmic anchor. There is a membrane spanning region of 28 amino acids
which contains 14 uncharged residues and 14 hydrophobic amino acids.
There are eight cysteine residues per subunit, four of which are clustered in
and around the transmembrane region. One or more of these cysteine residues
represents the site of disulphide bonding between the subunits. Finally, there
is a C-terminal region outside the cell of 70 000 daltons with an extracellular
trypsin-sensitive cleavage site, lys-arg-lys, at positions 128–130 and three
extracellular sites for asparagine-linked glycosylation, Asn-X-Ser/Thr, which
matches with the three N-linked carbohydrate chains in the mature receptor
(Figure 10.2).

Transferrin receptors are located on the surface membrane and in
intracellular vesicles within cells in culture and appear to have a similar
location in tissue sections. Most cell lines express transferrin receptors[61-63].
Similarly, normal as well as malignant tissues undergoing proliferation
express transferrin receptors[64-67]. These normal tissues include haematopoietic precursors in the bone marrow, seminiferous tubules in the testis as
well as basal epithelium of the skin, oesophagus and intestines. In addition,
transferrin receptors have been found on some tissues which either transport
iron or use it for specialized functions. These tissues include placental syncy-
tiotrophoblast, brain capillaries, anterior pituitary cells, Kupffer cells,
pancreatic islet cells, hepatocytes and kidney proximal tubules. The high
density of receptors on proliferating cells may reflect the additional iron
required for two daughter cells. In contrast to the mucin differentiation
antigen which is restricted to epithelial cells, the transferrin receptor is a
functional antigen present wherever increased proliferation or a special need

for iron is present. Interestingly, the monoclonal antibodies to transferrin receptor do not show identical binding to all the normal tissues noted above. Either epitopes are modified in some tissues by human transferrin saturation or there are biochemically distinct transferrin receptors in different human tissues. Further work will be needed to clarify this phenomenon.

More transferrin receptor is present on cell surfaces under conditions of iron deficiency (exposure to picolinic acid or desferoxamine) or active cell division[68]. Conversely, less surface transferrin receptor is present after exposure to phorbol diesters[69,70].

Growth inhibition can be produced by exposure of cells *in vitro* or *in vivo* to monoclonal antibodies which block transferrin binding to its receptor[71,72]. Similarly, exposure of cells to gallium which competes with iron for binding to transferrin causes arrest to cell proliferation. Thus, iron laden transferrin binding is a necessary event in cell proliferation for tumour cell lines.

Once transferrin containing 2 moles of Fe^{3+}/mole of transferrin is bound to the receptor, the complex aggregates over coated pits in the plane of the membrane. These clathrin-coated pits internalize and the vesicles lose their clathrin coats and migrate to a deeper endosomal compartment where the vesicle contents are exposed to low pH. This leads to dissociation of bound Fe^{3+} which enters the cytosol. The apotransferrin and transferrin receptor are then recycled to the cell surface. Apotransferrin is released and exchanged for more avidly bound transferrin. This process and subsequent cell division can be blocked by down-regulation of surface transferrin receptors by phorbol diester[69]. This agent acts to activate protein kinase C which phosphorylates cytoplasmic serines on the transferrin receptor causing internalization without return to the cell surface.

There are several clinical applications of monoclonal anitbodies reactive with the transferrin receptor. Immunohistologic studies may document a relationship between transferrin receptor density and malignant grade of breast tumours and other neoplasms. This may provide an easier test for the degree of tumour differentiation than thymidine labelling index or nuclear grade. Such an assay could be useful in predicting clinical behaviour.

Monoclonal antibodies to the transferrin receptor have been linked to peptide toxins and are extremely potent cytotoxins[71,73-78]. They are selective for transferrin receptor positive cells. In regional therapies for ovarian cancer, mesothelioma, bladder cancer and neoplastic meningitis they may provide a new useful therapeutic modality[79]. With the poor clearance of these large proteins from the body cavities one would anticipate minimal exposure of normal proliferating cells or other iron-requiring cells.

EGF receptor

An antigen present on a fraction of poorly differentiated breast tumours is the receptor for epidermal growth factor (EGF). Mouse monoclonal antibodies have been prepared to the vulvar carcinoma cell line, A431. A number of these antibodies bind the EGF receptor[80-85] including 101, EGFR1, 2G2, TL5, 29-1, 528, 225, 579, and 455.

The EGF receptor is a 175000 dalton glycoprotein with a polypeptide backbone of 138 000 daltons (about 1250 amino acids) and oligosaccharide side-chains of 37 000 daltons[84,86-89]. The antigen has three domains – an EGF binding domain external to the plasma membrane (about 710 amino acids), a transmembrane domain and a cytoplasmic tail with autophosphorylation sites (about 545 amino acids). The oligosaccharide contains mannose, galactose, N-acetylglucosamine and sialic acid[86]. The sialic acid participates in EGF binding[89]. The oncogene protein, v-erb-B, appears to be a truncated EGF receptor lacking the EGF binding site[84].

EGF receptors are found on the cell surface and within intracellular vesicles. A variety of normal and malignant cell lines express EGF receptors. About one-third of breast cell lines including MDA-MB231, BT 474, and BT 20 have at least 20 000 EGF receptor molecules per cell[90-92]. More differentiated breast tumour cell lines such as MCF7 and ZR75-1 have either few or no EGF receptors. When assayed either by binding of [^{125}I]EGF on membrane extracts or indirect immunoperoxidase assays of monoclonal antibodies to EGF receptor on frozen sections, about 35% of primary breast carcinomas show high levels of the antigen[93-95]. Tumours which lack oestrogen receptors, metastatic to axillary nodes, or exhibit high histologic grade tend to express EGF receptors. Similarly, metastatic breast tumour lesions are more frequently positive for EGF receptors than primary tumours. In addition to breast cancer, the antigen is found on a variety of neoplasms including squamous lung carcinomas, invasive bladder tumours and non-neural brain tumours[96,97]. A number of normal epithelial tissues express EGF receptors including the vas deferens, endometrium, endocervix, bladder, urethra, oral mucosa, oesophagus, hepatic bile ducts, bronchial epithelium, skin and thymic epithelium[98]. The antigen is localized to the basal epithelium in each organ. EGF is a 53 amino acid peptide with three internal disulphide bonds. The peptide folds spontaneously to its native conformation on oxidation–reduction[99]. EGF is produced in mice by the submaxillary gland. Its source in man is unknown. The peptide is found in the plasma (1 ng/ml) and in body secretions – urine, saliva, milk (30 ng/ml). The peptide binds to its receptor with a Ka of greater than 10^9 L/mol. Once EGF binds to its receptor a number of reactions occur[100]. The EGF–EGF receptor complex migrates on the cell surface to the region of coated pits where the complexes aggregate into groups of 8–50. The complexed receptor also triggers a phosphotyrosine kinase activity. The complexed receptor in the coated pits is then internalized into coated vesicles. The clathrin-coated vesicles uncoat and become endocytic vesicles. The EGF receptor complex travels with the vesicle to the peri-Golgi area where it again is associated with Golgi-coated vesicles. These distinct clathrin vesicles migrate to lysosomes where EGF and its receptor are metabolized. Physiologic consequences of receptor clustering and kinase activation can include either cell proliferation or differentiation, dependent on the cell type.

Several clinical applications have been proposed for monoclonal antibodies reactive with the EGF receptor. Immunoperoxidase staining of frozen sections of primary breast tumours with anti-EGF receptor monoclonal antibody EGFR1 identifies patients with a poor prognosis[95]. Such patients are at an increased risk of relapse and may need aggressive adjuvant treatment. Immunoperoxidase stains of lung cancer sections with EGFR1 have been used to distinguish small cell and non-small cell lung cancers[97]. Serotherapy of patients with EGF receptor-positive tumours may have clinical efficacy[101]. Monoclonal antibodies 528, 225, and 455 inhibited growth of human epidermoid tumour in nude mice. Finally, monoclonal antibodies to the EGF receptor or the EGF ligand itself may be covalently linked to peptide toxins. Such immunotoxins and ligand-toxins are potent cytotoxic agents for receptor positive cells[102–104]. Immunotoxins can be given intraventricularly to treat leptomeningeal breast or brain tumours and intravesically to treat superficial and invasive bladder carcinomas[79].

Breast carcinoma cells also have surface receptors for the peptide hormones somatomedin C[105] and prolactin[106] but there have been no reports of monoclonal antibodies to these receptors at the time of this review.

Oestrogen and progesterone receptors

The intracellular binding proteins for oestrogen and progesterone are called the oestrogen receptor and progesterone receptor, respectively, Rat monoclonal antibodies prepared to the human oestrogen receptor from the MCF7 breast tumour cell line include[107] D58, D75, D547, H221, H222, H226, F88, F344, G5, G13, H23, H142, H165. These antibodies recognize different antigenic determinants on the oestrogen receptor. Mouse monoclonal antibody to the hen oviduct progesterone receptor, 9B3-12, binds to the human progesterone receptor[108]. The rat monoclonal antibodies 9G10 and 3E8 prepared against the hen progesterone receptor react only with denatured chicken progesterone receptor B protein[109].

The oestrogen receptor is a single subunit with one oestrogen binding site and one DNA binding site[110]. The molecular weight is 60000–70000 daltons. Native oestrogen receptor may consist of multimers of the subunit. The nuclear form of the oestrogen receptor appears to be a homodimer with positive co-operativity of oestrogen binding. In contrast, the unactivated nuclear or cytoplasmic forms of the receptor consist of at least four subunits. All the oligomeric forms are dissociable with KCl. The cytoplasmic or unactivated form of the receptor appears to be phosphorylated. While the oestrogen binding site and DNA binding site are at opposite ends of the polypeptide, in the native conformation they are spatially close together. Highly conserved determinants on the oestrogen receptor are close to the DNA or oestrogen binding sites[101]. The association of the oestrogen receptor with oestrogen leads to an increase in its affinity for DNA.

The human progesterone receptor consists of two dissimilar polypeptides in equimolar amount of 83000 daltons and 115000 daltons called proteins A and B, respectively[111]. The A protein binds DNA and the A and B proteins bind progesterone. There is a phosphorylation site near the carboxyl-terminal end of protein B. Once the receptor has been activated and transformed by progestin treatments, its subunit structure and size is unchanged but it binds DNA more avidly.

The oestrogen receptor is confined to the nucleus in receptor positive cells[112]. Related immunohistologic studies for the progesterone receptor have

Carcinoembryonic antigen

CEA or carcinoembryonic antigen is a 180000 dalton glycoprotein found originally in tumours of the gastrointestinal tract but subsequently discovered in a large number of different tumours and in some fetal and normal adult tissues[132]. Mouse monoclonal antibodies have been prepared to at least six distinct epitopes on CEA[133-146]. Molecules immunologically related to, if not identical, to CEA have been found in breast tumours and in the serum of patients with breast cancer[147,148].

CEA contains a polypeptide chain of 70000-80000 daltons with 575-829 amino acids and six intrachain cystine disulphide bonds[149]. 30 N-terminal residues have been sequenced by the standard Edman procedure[150]. This peptide lacks methionine residues. The CEA protein has been digested with trypsin and a limited number of the tryptic peptides have been sequenced[151]. The isoelectric point is 3-4[152]. All of the carbohydrate which represents 50% of the molecule is N-acetylglucosamine, mannose, galactose, fucose, sialic and neuraminic acid. The carbohydrate is organized in oligosaccharide units of 4-9 monosaccharide residues attached to between 51 and 124 sites on the protein. The only attachment is a N-glycosidic linkage to asparagine[153]. Most of the antigenic epitopes appear to depend on the protein tertiary structure and are not carbohydrate related. The mRNA for CEA has been isolated and the complete amino acid sequence for CEA should soon be available[154]. The *in vitro* translation product for this mRNA is an 85000 dalton polypeptide.

CEA is found on the surface membrane of normal and malignant cells including mammary cells[155]. It appears to be a member of a family of related epithelial glycoproteins which includes NCA, NCA-2, TEX, BGP-I and NFA1. CEA appears to have distinct epitopes for monoclonal antibodies as well as a unique primary sequence. The function of the members of this protein family is unknown.

Applications of monoclonal antibodies to CEA include immunohistology of primary breast carcinomas. Both benign breast lesions (25-65%) and malignant breast tumours (60-70%) show positivity using immunostaining[153]. While some reports suggested prognostic significance to the presence or absence of immunostaining with anti-CEA antibody, this could not be confirmed in a large ECOG study[156].

Sandwich monoclonal immunoassays using two distinct determinants on CEA have been developed to supplement and perhaps improve the results using polyclonal radioimmunoassays. Circulating CEA is found in 9% of Stage I, 23% of Stage II, 45% of Stage III and 58% of Stage IV patients[157]. Patients with lung or visceral involvement have more frequent elevations of CEA than patients with only soft tissue involvement[157]. Patients with greater bulk of metastatic disease have higher levels. Unfortunately, CEA is a poor screening test for breast cancer with low sensitivity and specificity[158].

While CEA levels do correlate with other tests for staging, they fail to provide independent prognostic information[157]. When patients are monitored serially, a rising CEA can sometimes precede recurrence, but CEA generally rises concomitantly with overt disease. Elevations of CEA with occult disease are often in the range associated with benign conditions. A large prospective study failed to confirm the utility of CEA for monitoring breast cancer patients[159]. Response to therapy was readily monitored by history, physical examination and intermittent radiologic evaluations. The most useful application of CEA immunoassays may be in the screening of CSF in patients with suspected carcinomatous meningitis. Positive CSF assays had a high correlation with eventual carcinomatous pleocytosis[157].

Monoclonal antibodies to CEA have been fragmented with proteases and labelled with radioiodine and injected into patients with a variety of neoplasms. With the use of rectilinear or SPECT scanning tumour localization has been demonstrated[160]. As yet, it is not clear how this will aid in the management of patients with metastatic breast cancer.

Potentially toxic substances including cytotoxic drugs, radiotherapeutic nuclides or toxins can be attached to monoclonal antibodies to CEA and administered to patients with metastatic breast cancer. *In vitro* and animal model studies have been reported using 11-285.14-vindesine[161] and C19-RTA[162].

Secreted or shed antigens

In addition to the mucins, CEA and the oestrogen-regulated 52 000 dalton glycoprotein there are several other breast cancer-associated antigens which have been detected in human serum.

Three monoclonal antibodies to human breast milk (67D11, 115H10 and 115C2) exhibited similar cellular reaction patterns[163-165], but the antibodies do not cross-block. The antigenic epitopes were named Mam-3a, Mam-3b and Mam-3c. The Mam-3c epitope has recently been characterized[166] as lacto-N-difucohexaose II. This is a combination of type 1 and type 2 based fuco-oligosaccharides. It is not known whether the backbone for this epitope is a glycolipid or glycoprotein. Using a modified low pH ELISA assay women with breast cancer were found to have elevated Mam-3 antigen levels in their serum[167]. 83% of breast cancer patients had elevated levels compared to only 5% of controls. This monoclonal immunoassay of serum may provide a screening test or monitoring test for breast cancer. Immunoperoxidase assay of paraffin sections of primary breast carcinoma with the 115H10 monoclonal antibody to Mam-3b revealed reactivity with 54% of tumours[168]. These patients with Mam-3b epitope had an improved disease-free survival compared to those without Mam-3b. However, the presence of Mam-3b does not add significant prognostic information.

Another monoclonal antibody to breast milk, Mc3, detects a breast cancer-associated antigen shed into serum[169]. The antigen is a 46 000 dalton glycoprotein. It is detected on the surface of breast tumour cell lines but not on cell lines derived from other tissues. By using a sandwich radioimmunoassay with Mc3 coated on beads, the antigen was detected in the sera of breast cancer patients. As with Mam-3, the Mc3 antigen may be useful in the early detection of breast cancer or in monitoring the response to treatments of patients with metastatic breast cancer.

The monoclonal antibody 24-17.2 was prepared against the MCF7 breast tumour cell line[53]. This antibody recognizes a 100 000 dalton protein present on the surface of breast tumour cell lines but not on cell lines of non-breast origin. Using an indirect immunofluorescence assay on frozen tissue sections, the antigen was detected in malignant breast cancer tissue but not on colon, lung, kidney, thymic or oral cancer. Normal tissues containing the antigen included pancreatic acini, hepatic bile ducts, renal tubules, salivary gland epithelium, prostate epithelium, bronchial epithelium and normal breast epithelium. While the breast tumour cell lines and normal epithelium show surface membrane antigen, breast carcinomas show high levels of cytoplasmic antigen. Binding inhibition assays showed the presence of antigen in sera of patients with advanced breast carcinoma but not in normal human serum. Since 24-17.2 fails to react with non-breast tumours, it may be useful in categorizing tumours of unknown origin. As with the other antigens found in sera, the 24-17.2 antigen may lead to a serum screening or monitoring assay.

The milk proteins, casein, a-lactalbumin and lactoferrin are unique products of fully differentiated mammary epithelium but do not appear to be synthesized or secreted by breast carcinoma cells. Monoclonal antibodies recently made against casein (F20.1, F20.4, F20.10, F20.14) may permit retesting for this marker in breast cancer frozen sections and sera[170].

Other breast cancer-associated antigens which have been characterized

The mouse IgG1 monoclonal antibody 10-3D2 binds a 126 000 dalton phosphoglycoprotein found in membrane extracts of the breast tumour cell line[171] BT20. The antigen is phosphorylated at serines or threonines and is located both on cell surface membrane and in the cytoplasm. The antigen is found on all breast tumour cell lines and several other tumour cell lines. When labelled with [^{111}In]DTPA the antibody localizes to BT20 breast tumour xenografts in nude mice[172]. Hence, it may be useful in radioimmunoimaging.

Monoclonal antibody B6.2 was prepared against membrane extracts of breast carcinoma metastases[9]. It recognizes a 90 000 dalton protein on the cell surface of three breast tumour cell lines[173]. The antigen is a normal cross-reacting antigen (NCA)[174]. NCA is a glycoprotein containing homologous regions with CEA[175]. NCA is present in various normal tissues including lung, spleen and on the surface of circulating granulocytes. The antigen is present on 75% of primary and metastatic breast carcinomas. However, there is marked heterogeneity in individal tumours for expression of the antigen. This may be due to the expression of either the epitope or antigen only during S phase[176]. While radioiodinated B6.2 localizes to breast tumour xenografts in nude mice, human radioimmunoimaging with B6.2 has not been as successful[174,177]. Metastases could be imaged in only one of 13 patients. Non-specific binding to peripheral granulocytes followed by dehalogenation may have prevented effective localization. Similar lack of success with tumour-specific imaging has occurred using an anti-CEA monoclonal antibody which reacts with a CEA-like (non-NCA) antigen on peripheral granulocytes[178]. Because of the large doses used in this latter case, there was significant toxicity associated with rapid clearance of the circulating granulocytes including fever, rigors, and emesis.

The monoclonal antibody B14B8 made against breast carcinoma ascites cells recognized a 70000–90000 dalton membrane protein which is not present in human milk[179]. The antigen is localized to the cell surface and is found on several breast tumour cell lines. 75% of primary breast tumours show reactivity while no reactivity was seen with normal breast.

Among a large panel of monoclonal antibodies to breast cancer-associated antigens prepared at The Cetus Corporation, a number of highly breast cancer selective monoclonal antibodies including 741F8, 520C9 and 454C11 bound to distinct epitopes on a 210000 dalton surface glycoprotein[8]. The most selective epitopes on this antigen were not present on any normal tissue examined. The antigen was present in 60% of breast tumour cell lines and primary tumours. The antigen appears to internalize from the cell surface, although at a rate slower than that observed for the transferrin receptor[180]. Ricin A-chain conjugates with several of the monoclonals to this antigen were extremely potent and selective with killing of target breast tumour cell lines at less than 1 nmol/l concentration[76]. The monoclonal antibodies to this antigen may be useful for immunotoxin therapy of appropriate antigen-positive patients.

The monoclonal antibody MBr1 prepared against MCF7 cell line identifies a glycosphingolipid on breast cancer cell lines and breast milk epithelial cells[181] (Figure 10.3). The antigen[182,183] is: Fucα1→2Galβ1→3Galnacβ1→3Galα1→4Galβ1→4Glcβ1→1Cer. The antigenic epitope is found on the

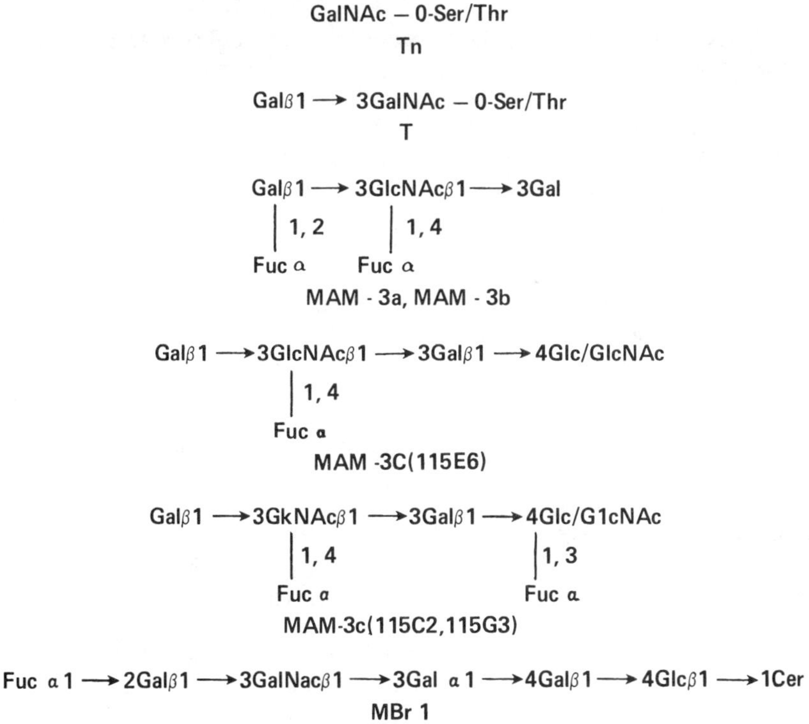

GalNAc – 0-Ser/Thr

Tn

Galβ1 ⟶ 3GalNAc – 0-Ser/Thr

T

Galβ1 ⟶ 3GlcNAcβ1 ⟶ 3Gal
   | 1, 2 | 1, 4
  Fuc α Fuc α

MAM - 3a, MAM - 3b

Galβ1 ⟶ 3GlcNAcβ1 ⟶ 3Galβ1 ⟶ 4Glc/GlcNAc
   | 1, 4
  Fuc α

MAM -3C(115E6)

Galβ1 ⟶ 3GkNAcβ1 ⟶ 3Galβ1 ⟶ 4Glc/G1cNAc
   | 1, 4 | 1, 3
  Fuc α Fuc α

MAM-3c(115C2,115G3)

Fuc α1 ⟶ 2Galβ1 ⟶ 3GalNacβ1 ⟶ 3Gal α1 ⟶ 4Galβ1 ⟶ 4Glcβ1 ⟶ 1Cer

MBr 1

Figure 10.3 The monoclonal antibody MBr1

181

apical membrane of resting and lactating breast as well as in breast milk fat globules. The antibody reactivity is found on the cytoplasm of poorly differentiated breast carcinoma cells[184]. Normal tissues with reactivity by immunoperoxidase assays include pancreatic acini, salivary gland, epithelium, renal tubules, prostate epithelium, sweat and sebaceous glands and seminal vesicle, epididymis and endometrial epithelium.

Monoclonal antibody 323A3 binds a 43000 dalton glycoprotein on the surface of MCF7 cell line in culture[185]. The antigen is present on the surface of 76 of 128 primary and six of eight metastatic breast cancers. It is also found on normal colon and kidney tubules. When 323A3 is linked to ricin A-chain the resulting immunotoxin is toxic to breast tumour cell lines *in vitro* at less than 1 nmol/L concentration[186]. Monoclonal antibodies to this antigen may be useful in therapy as toxin conjugates in antigen-positive breast cancer patients.

Several other breast cancer-associated antigens have been defined by monoclonal antibodies. McR2 is a rat monoclonal antibody to a 70000 dalton glycoprotein in breast milk fat globules[7]. gp70 expression in breast cancers and normal tissues has not been reported. 41B4 is a mouse monoclonal IgG1 antibody to an intracellular 230000 dalton protein present in the majority of breast carcinomas and expressed only on several normal tissue substructures, i.e. sweat gland, normal breast epithelium and tonsillar epithelium[8].

Monoclonal antibodies to breast cancer for which epitope and antigen are unknown

3E1-2 is a mouse IgM monoclonal antibody prepared by immunizing mice with a single cell suspension of a primary ductal-type breast carcinoma[187]. The antibody reacted with 37 of 37 breast tumours although six of 37 had <60% of malignant cells stained. Normal tissues reactive with 3E1-2 include normal breast tissue, renal distal tubule, skin sweat glands, urinary bladder, cervical epithelium, endometrial epithelium, thyroid epithelium, hepatic biliary ducts, pancreatic acini, pancreatic islets and some lung alveolar cells. The antigen appears to be present in the cytoplasm and on the cell surface of different breast tumours. Sera from breast carcinoma patients but not normal sera were able to inhibit the binding of 3E1-2 to a kidney membrane preparation. Based on this finding, a serum test has been developed which detects circulating 3E1-2 antigen in the blood. The test yields abnormal levels in less than 2% of normal and over 80% of primary breast cancer patients and over 90% of patients with metastatic breast cancer. Additionally, the 3E1-2 antibody has been radioiodinated with ^{131}I and used to image axillary metastases after intralymphatic injection in patients with stage II breast cancer[52,188]. Patients with non-palpable, <1 cm nodes with histologic metastases have been successfully imaged and contain four-fold as much specific [^{131}I]3E1-2 as ^{125}I-labelled control antibody. Thus, 3E1-2 may be useful both for serum detection and monitoring of breast cancer and for staging by axillary radioimmunolymphoscintigraphy.

Immunization of mice with MCF7 cell lines was used[189] to generate the

IgG1 monoclonal antibodies 3B18 and 15A8. 3B18 reacts with 27 of 31 human mammary carcinomas and does not react with any normal human tissue and reacts with only one of 19 other cancers. It binds a cytosol antigen which is not identified. 3B18 may be useful in immunohistology to recognize premalignant breast lesions and to identify a breast origin to an adeno-carcinoma of unknown primary. 15A8 reacts with 28 of 31 human mammary carcinomas and reacts with a number of normal tissues. These normal tissues include breast epithelium, renal proximal tubule, skin, oesophagus and salivary gland epithelium. The 15A8 antigen is localized to the cell surface. The antibody reacts with several non-breast tumours including lung, cervix, colon and prostate carcinoma. *In vitro* 15A8 inhibits breast cancer cell replication and, thus, it may have therapeutic potential.

MBE6 is a human IgM monoclonal antibody obtained from a human–mouse hybridoma[5]. Draining axillary lymph node cells from a patient with primary breast carcinoma were used for fusion. The antibody binds 54 of 67 primary breast cancers, 100% of metastatic breast cancer lesions and 14% of benign breast lesions[190]. There was no specific normal tissue reactivity with 11 normal tissues. Reactivity was observed with lung, colon and medullary thyroid carcinomas.

Additional human (e.g. YBDO47) and murine (e.g. BT.6F9) monoclonal antibodies have been prepared against breast cancer tissue but very little characterization had been done[191-195].

Conclusions regarding breast cancer-associated antigens

There are several immunodominant antigens on breast carcinoma cells defined by monoclonal antibodies. Most of these antibodies react with a substantial fraction of human breast carcinomas both primary and metastatic. None of the antigens recognized by monoclonals appears to be absolutely tumour-specific. Antigen expression is usually observed on subsets of adult or fetal epithelia. Except in the case of the transferrin receptor, the function of these breast cancer-associated antigens is unknown. Nevertheless, characteristics of some of these antigens make them candidates for several clinical applications. Antigens which are secreted or shed by breast tumour cells appear to be present in the sera of breast cancer patients but not in the sera of control subjects. These antigens may be useful in preparing serum screening or monitoring tests for breast cancer. Antigens which are on the cell surface of the majority of breast tumours and which are not shed may be excellent targets for axillary immunolymphoscintigraphy. Antigens which internalize from the cell surface rapidly into endocytic vesicles appear to be the best targets for antibody toxin conjugates. Such immunotoxins may be useful in the therapy of patients with antigen-positive tumours, particularly when the tumour is confined to regional sites such as the subarachnoid or pleural space. Oestrogen-regulated antigens detected by immunoassays of cytosol extracts or tissue sections may provide additional information regarding the response of metastatic breast cancer to hormonal manipulation.

early operable breast cancer, patients with small primary tumours and nodal metastases were more immunosuppressed than patients without nodal metastases[217]. Because of the small tumour burden (T1) in these patients, the authors hypothesized the existence of a primary patient-related immuno-suppression distinct from the secondary tumour-related immunosuppression of advanced breast cancer.

Pretreatment immune parameters have been evaluated as independent prognostic factors in breast cancer. DNCB skin test reactivity has had prognostic value for patients with certain solid tumours[220]. Breast cancer patients with strong DNCB reactivity have had significantly prolonged survival[221]. When delayed cutaneous reactivity to five recall skin test antigens and to KLH were tested for prognostic value in metastatic breast cancer, only reactivity with KLH was predictive for response to systemic therapy and survival following chemotherapy[222]. In two additional studies which measured recall or DNCB skin test reactivity and *in vitro* mitogen reactivity[223,224], the more immunocompetent patients had a lower incidence of recurrence, increased disease-free period, and prolonged survival. Krown *et al.*[211] also found that DNCB reactivity correlated with extent of disease in breast cancer patients at the time of initial diagnosis, but when patients with positive or negative DNCB response were compared there was no significant difference in the incidence of recurrence at 2 years following mastectomy. In contrast to the expectation that immunocompetent patients would enjoy prolonged disease-free survival, DNCB-reactive patients with positive lymph nodes experienced earlier recurrence. Survival was significantly prolonged for DNCB-reactive patients only when both primary operable and advanced breast cancer patients were considered together, not when considered separately. The authors concluded that DNCB reactivity failed to add prognostic information beyond that provided by clinical and pathological tumour stage. In several recent studies[212] with long-term follow-up of 5–11 years, neither DNCB or PPD[223] reactivity in early breast cancer patients correlated with disease-free survival.

Pretreatment lymphocyte levels may or may not have prognostic significance in breast cancer[224]. Significantly higher pretreatment lymphocyte levels in early breast cancer patients have correlated favourably with disease-free status at 5 years[225–227]. In contrast, several recent studies found that higher absolute or T-lymphocyte levels correlated negatively with prognosis. After 3.5–9.5 years of follow-up, pretherapy lymphocyte counts were significantly higher in patients with three or more positive lymph nodes compared to patients with 0–2 positive lymph nodes[228]. Absolute lymphocyte counts within these groups were not predictive of recurrence. A T-lymphocyte level of >63% was, however, significantly associated with earlier recurrence. In a separate study, patients who developed recurrence within 5–10 years had significantly higher pretherapy lymphocyte counts[212]. Sequential post-treatment studies of immune parameters for 5 years in the same patients revealed no clinically useful change in immunocompetence immediately before recurrence.

Decreased immunoglobulin levels have been associated with a good prognosis in one study[229] but not in another[212]. Operable primary breast cancer patients with low presurgical IgM concentrations or patients with low presurgery IgG and oestrogen receptor-positive tumours had significantly improved survival[229]. When IgM and IgE levels, allergen-specific IgE scores, and oestrogen receptor status were combined in a single index, the index was more prognostic than any of the individual components and could define patient groups with significantly different survival times within individual clinical stages and within the lymph node-negative or -positive patients. In another report, individual pretherapy serum immunoglobulin concentrations (IgG, IgM, IgA) had no prognostic value[212].

Although tests which have been used to measure general immuno-competence have provided statistical correlation with tumour burden at presentation, these parameters have been disappointing as prognostic indicators for the individual breast cancer patient[230]. Most studies of immune status in breast cancer patients agree that immunocompetence declines at later stages of the disease when tumour burden increases. Many patients with early breast cancer retain a high degree of immunocompetence by many methods of evaluation with lack of delayed hypersensitivity response to DNCB being the most consistent abnormality. Consequently, one might predict that in patients with early stages of breast cancer, a failure to respond immunologically to tumour-associated antigens should not be due to a lack of general immunocompetence.

Evidence for an antibreast cancer immune response

Histological studies[231] have documented infiltration of primary breast cancers by lymphocytes. Medullary breast cancer, an infrequent histological type, is associated with a more favourable prognosis than the more prevalent infiltrating ductal breast cancer[232]. Characteristically, the medullary cancers contain poorly differentiated tumour cells but are infiltrated by large numbers of lymphocytes. Accumulation of histiocytes in the sinusoids of the axillary lymph nodes of breast cancer patients has correlated positively with long-term survival[233,234]. Lymphocytic infiltration in the tumour and reactive changes in the axillary lymph nodes predicted improved 15-year survival[235]. Several studies, however, failed to confirm the association of lymphoid infiltration of the primary tumour with improved survival[236] or found the association only for patients with poorly differentiated tumours[237].

Although lymphoid infiltration has often been cited as evidence for an antitumour immune response, it is circumstantial evidence at best since there is little information regarding the functional significance of the infiltrating lymphocytes. Infiltrating lymphocytes might not affect or might even stimulate tumour growth[198]. Monoclonal antibodies are now available which recognize differentiation antigens on human lymphocytes. Different monoclonal reagents can discriminate B, T and null cells as well as T-cell subsets with differing function. Several studies have phenotyped the lymphocytes infiltrating primary breast cancers using frozen sections stained by an immunoperoxidase technique.

Most of the mononuclear cells which infiltrate breast cancers express T-cell differentiation antigens[238-242]. Prevalence of the helper/inducer T-lymphocyte subset and the cytotoxic/suppressor T-lymphocyte subset varied from study to study. In two reports[240,242] helper/inducer T-cells predominated, whereas cytotoxic/suppressor cells were more prevalent in a third study. Bahn and DesMarias[238] noted that T-lymphocytes in aggregates were predominantly of the helper/inducer subset, whereas diffusely scattered T-lymphocytes were more often of the cytotoxic/suppressor phenotype. Direct lymphocyte-tumour cell contact was infrequent except in medullary cancer. Infiltrating lymphocytes were found in the tumour stroma or in connective tissue surrounding tumour nodules, rather than within nests of tumour cells. Biologically, this may be important in that direct contact between tumour cells and lymphocytes is required for tumour cell killing at least when measured *in vitro*.

Development of a specific cellular immune response generally requires the activation of T-cells following contact with specific antigen. Antigen stimulation can be associated with the expression of 'activation' antigens by T-lymphocytes. In several studies, a subset of infiltrating T-cells has expressed antigens associated with lymphocyte activation. In one report, about 10–30% of the total number of T-lymphocytes in breast cancers were positive for the activation antigens TAC (interleukin 2 receptor) and HLA DR, whereas lymphocytes positive for these antigens were only rarely observed in normal breast tissue[241]. In most cases, there were few monocytes, NK cells or B-cells[238-242]. A few heavily T-cell infiltrated cases contained moderate numbers of B-cells often arranged in follicles surrounded by T-cells[239]. Cells which stained with the anti-T10 monoclonal antibody had the morphology of plasma cells and were variable in number. Interestingly, medullary cancers had many T10 positive cells[238].

The intensity of T-cell infiltration varied widely from tumour to tumour. Using an arbitrary scale to score intensity of infiltration, 40% of tumours had sparse to slight infiltration, 40% had moderate infiltration and 25% were intensely infiltrated[238]. Intensity of T-lymphocyte infiltration has correlated with tumour cell expression of Class I major histocompatibility antigens in melanoma[243]. Breast cancers vary substantially in expression of Class I and Class II HLA antigens. Depending on the study, 40–95% of breast cancers have expressed HLA Class I antigens[238-240,242]. Expression of HLA Class II (DR) antigens was less prevalent ranging from 0 to 40% of tumours[238-240,242]. Only one of three studies[238-240] found a correlation between intensity of T-cell infiltration and Class I HLA expression on breast cancer cells. A fourth study observed dense T-cell infiltration only in areas with DR-positive tumour cells[242].

Suspensions of leukocytes from axillary lymph nodes and peripheral blood of breast cancer patients were phenotyped by flow cytometric analysis of two colour immunofluorescence[244]. DR-positive T-lymphocytes of both helper/inducer and cytotoxic/suppressor subsets were more frequent in peripheral blood of node-positive Stage II breast cancer patients than in node-negative Stage I patients. Between the two stages there was no difference in the frequency of T-cells, T-cell subsets or B-cells in peripheral blood. Lymph node cells from Stage I patients had significantly more helper/inducer (leu 3+) T-cells than lymph node cells from Stage II patients. This was due to a decrease in Stage II patients of leu 3[+] cells lacking the leu 8 marker which is found on T-helper cells. Lymph node cells from Stage II patients had significantly elevated proportions of Leu 12[+] B cells, cytotoxic/suppressor T-cells, activated DR-positive T-cells of both helper/inducer and cytotoxic suppressor subsets, and Leu 7[+] 11[+] natural killer cells. Changes observed in lymph node cell subsets, including expression of activation antigens, were thought to be related to metastasis of breast cancer cells to the regional nodes[244].

In summary, histological studies of mononuclear cells infiltrating primary breast cancers have identified T lymphocytes as the predominant leukocyte. Heterogeneity has been observed among different tumours with regard to the intensity of the infiltrate, the proportion of T-cells and the prevalence of T-lymphocyte subsets. Direct contact between tumour cells and T-cells has not been frequently observed. Breast cancer epithelial cells had variable expression of Class I and II HLA antigens, and there is controversy as to whether intensity of T-cell infiltration correlates with tumour cell HLA expression. When tumour cells metastasize, the proportion of helper/inducer cells may decline in regional lymph nodes and activated T-cells may recur locally and in the peripheral blood. B-cells and NK cells may also decrease within affected nodes. Whether or not changes in lymphocyte populations reflect specific recognition of tumour-associated antigens cannot be determined from these studies, nor is it known whether T or NK cells actually affect tumour growth.

In vivo responses to breast cancer

A number of studies have attempted to demonstrate specific immunologic reactivity with breast tumour-associated antigens. Skin tests with crude extracts of autologous breast cancer tissue produced delayed hypersensitivity reactions in about 25% of breast cancer patients[245,246]. Approximately one-half of the patients who responded to autologous tumour extracts also responded to allogeneic extracts[245]. Similarly, using fixed cryostat sections of autologous tissue in an *in vivo* skin window technique, 40% of breast cancer patients showed cellular hypersensitivity to malignant sections compared with 10% reactivity to benign sections[247]. The crude breast cancer extracts used for *in vivo* skin tests were not well characterized for specificity and some normal tissue extracts also elicited reactions, particularly at high protein concentrations[248]. Some of the observed skin test reactivity was ascribed to a tissue-associated antigen since breast cancer patients responded to extracts of both tumour and normal breast tissue[249,250].

Subsequent studies tested fractions separated from crude antigen extracts in an attempt to improve specificity. Hollinshead *et al.*[251] found two antigens with skin test reactivity after separation of tumour membrane extracts by gel filtration and polyacrylamide gel electrophoresis. One antigen which produced skin reactions in patients with localized or metastatic breast cancer was present in breast cancer extracts, but not normal breast extracts. The second antigen elicited skin test reactivity in patients with localized breast cancer and was found in membrane extracts of both breast cancer and benign

189

breast tissue[251]. The number of patients who could be tested with extracts from breast tumours was limited. Both reactivity and specificity for breast cancer varied among different extracts prepared in the same manner[252].

Breast cancer cell lines (e.g. MCF-7) have been evaluated as a renewable source of skin test antigens. One subfraction (2a) isolated from an extract of the MCF-7 cell line by gel filtration and polyacrylamide gel electrophoresis produced significantly more delayed cutaneous reactions in breast cancer patients than in patients with other cancers[252]. Unfractionated extracts prepared from vesicular stomatitis virus-infected MCF-7 cells were more potent skin test antigens than extracts from uninfected MCF-7 cells[253].

Generally, it has been difficult to evaluate the specificity of skin test preparations containing complex mixtures of antigens. The Thomsen–Friedereich ('T') antigen is, however, one well defined breast carcinoma-associated determinant which can be prepared by desialation of MN antigens from human erythrocytes and which has been used to skin test breast cancer patients[31]. T antigen is the immediate precursor of MN blood group antigens and is found on 95% of carcinomas but not on normal tissues. Purified T antigen elicited delayed type hypersensitivity responses in 96 of 108 patients with infiltrating ductal breast cancer, in only 11 of 144 patients with benign breast disease, and in 0 of 85 normal individuals. Positive reactions were also elicited in patients with carcinomas originating at other sites including lung, pancreas and colon[31].

Delayed cutaneous reactions using both crude and more purified preparations of breast tumour-associated antigen are compatible with the existence of a cell-mediated immune response. With the exception of T antigen, however, delayed cutaneous reactivity could not be evaluated in healthy individuals because of the possibility of transferring oncogenic materials. To avoid this ethical dilemma, cell-mediated and humoral immunity to breast tumour-associated antigens have been investigated *in vitro*.

Measurement of specific immune responses *in vitro*

Assessment of tumour immunity *in vitro* has permitted different investigators to test sera or cells both from cancer patients and from apparently healthy donors. *In vitro* assays of tumour immunity have not, however, always correlated with *in vivo* assessment of tumour immunity in animal models[254,255]. A major problem common to *in vitro* tests of tumour immunity as well as the *in vivo* skin testing described above has been the limited availability of breast cancer cells an normal breast epithelial cells. Auto-logous tumour cells may be the only appropriate antigen source for assays of antitumour T-lymphocyte responses restricted by autologous major histocompatibility antigens. Use of allogeneic cells or cell lines may result in detection of anti-HLA reactivity. Antibody or cell-mediated responses to unique tumour specific antigens not shared by other breast cancers would also only be detected on the autologous tumour cells. There is a need for improved culture methods for solid tumour cells[256]. Short-term culture methods have been described for both normal and breast cancer epithelial cells[257]. Establishment of cell lines, however, can rarely be achieved and most often occurs with highly metastatic tumour cells from pleural effusions or from skin nodules which probably represent only a subpopulation of the original primary tumour. Aside from selection of subpopulations, *in vitro* culture may also result in loss of surface antigens or acquisition of surface antigens from serum supplements. Cultured tumour cells can also be more susceptible than freshly isolated cells to the cytotoxic effects of leukocytes from normal donors[258].

In vitro assessment of humoral immunity to breast cancer

Early studies reported that serum antibodies from breast cancer patients could bind to fixed cancer cells when measured by indirect immuno-fluorescence[259,260]. About half of sera from different breast cancer patients reacted with both surface and intracellular antigens of fresh autologous or allogeneic breast tumour cell suspensions[261]. Up to 25% of the positive sera also reacted with fixed lung or colon carcinoma cells. Approximately 15% of sera from controls matched for parity and age reacted with fixed breast cancer cells as did sera from patients with benign conditions and other malignant diseases. Absorption with normal breast or other normal tissue failed to remove reactivity from breast cancer sera[261,262].

More recently, antibodies in 30 of 324 (9%) breast cancer sera bound to glutaraldehyde fixed breast cancer cells lines when measured by radioimmuno-assay. Only two sera, however, failed to react with an assortment of other normal and malignant cell lines. Reactivity was not reduced after absorption with normal cells or with heterophile antigens[263]. Using an immune adherence assay to detect complement fixing antibodies, 55 of 353 (16%) breast cancer sera preabsorbed with bovine erythrocytes were reactive[264] with an established breast cancer cell line (MDA-MB-436). Only ten sera remained positive after absorption with a B-cell line autologous to MDA-MB-436 and all the remaining activity was absorbed with fetal tissues or cell lines expressing oncofetal antigens. Reactivity of the breast cancer sera with several other breast cancer cell lines could also be attributed to reactivity with oncofetal antigens or HLA antigens. Most of the serological studies performed to date have not utilized such extensive absorption to characterize reactivity found in breast cancer sera and not all studies have examined reactivity with autologous cells primarily due to the constraints of limited tumour cell availability. No breast cancer antigens have been described which are analogous to the antigens of some melanomas or renal cell carcinomas[196] that are restricted only to autologous tumour cells.

Springer *et al.*[265] observed that naturally occurring anti-T agglutinins induced by cross-reacting determinants on gut bacterial flora were severely depressed in about 20% of breast cancer patients compared with <5% of controls of similar age. The level of anti-T agglutinins increased in 66% of breast cancer patient sera following mastectomy, whereas only 3% of patients undergoing breast biopsy for benign breast disease had similar increases. Depression of anti-T antibody levels might be due to absorption of antibody by tumour cells prior to mastectomy. Alternatively, the tumour might exert

organ-related reactivity detected in LAI assays was not restricted by HLA. Aside from these MHC determinants, the epitopes recognized in LAI have not been well characterized.

Mixed lymphocyte tumour cell reactions

Several *in vitro* assays have been used to evaluate direct lymphocyte reactivity to intact tumour cells. Initial results showed that both autologous and allogeneic lymphocytes from breast cancer patients were cytotoxic or inhibited the growth of breast tumour cells but not skin fibroblasts from tumour patients[295,296]. Serum from most breast tumour-bearing patients inhibited the cytotoxic reactivity of lymphocytes[297]. Other investigators, however, have observed reactivity in lymphocytes from normal individuals in microtoxicity assays and found it more difficult to discern specific reactivity of cancer patients[298,299]. The lack of normal breast epithelial cell controls has also hampered analysis of the specificity for the cytotoxic reactions[248]. Naturally occurring cytotoxic effectors or 'natural killer' (NK) cells were soon recognized in the blood and lymphoid organs of normal individuals and cancer patients[300].

The demonstration of major histocompatibility restriction of cytotoxic T-lymphocyte killing of virus injected targets[200] and evidence of MHC-restricted immunity in animal tumour models[301,302] suggested that HLA-restricted reactivity to breast tumour antigens would be missed unless autologous breast tumour cells were used as targets. In subsequent studies, responses of breast cancer patients to fresh autologous tumour cells were analysed in mixed lymphocyte tumour cell proliferation assays (MLTC) and in short-term lymphocyte cytotoxicity assays. The use of uncultured tumour cells was advantageous since they resisted damage by NK cells in normal unfractionated leukocytes[303].

Assays of T-lymphocyte proliferation in response to tumour-associated antigens may be especially relevant since recent studies have demonstrated that proliferating T-helper/inducer cells can transfer tumour-rejection immunity in animals[243]. Proliferating helper/inducer T-cells are known to release lymphokines which recruit and activate both specific cytotoxic T-cells and non-specific effectors such as monocytes and NK cells. Blood lymphocytes from about 35% of patients with cancers from different primary sites had cytotoxic reactive T-cells. In only 7% of patients could cytotoxic reactions be demonstrated against allogeneic tumour cells matched for site and histology[258]. Lymphocytes from approximately 70% of cancer patients proliferated in the presence of autologous tumour cells[255]. Lymphocytes from the peripheral blood and/or separated from the dissociated primary tumour of six breast cancer patients were stimulated by autologous tumour cells in 7/9 MLTC tests[304]. Lymphoproliferative responses were also observed to MMTV[305,306] and hypotonic membrane preparations of autologous breast tumours[307]. Patients with positive responses to autologous membrane preparations had a significantly longer disease-free survival after a 3-year follow-up[307]. Although T antigen induced delayed hypersensitivity *in vivo* and LMI and LAI responses *in vitro*, there was no *in vitro* lymphoproliferation to T antigen[308].

194

Reactivity in MLTC reactions may or may not indicate a response to tumour-specific antigens. T-cells can be stimulated by autologous DR antigens on normal B-cells or monocytes in the autologous mixed lymphocyte reaction (AMLR)[309]. AMLR reactivity requires purified responding T-cells and purified stimulator cells for optimal detection whereas MLTC reactions occur without fractionation of responder lymphocytes[258]. Tumour-derived lymphocytes and macrophages have not elicited MLTC reactions[310]. Even if contaminating leukocytes are removed from stimulating autologous tumour cells, however, tumour cells themselves can express DR antigens. Consequently, DR-positive and DR-negative tumour cell variants and/or cloned responder T-lymphocytes will be needed to define the specificity of the reaction. In addition, controls from benign tissue will be critical. Some positive reactions have been observed with stimulator cells from normal tissues[311]. Even if the corresponding normal tissue is available, it may not be an appropriate control since the tumour cell population may reflect transformation of a minor subpopulation of cells in the normal tissue[255]. For detection of tumour-specific antigens not found on the normal counterpart, the subpopulation of normal cells would need to be purified to provide a control directly comparable to the tumour cells.

Recent advances in recombinant DNA technology should permit more precise analysis of determinants recognized in the MLTC. The discovery and cloning of interleukin-2(IL-2; T-cell growth factor) have made it possible to expand tumour-reactive lymphocytes for further analysis[312]. Lymphocytes placed directly into culture with IL-2 or mitogens become broadly cytotoxic for fresh autologous or allogeneic tumour cells or lines and have been called lymphokine activated killer cells (LAK cells)[313]. NK cells can also be expanded by treatment with IL-2[304]. T-cell clones have been described with proliferative or cytotoxic reactivity to autologous lymphoma[314], melanoma[315,316] and lung colon cancers[304]. Some human T-cell clones failed to continue proliferating after 12 weeks in culture[304]. Limited availability of autologous tumour cells also hampers cloning attempts since T-cell clones require periodic exposure to antigen besides IL-2. T-lymphoblasts activated in MLTC and first separated from non-blast cells before culture in IL-2 retained specific cytotoxic activity for autologous tumour cells with little activity for allogeneic tumours of the same site or NK-sensitive target cells. Proliferative activity of the cultured T-cells was observed with both autologous and allogeneic breast tumour stimulator cells[310]. When assays were performed by limiting dilution analysis, lymphocytes which proliferated in the presence of IL-2 were more numerous in lymphocytes infiltrating the tumour than in peripheral blood suggesting that this population was activated *in vivo*[317].

Demonstration of autologous tumour-reactive lymphocytes *in vitro* in humans points to the existence of tumour-specific or tumour-associated antigens which are immunogenic in the autologous host. Continued improvement in techniques available for the growth of T-cells and tumour cells should make it possible to define the specificity of reactivity observed in MLTC and cytotoxicity assays. Whether these antigens function as tumour rejection antigens *in vivo* is unknown.

Suppressor cells

Leukocytes with suppressive activity can be responsible for depressed reactivity to tumour-associated antigens or other antigens in cancer patients[318]. Tumour-specific suppressor cells analogous to those described in murine systems which interfere with effective antitumour immunity[319] have not been found in humans. Non-specific suppressor cells with the characteristics of monocytes have been found in breast cancer patients which inhibit proliferative responses to PPD and PHA[320]. One mechanism of immunosuppression by non-specific suppressor monocytes is the release of prostaglandins. Addition of indomethacin, a prostaglandin synthesis inhibitor, enhanced proliferation to mitogens[321] and macrophage-mediated tumour cell cytotoxicity[322] in breast cancer patients. In a study of 38 lung and breast cancer patients, about 50% of patients had suppressor cells which inhibited proliferative responses to mitogens or alloantigen. Of the six breast cancer patients with demonstrable suppressor cells, two had adherent esterase-positive suppressor cells and four had non-adherent suppressor cells[323]. Suppressor activity for alloantigen proliferation in patients with early breast cancer was associated with ferritin$^+$ T-lymphocytes[324]. Leukocytes infiltrating breast cancers had suppressive activity for peripheral blood leukocyte responses to PHA and for MLTC responses to autologous tumour cells[325]. It is not known whether the human suppressor cells found *in vitro* assays interfere with effective human antitumour responses *in vivo*.

Conclusions regarding the immune response to breast cancer

Immunocompetence appears to be well preserved in many patients with early breast cancer. In advanced disease, development of delayed cutaneous reactivity and other T-cell-mediated responses may be impaired. Among the leukocytes which infiltrate human breast cancers, T-cells are observed most frequently. The intensity of T-cell infiltrates varies substantially from tumour to tumour. Direct contact between T-lymphocytes and tumour cells is uncommon. Activated T-cells can be observed within regional lymph nodes and in the peripheral blood of breast cancer patients. A fraction of breast cancer patients will have antibodies which react with breast cancer-associated antigens. Whether any of these antigens is tumour-specific remains in doubt. Tumour cells or extracts can evoke delayed cutaneous reactivity, leukocyte migration inhibition, leukocyte adherence inhibition, cell-mediated cytotoxicity and lymphocyte proliferation. In contrast to studies with xenogeneic murine monoclonal antibodies, the antigens responsible for autologous reactivity have not been well defined. In assessing specific immunocompetence it will be important to take into account the activity of suppressor cells. To date only non-specific suppressors have been documented among leukocytes from breast cancer patients. In some cases, immunosuppression appears to be mediated by prostaglandin-producing leukocytes and can be abrogated with indomethacin.

IMMUNOTHERAPY OF BREAST CANCER

Active immunotherapy with immunostimulants, immunorestorative agents and tumour cell vaccines

Local immunotherapy

Direct intralesional injection of the tuberculosis vaccine Bacillus Calmette-Guérin (BCG) has produced regression of cutaneous metastases from malignant melanoma in 60% of patients treated[326]. In approximately 15% of melanoma patients, non-injected lesions have also regressed. Despite these encouraging results with cutaneous disease, lymph node metastases have responded less frequently and there are only anecdotal cases where clinically apparent visceral metastases of malignant melanoma have regressed following local immunotherapy. A similar approach has been applied to the management of chest wall recurrence and other cutaneous metastases from breast carcinomas. If the results of five studies are combined, injected lesions regressed in 42% of 50 patients whereas non-injected lesions failed to respond[327-331]. In the largest single series which included 20 patients, only three partial responses were observed[330]. Among patients whose tumours did regress, PPD sensitivity was present prior to treatment or developed following exposure to the organisms. Given the relative immunocompetence of breast cancer patients, it is likely that breast carcinomas are somewhat less susceptible to the 'bystander' killing exerted by a local inflammatory response to BCG.

The alkylating agent, nitrogen mustard, is directly cytotoxic for tumour cells, but can also act as a contact allergen. Approximately 75% of breast cancer patients can be sensitized to nitrogen mustard. Local treatment of cutaneous breast cancer metastases with nitrogen mustard produced complete regression in five of ten cases[332]. Development of contact sensitivity was observed in each of the responders. Using topical application of the contact allergen dinitrochlorobenzene, local tumour regression could also be produced in three of eight breast cancer patients[333]. While local antitumour activity is of interest, the major clinical problem in breast cancer is systemic control of micrometastatic disease within viscera.

Systemic therapy with BCG and Corynebacterium parvum

Considering the local activity of BCG against melanoma and other solid tumours, a number of trials were undertaken to evaluate possible systemic antitumour activity of the immunostimulant[334-338]. In many of these trials, BCG was administered by scarification at a site distant from the primary tumour or clinically apparent metastatic disease. Early reports from the M.D. Anderson Hospital suggested that the addition of BCG to combination chemotherapy with 5-fluorouracil, adriamycin and cyclophosphamide (FAC) prolonged overall survival[334-337]. In general, however, these studies were historically controlled and have not been confirmed in prospective trials[338]. Similarly, early trials with *Corynebacterium parvum* and *C. granulosum* indicated that treatment with these agents would prolong survival of patients with advanced solid tumours when used alone or in combination with chemo-therapy[339-343]. Subsequent studies have not confirmed the efficacy of *C. parvum*[344,345] and have documented increased toxicity[346-348], particularly when the immunostimulant is used in combination with cytotoxic drugs[346].

Judging from experiments in animal systems, immunotherapy is likely to be most effective in an adjuvant setting when only a small number of tumour cells remain following conventional treatment with surgery, radiation or cytotoxic chemotherapy. In several large, concurrently controlled adjuvant studies, no significant effect has been exerted by BCG, the methanol extraction residue of BCG (MER) or *C. parvum*[344,349-353].

Interestingly, there is one trial with 4 years of follow-up where the administration of the synthetic polyribonucleotide, poly-A/poly-U, has prolonged disease-free survival and overall survival following mastectomy[345,355]. This report requires confirmation, but is the most promising result with active non-specific immunotherapy. Administration of poly-A/poly-U is associated with a transient increase in circulating NK and T-cells[356]. Interferon cannot be detected in serum, but levels of 2,5 oligoadenylate synthetase are increased in leukocytes[356].

Immunorestoration with levamisole

The low molecular weight antihelmintic drug levamisole is capable of augmenting monocyte, macrophage and T-cell function in animals and in patients who are immunosuppressed[357]. Attempts have been made to utilize this immunorestorative activity in adjuvant trials[358-366]. One early report from Argentina tested the adjuvant activity of levamisole following radiotherapy for stage III breast carcinoma[358]. At 30 months, 95% of patients who received levamisole were alive whereas only 35% of controls still survived. Three trials in advanced breast cancer suggested that levamisole could improve response rates to combination chemotherapy and prolong survival[363,365,366]. Several subsequent studies have, however, failed to confirm these early promising results[359-361,364]. Consequently, at the present time there is no convincing evidence that BCG, MER, *C. parvum* or levamisole contribute significantly to the management of breast cancer.

Tumour cell vaccines

Whole tumour or tumour cell extracts have been administered alone or in combination with immunostimulants. At least three trials have utilized autologous tumour cells[367-369]. One investigator coupled rabbit immuno-globulin to autologous tumour and administered the derived cells to patients in Freund's incomplete adjuvant[367]. None of six breast cancer patients responded objectively to treatment, although one patient did have stable disease for a year without cytotoxic or hormonal therapy. In a pilot study, autografts of irradiated tumour cells were given to 16 patients following simple mastectomy for Stage II or Stage III disease. 11 of the 16 survived disease-free for 4–7 years[368].

Another report deals with more complex therapy in which patients received extracts of allogeneic tumour or a subcellular fraction from these extracts[370]. In some cases, leukocytes were transferred between patients who had been immunized with tumour extracts. In patients receiving extracts alone, three of 19 had objective regression of measurable disease. Among patients who received both allogeneic leukocytes and tumour cell vaccine, 12 of 42 responded. Based upon this experience, 78 patients have been enrolled in a single arm adjuvant trial in which allogeneic breast tumour extracts have been administered following modified radical mastectomy[371]. 5-year disease-free survival among 39 node-negative patients has been 94%, whereas that among 39 node-positive patients has been 70%. Without larger, concurrently controlled trials, clinical observations with tumour cell vaccines are difficult to interpret.

Interferons and other mediators

The interferons constitute a family of proteins synthesized by mammalian cells in response to viral infection. In addition to antiviral activity, interferons possess the ability to inhibit cell proliferation and to modulate immune responses. Three types of interferons have been identified: α (leukocyte-derived), β (fibroblast-derived) and γ (immune). α-interferons have exerted antitumour reactivity against several lymphoreticular and haematopoietic malignancies including hairy cell leukaemia, follicular non-Hodgkin's lymphoma, multiple myeloma and chronic granulocytic leukaemia. Responses have also been observed in melanoma, renal cell carcinoma and Kaposi's sarcoma, but the utility of treatment with interferon for other solid tumours remains to be defined. Incubation with α-interferon can inhibit growth of breast tumour cell lines in culture[372]. Administration of α-interferons can also retard growth of breast cancer heterografts in nude mice[372].

Two early studies using partially purified α-interferon derived from virus-infected human leukocytes produced objective responses in 11 of 40 evaluable patients (27.5%)[373,374]. Subsequent trials with highly purified lymphoblastoid interferon produced by cell lines and α interferon produced by *E. coli* using recombinant DNA techniques have proven less promising with only five objective responses (4%) among 125 patients treated[375-382]. Responses to the purified interferons have been partial and generally short lived. Success in the earlier trials may relate to several factors. Recombinant technology selects only one from more than a dozen α-interferon genes which may be expressed in virus-infected leukocytes. Alternative forms of α-interferon may be important for inhibiting tumour growth. Impure preparations of interferon may contain other mediators which contribute to antitumour activity. Patient selection may be important in that one of the two early trials excluded patients who had had extensive prior cytotoxic chemotherapy, whereas trials with lymphoblastoid and recombinant preparations have been performed, for the most part, in patients who have failed both hormonal therapy and chemotherapy.

Treatment with recombinant interferons has been associated with the same

platelet fragments. Many of these populations are decreased in cancer patients, particularly following cytotoxic chemotherapy. Circulating immune complexes can also interfere with Fc receptor function. Two antibodies directed against high molecular weight glycoproteins, F36/22 and M7/105, can destroy human breast cancer cells in the presence of murine or human complement. Both can inhibit growth of human breast cancer heterografts in nude mice[17]. F(ab')$_2$ fragments were inactive consistent with either complement-mediated or antibody-dependent cell-mediated cytotoxicity. Intact antibodies were not particularly effective in ADCC *in vitro* supporting the possible importance of complement-mediated cytotoxicity.

To improve tumour cell killing, monoclonal antibodies have been conjugated with radionuclides, drugs or plant toxins. Conjugation with the first may permit bystander killing of adjacent cells which can be an advantage in compensating for a lack of antigen expression by individual cells within a tumour. Emission of radioactivity does, however, continue during the interval before antibody binds to the tumour and while the radionuclide is being excreted. Normal tissues including the bone marrow are irradiated by circulating radionuclide conjugates. Drugs and toxins kill individual cells to which they have bound and this should provide greater specificity. Antigen-negative cells may, however, evade tumour cell killing.

The substantial number of antigenic determinants defined by monoclonal antibodies might provide useful targets for delivery of isotopes, drugs or toxins. Many of the plant toxins inhibit protein synthesis at the level of ribosomes. Consequently, their activity depends upon translocation into the appropriate cytoplasmic compartment within the cell. In the case of radio-nuclide conjugates, internalization may not be required, depending upon the particular isotopes utilized.

Radionuclide conjugates have been prepared with a number of monoclonal reagents directed againt human breast cancer including F3622, B6.2, B72.3, 115D8, L1CR-LON-M8, HMF61, HMFG2, 10-3D2, 3E1.2 and DF3[49-52,172,397,398]. Radionuclide conjugates have usually been prepared[51,397] with ^{131}I, although the 10-3D2 and M8 antibodies have been conjugated[50,172] with [111]In. Optimal tumour tissue ratios have generally been obtained with F(ab')$_2$ fragments rather than with intact immunoglobulins[172,397]. Imaging of nodules as small as 0.4 cm has been achieved in nude mouse heterograft models without computer subractions[397]. In one clinical study the 3E1.2 antibody labelled with ^{131}I has been used to image axillary lymph nodes after intralymphatic injection[52]. Uptake was optimal at 16–24 hours. Tumour was appropriately localized in seven instances with palpable nodes and in two instances in which nodes were not palpable. The therapeutic activity of radionuclide conjugates has not been demonstrated.

In the case of immunotoxins, three groups have reported preparation of anti-breast immunotoxins using ricin A-chain[76,399,400]. Some of the most extensive work has been performed at the Cetus Corporation[76]. Some 85 antibodies were used to prepare ricin A-chain (RTA) conjugates. 24 of these reagents proved to be effective immunotoxins with 21 specifically toxic at ≤ 1 nmol/L. Affinity of the antibody, antigen copy number and internaliza-tion of antigen all seemed important factors in preparing effective immunotoxins. Several of these antibodies have also been conjugated to *Pseudomonas* exotoxin. In some cases, the *Pseudomonas* exotoxin seemed superior to ricin A-chain in destroying ovarian tumour targets which also bore the breast tumour-associated determinants[74].

To date, clinical trials with immunotoxins directed against breast cancer have not been performed. Recent results with melanoma (Chapter 8) suggest that ricin A-chain monoclonal conjugates can be given with tolerable toxicity. Considering potential difficulties in prompt localization to tumours outside the vascular compartment, regional applications of monoclonal antibodies are most likely to be effective in the short term. Intratumour injection of radionuclide conjugates might be attempted. In addition, conjugates may prove useful in the control of malignant effusions and meningeal metastases when injected via the intrapleural, intraperitoneal or intrathecal routes.

Autologous bone marrow transplantation has been utilized in patients with breast cancer[401]. Using multiple high dose alkylating agents, complete responses of visceral metastases have been observed in 60% of premenopausal patients undergoing treatment for visceral metastases from ER-negative tumours. The number of patients for whom autologous transplantation would be appropriate may be limited by contamination of bone marrow with metastatic tumour cells. Two groups have utilized monoclonal antibodies to detect contaminating tumour in bone marrow by indirect immunofluorescence[43,44,402]. Multiple monoclonal antibodies have proven superior to individual reagents for detecting residual tumour cells[402]. Our own studies have documented that the use of multiple monoclonal antibodies in combination can detect as few as one tumour cell in 10 000 haematopoietic precursors. A recent report with an abrin immunotoxin suggests that breast tumour cells can be purged effectively from bone marrow without affecting the ability of marrow to engraft[403]. Given the ability to detect contaminating tumour cells and to remove them effectively, autologous bone marrow transplantation might be extended to a larger number of patients.

Conclusions regarding immunotherapy

Despite a substantial amount of clinical investigation, immunological techniques have had relatively little impact upon the management of human breast cancer. Direct intralesional injection of BCG, dinitrochlorobenzene or IL-2 treated cells has exerted local antitumour activity. Although systemic activity may have been observed using immunostimulants in some trials, most well controlled studies have failed to show therapeutic advantage to the use of BCG, *C. parvum* and levamisole. Early studies with crude preparations of leukocyte interferon suggested that as many as 25% of breast cancer patients might respond. Using two different clones of recombinant interferon very few responses have been observed. The highly purified mediators obtained by recombinant DNA technology offer the promise, however, of a more rational approach to immunotherapy. One of the most promising areas for further investigation is the use of monoclonal antibodies which bind to a number of well defined determinants on the tumour cell surface. Conjugation of antibodies with radionuclides, drugs or toxins may permit more selective delivery of these agents to breast cancer cells. A number of obstacles have been identified in the use of murine monoclonal antibodies *in vivo* and these are least likely to be a problem when monoclonals are used for regional therapy or for removing malignant cells from bone marrow. Successful use in these settings may point the way to more effective systemic therapy.

ACKNOWLEDGEMENTS

The outstanding assistance of Mrs Nancy Holmes and Mrs Peggy Haythorn is gratefully acknowledged.

References

1. Kohler, G. and Milstein, C. (1975). Continuous cultures of fused cells secreting antibody of predefined specificity. *Nature (London)*, **256**, 494–7
2. Papsidero, L., Croghan, G., O'Connell, M., Valenzuela, L., Nemoto, T. and Chu, T. (1983). Monoclonal antibodies (F36/22 and M7/105) to human breast carcinoma. *Cancer Res.*, **43**, 1741–7
3. Kufe, D., Inghirami, G., Abe, M., Hayes, D., Justi-Wheeler, H. and Schlom, J. (1984). Differential reactivity of a novel monoclonal antibody (DF3) with human malignant versus benign breast tumours. *Hybridoma*, **3**, 223–32
4. Taylor-Papdimitriou, J., Peterson, J., Arklie, J., Burchell, J., Ceriani, R. and Bodmer, W. (1981). Monoclonal antibodies to epithelium-specific components of the human milk fat globule membrane: production and reaction with cells in culture. *Int. J. Cancer*, **28**, 17–21
5. Schlom, J., Wunderlich, D. and Teramoto, Y. (1980). Generation of human monoclonal antibodies reactive with human mammary carcinoma cells. *Proc. Natl. Acad. Sci. USA*, **77**, 6841–5
6. Hilkens, J., Buijs, F., Hilgers, J., Hageman, P., Calafat, J., Sonnenberg, A. and Van der Valk, M. (1984). Monoclonal antibodies against human milk-fat globule membranes detecting differentiation antigens of the mammary gland and its tumors. *Int. J. Cancer*, **34**, 197–206
7. Ceriani, R., Peterson, J., Lee, J., Moncada, R. and Blank, E. (1983). Characterization of cell surface antigens of human mammary epithelial cells with monoclonal antibodies prepared against human milk fat globule. *Somat. Cell Genet.*, **9**, 415–27
8. Frankel, A., Ring, D., Tringale, F. and Hsieh-Ma, S. (1985). Tissue distribution of breast cancer-associated antigens defined by monoclonal antibodies. *J. Biol. Resp. Mod.*, **4**, 273–86
9. Colcher, D., Hand, P., Nuti, M. and Schlom, J. (1981). A spectrum of monoclonal antibodies reactive with human mammary tumor cells. *Proc. Natl. Acad. Sci. USA.*, **78**, 3199–203
10. Foster, C., Edwards, P., Dinsdale, E. and Neville, A. (1982). Monoclonal antibodies to the human mammary gland. *Virchows. Arch.*, **394**, 279–93
11. Ellis, I., Robins, R., Elston, C., Blamey, R., Ferry, B. and Baldwin, R. (1984). A monoclonal antibody, NCRC 11, raised to human breast carcinoma. *Histopathology*, **8**, 501–16
12. Ashall, F., Bramwell, M. and Harris, H. (1982). A new marker for human cancer cells. 1. The Ca antigen and the CA1 antibody. *Lancet*, **2**, 1–11
13. Foster, C., Dinsdale, E., Edwards, P. and Neville, A. (1982). Monoclonal antibodies to the human mammary gland. *Virchows. Arch.*, **394**, 295–305
14. Johnson, V., Schlom, J., Paterson, A., Bennett, J., Magnani, J. and Colcher, D. (1986). Analysis of a human tumor-associated glycoprotein (TAG-72) identified by monoclonal antibody B72.3. *Cancer Res.*, **46**, 850–7
15. Price, M., Edwards, S., Owainati, A., Bullock, J., Ferry, P., Robins, R. and Baldwin, R. (1985). Multiple epitopes on a human breast-carcinoma-associated antigen. *Int. J. Cancer*, **36**, 567–74
16. Nuti, M., Teramoto, Y., Mariani-Costantini, R., Hand, P., Colcher, D. and Schlom, J.

(1982). A monoclonal antibody (B72.3) defines patterns of distribution of a novel tumor-asociated antigen in human carcinoma cell populations. *Int. J. Cancer*, **29**, 539–45

17. Capone, P., Papsidero, L., Croghan, G. and Chu, T. (1983). Experimental tumoricidal effects of monoclonal antibody against solid breast tumors. *Proc. Natl. Acad. Sci. USA*, **80**, 7328–32

18. Capone, P., Papsidero, L. and Chu, T. (1984). Relationship between antigen density and immunotherapeutic response elicited by monoclonal antibodies against solid tumors. *J. Natl. Cancer Inst.*, **72**, 673–7

19. Ormerod, M., McIlhinney, J., Steele, K. and Shimizu, M. (1985). Glycoprotein PAS-O from the milk fat globule membrane carriers antigenic determinations for epithelial membrane antigen. *Mol. Immunol.*, **22**, 265–9

20. Sekine, H., Ohno, T. and Kufe, D. (1985). Purification and characterization of a high molecular weight glycoprotein detectable in human milk and breast carcinomas. *J. Immunol.*, **135**, 3610–15

21. Feizi, T., Gooi, H., Childs, R., Picard, J., Uemura, K., Loomes, L., Thorpe, S. and Hounsell, E. (1984). Tumor-associated and differentiation antigens on the carbohydrate moieties of mucin-type glycoproteins. *Biochem. Soc. Trans.*, **12**, 591–6

22. Arklie, J., Taylor-Papdimitriou, J., Bodmer, W., Egan, M. and Millis, R. (1981). Differentiation antigens expressed by epithelial cells in the lactating breast are also detectable in breast cancers. *Int. J. Cancer*, **28**, 23–9

23. Wilkinson, M., Howell, A., Harris, M., Taylor-Papdimitriou, J., Swindell, R. and Sellwood, R. (1984). The prognostic significance of two epithelial membrane antigens expressed by human mammary carcinomas. *Int. J. Cancer*, **33**, 299–304

24. Burchell, J., Durbin, H. and Taylor-Papdimitriou, J. (1983). Complexity of expression of antigenic determinants, recognized by monoclonal antibodies HMFG-1 and HMFG-2, in normal and malignant human mammary epithelial cells. *J. Immunol.*, **131**, 508–13

25. Springer, G., Desai, P., Robinson, M., Tegtmeyer, H. and Scanlon, E. (1986). The fundamental and diagnostic role of T and Tn antigens in breast carcinoma at the earliest histologic stage and throughout. *Prog. Clin. Biol. Res.*, **204**, 47–70

26. Rittenhouse, H., Manderino, G. and Hass, G. (1985). Mucin-type glycoproteins as tumor markers. *Lab. Med.*, **16**, 556–60

27. Ormerod, M., Steele, K., Westwood, J. and Mazzini, M. (1983). Epithelial membrane antigen: partial purification, assay and properties. *Br. J. Cancer*, **48**, 533–51

28. Croghan, G., Papsidero, L., Valenzuela, L., Nemoto, T., Penetrante, R. and Chu, T. (1983). Tissue distribution of an epithelial of tumor-associated antigen recognized by monoclonal antibody F36/22. *Cancer Res.*, **43**, 4980–8

29. Abe, M. and Kufe, D. (1984). Sodium butyrate induction of milk-related antigens in human MCF-7 breast carcinoma cells. *Cancer Res.*, **44**, 4574–7

30. Hand, P., Colcher, D., Salomon, D., Ridge, J., Noguchi, P. and Schlom, J. (1985). Influence of spatial configuration of carcinoma cell populations on the expression of a tumor-associated glycoprotein. *Cancer Res.*, **45**, 833–40

31. Springer, G. (1984). T and TN, general carcinoma autoantigens. *Science*, **224**, 1198–206

32. Springer, G., Cheingsong-Popov, R., Schirrmacher, V., Desai, P. and Tegtmeyer, H. (1983). Proposed molecular basis of murine tumor cell–hepatocyte interaction. *J. Biol. Chem.*, **258**, 5702–6

33. Hayes, D., Sekine, H., Ohno, T., Abe, M., Keefe, K. and Kufe, D. (1985). Use of murine monoclonal antibody for detection of circulating plasma DF3 antigen levels in breast cancer patients. *J. Clin. Invest.*, **75**, 1671–8

34. Linsley, P., Ochs, V., Horn, D., Brown, J., Ring, D. and Frankel, A. (1986). Identification of monoclonal antibodies which recognize antigens elevated in sera from breast cancer patients. *Cancer Res.*, In press

35. Hilkens, J., Kroezen, V., Buijs, F., Hilgers, J., van Vliet, M., de Voogd, W., Bonfrer, J. and Bruning, P. (1985). Mam-6, a carcinoma associated marker: preliminary characterization and detection in sera of breast cancer patients. In Ceriani, R. (ed.) *Monoclonal Antibodies and Breast Cancer*. pp. 28–42. (Boston: Martinus Nijhoff)

36. Papsidero, L., Nemoto, T., Croghan, G. and Chu, T. (1984). Expression of ductal carcinoma antigen in breast cancer sera as defined using monoclonal antibody F36/22. *Cancer Res.*, **44**, 4653–7

37. Papsidero, L., Croghan, G., Johnson, E. and Chu, T. (1984). Immunoaffinity isolation of

205

ductal carcinoma antigen using monoclonal antibody F36/22. *Mol. Immunol.*, **21**, 955–60

38. Hilkens, J., Kroezen, V., Bonfrer, J., De Jong-Bakker, M. and Bruning, P. (1986). Mam-6, a new serum marker for breast cancer monitoring. *Cancer Res.*, In press

39. Bast, R., Klug, T., St. John, E., Jenison, E., Niloff, J., Lazarus, H., Berkowitz, R., Leavitt, T., Griffiths, T., Parker, L., Zurawski, V. and Knapp, R. (1983). A radioimmuno-assay using a monoclonal antibody to monitor the course of epithelial ovarian cancer. *N. Engl. J. Med.*, **309**, 883–7

40. Sekine, H., Hayes, D., Ohno, T., Keefe, K., Schaetzl, E., Bast, R., Knapp, R. and Kufe, D. (1985). Circulating DF3 and CA125 antigen levels in serum from patients with epithelial ovarian carcinoma. *J. Clin. Oncol.*, **3**, 1355–63

41. Epenetos, A., Taylor-Papdimitriou, J., Curling, M., Canti, G. and Bodmer, W. (1982). Use of the two epithelium-specific monoclonal antibodies for diagnosis of malignancy in serous effusions. *Lancet*, **2**, 1004–6

42. To, A., Coleman, D., Dearnaley, D., Ormerod, M., Steel, K. and Neville, A. (1981). Use of antisera to epithelial membrane antigen for the cytodiagnosis of malignancy in serous effusions. *J. Clin. Pathol.*, **34**, 1326–32

43. Redding, W., Monaghan, P., Imrie, S., Ormerod, M., Gazet, J.-C., Coombes, R., Clink, H., Dearnaley, D., Sloane, J., Powles, T. and Neville, A. (1983). Detection of micro-metastases in patients with primary breast cancer. *Lancet*, **2**, 1271–4

44. Coombes, R. (1986). Personal communication

45. Coakham, H., Brownell, B., Harper, E., Garson, J., Allan, P. and Kemshead, J. (1984). Use of monoclonal antibody panel to identify malignant cells in cerebrospinal fluid. *Lancet*, **1**, 1095–8

46. Gatter, K., Abdulaziz, A., Beverley, P., Corvalan, J., Ford, C., Lane, E., Mota, M., Nash, J., Pulford, K., Stein, H., Taylor-Papdimitriou, J., Woodhouse, C. and Mason, D. (1982). Use of monoclonal antibodies for the histopathological diagnosis of human malignancy. *J. Clin. Pathol.*, **35**, 1253–67

47. Gatter, K. and Mason, D. (1982). The use of monoclonal antibodies for histopathologic diagnosis of human malignancy. *Sem. Oncol.*, **9**, 517–25

48. Ellis, I., Hinton, C., MacNay, J., Elston, C., Robins, A., Owainati, A., Blamey, R., Baldwin, R. and Ferry, B. (1985). Immunocytochemical staining of breast carcinoma with the monoclonal antibody NCRC11: a new prognostic indicator. *Br. Med. J.*, **290**, 881–3

49. Rainsbury, R., Westwood, J., Coombes, R., Neville, A., Ott, R., Kalirai, T., McCready, V. and Gazet, J.-C. (1983). Location of metastatic breast carcinoma by a monoclonal antibody chelate labelled with indium-111. *Lancet*, **2**, 934–8

50. Haisma, H., Goedemans, W., de Jong, M., Hilkens, J., Hilgers, J., Dullens, H. and Den Otter, W. (1984). Specific localization of In-111-labeled monoclonal antibody versus 67-Ga-labeled immunoglobulin in mice bearing human breast carcinoma xenografts. *Cancer Immunol. Immunother.*, **17**, 62–5

51. Epenetos, A., Mather, S., Granowska, M., Nimmon, C., Hawkins, L., Britton, K., Shepherd, J., Taylor-Papdimitriou, J., Durbin, H., Malpas, J. and Bodmer, W. (1982). Targeting of iodine-123-labelled tumour-associated monoclonal antibodies to ovarian, breast, and gastrointestinal tumours. *Lancet*, **2**, 999–1004

52. Thompson, C., Stacker, S., Salehi, N., Lichtenstein, M., Leyden, M., Andrews, J. and McKenzie, I. (1984). Immunoscintigraphy for detection of lymph node metastases from breast cancer. *Lancet*, **2**, 1245–7

53. Thompson, C., Jones, S., Whitehead, R. and McKenzie, I. (1983). A human breast tissue-associated antigen detected by a monoclonal antibody. *J. Natl. Cancer Inst.*, **70**, 409–19

54. Lebman, D., Trucco, M., Bottero, L., Lange, B., Pessano, S. and Rovera, G. (1982). A monoclonal antibody that detects expression of transferrin receptor in human erythroid precursor cells. *Blood*, **59**, 671–8

55. Gross, H.-J. (1985). A monoclonal antibody D51 recognizes the transferrin-receptor structure. *Blut*, **51**, 117–22

56. Sutherland, R., Delia, D., Schneider, C., Newman, R., Kemshead, J. and Greaves, M. (1981). Ubiquitous cell-surface glycoprotein in tumor cells is proliferation-associated receptor for transferrin. *Proc. Natl. Acad. Sci. USA*, **78**, 4515–19

57. Trowbridge, I. and Omary, M. (1981). Human cell surface glycoprotein related to cell

proliferation is the receptor for transferrin. *Proc. Natl. Acad. Sci. USA*, **78**, 3039–43

58. Seligman, P. (1985). Structure and function of the transferrin receptor. *Prog. Hematol.*, **13**, 131–47

59. McLelland, A., Kuhn, L. and Ruddle, F. (1984). The human transferrin receptor gene: genomic organization, and the complete primary structure of the receptor deduced from a cDNA sequence. *Cell*, **37**, 267–74

60. Schneider, C., Owen, M., Banville, D. and Williams, J. (1984). Primary structure of human transferrin receptor deduced from the mRNA sequence. *Nature (London)*, **311**, 675–8

61. Haynes, B., Hemler, M., Cotner, T., Mann, D., Eisenbarth, G., Strominger, J. and Fauci, A. (1981). Characterization of a monoclonal antibody (5E9) that defines a human cell surface antigen of cell activation. *J. Immunol.*, **127**, 347–51

62. Galbraith, G., Galbraith, R. and Faulk, W. (1980). Transferrin binding by human lymphoblastoid cell lines and other transformed cells. *Cell Immunol.*, **49**, 215–22

63. Omary, M., Trowbridge, I. and Minowada, J. (1980). Human cell-surface glycoprotein with unusual properties. *Nature (London)*, **286**, 888–91

64. Gatter, K., Brown, G., Strowbridge, I., Woollston, R. -E. and Mason, D. (1983). Transferrin receptors in human tissues: their distribution and possible clinical relevance. *J. Clin. Pathol.*, **36**, 539–45

65. Faulk, W., Hsi, B. -L. and Stevens, P. (1980). Transferrin and transferrin receptors in carcinoma of the breast. *Lancet*, **2**, 390–2

66. Shindelman, J., Ortmeyer, A. and Sussman, H. (1981). Demonstration of the transferrin receptor in human breast cancer tissue, potential marker for identifying dividing cells. *Int. J. Cancer*, **27**, 329–34

67. Jefferies, W., Brandon, M., Hunt, S., Williams, A., Gatter, K. and Mason, D. (1984). Transferrin receptor on endothelium of brain capillaries. *Nature (London)*, **312**, 162–3

68. Testa, U., Louache, F., Titeux, M., Thomopoulos, P. and Rochant, H. (1985). The iron-chelating agent picolinic acid enhances transferrin receptors expression in human erythroleukemic cells lines. *Br. J. Haematol.*, **60**, 491–502

69. May, W., Sahyoun, N., Jacobs, S., Wolf, M. and Cuatrecasas, P. (1985). Mechanism of phorbol diester-induced regulation of surface transferrin receptor involves the action of activated protein kinase C and an intact cytoskeleton. *J. Biol. Chem.*, **260**, 9419–26

70. Sager, P., Brown, P. and Berlin, R. (1984). Analysis of transferrin recycling in mitotic and interphase HeLa cells by quantitative fluorescence microscopy. *Cell*, **37**, 275–82

71. Trowbridge, I. and Domingo, D. (1981). Anti-transferrin receptor monoclonal antibody and toxin–antibody conjugates affect growth of human tumour cells. *Nature (London)*, **294**, 171–3

72. Lesley, J. and Schulte, R. (1984). Selection of cell lines resistant to anti-transferrin receptor antibody: evidence for a mutation in transferrin receptor. *Mol. Cell. Biol.*, **4**, 1675–81

73. Lesley, J., Domingo, D., Schulte, R. and Trowbridge, I. (1984). Effect of an anti-murine transferrin receptor–ricin A conjugate on bone marrow stem and progenitor cells treated *in vitro*. *Exp. Cell. Res.*, **150**, 400–7

74. Pirker, R., Fitzgerald, D., Hamilton, T., Ozols, R., Willingham, M. and Pastan, I. (1985). Anti-transferrin receptor antibody linked to *Pseudomonas* exotoxin as a model immunotoxin in human ovarian carcinoma cell lines. *Cancer Res.*, **45**, 751–7

75. Akiyama, S. -I., Seth, P., Pirker, R., Fitzgerald, D., Gottesman, M. and Pastan, I. (1985). Potentiation of cytotoxic activity of immunotoxins on cultured human cells. *Cancer Res.*, **45**, 1005–7

76. Bjorn, M., Ring, D. and Frankel, A. (1985). Evaluation of monoclonal antibodies for the development of breast cancer immunotoxins. *Cancer Res.*, **45**, 1214–21

77. Ramakrishnan, S., Uckun, F. and Houston, L. (1985). Anti-T cell immunotoxins containing pokeweed anti-viral protein: potential purging agents for human autologous bone marrow transplantation. *J. Immunol.*, **135**, 3616–22

78. Ramakrishnan, S. and Houston, L. (1984). Inhibition of human acute lymphoblastic leukemia cells by immunotoxins: potentiation by chloroquine. *Science*, **223**, 58–61

79. Frankel, A. (1985). Antibody-toxin hybrids: a clinical review of their use. *J. Biol. Resp. Mod.*, **4**, 437–46

estrogen-regulated breast cancer protein by monoclonal antibody affinity chromatography. *Endocrinology*, **113**, 415–17

124. Ciocca, D., Adams, D., Bjercke, R., Edwards, D. and McGuire, W. (1982). Immunohistochemical detection of an estrogen-regulated protein by monoclonal antibodies. *Cancer Res.*, **42**, 4256–8

125. Ciocca, D., Adams, D., Edwards, D., Bjercke, R. and McGuire, W. (1983). Distribution of an estrogen-induced protein with a molecular weight of 24000 in normal and malignant human tissues and cells. *Cancer Res*, **43**, 1204–10

126. Adams, D. and McGuire, W. (1985). Quantitative enzyme-linked immunosorbent assay for the estrogen-regulated Mr 24000 protein in human breast tumors. Correlation with estrogen and progesterone receptors. *Cancer Res.*, **45**, 2445–9

127. Ciocca, D., Asch, R., Adams, D. and McGuire, W. (1983). Evidence for modulation of a 24K protein in human endometrium during the menstrual cycle. *J. Clin. Endocrinol. Metab.*, **57**, 496–9

128. Hendler, F., Yuan, D. and Vitetta, E. (1981). Characterization of a monoclonal antibody to human breast cancer cells. *Trans. Assoc. Am. Phys.*, **94**, 217–24

129. Yuan, D., Hendler, F. and Vitetta, E. (1982). Characterization of a monoclonal antibody reactive with a subset of human breast tumours. *J. Natl. Cancer Inst.*, **68**, 719–28

130. Hendler, F. and Yuan, D. (1985). Relationship of monoclonal antibody binding to estrogen and progesterone receptor content in breast cancer. *Cancer Res.*, **45**, 421–9

131. Hendler, F. and House, D. (1985). Presence of breast cancer antigens in univoled axillary lymph nodes. *Cancer Res.*, **45**, 3364–73

132. Gold, P. and Freedman, S. (1965). Demonstration of tumor-specific antigens in human colonic carcinomata by immunological tolerance and absorption techniques. *J. Exp. Med.*, **121**, 439–62

133. Koprowski, H., Steplewski, Z., Mitchell, D., Herlyn, M., Herlyn, D. and Fuhrer, P. (1979). Colorectal carcinoma antigens detected by hybridoma antibodies. *Somat. Cell. Genet.*, **5**, 957–72

134. Accolla, R. S., Carrel, S. and Mach, J. -P. (1980). Monoclonal antibodies specific for carcinoembryonic antigen and produced by two hybrid cell lines. *Proc. Natl. Acad. Sci. USA*, **77**, 563–6

135. Haskell, C. M., Buchegger, F., Schreyer, M., Carrel, S. and Mach, J. -P. (1983). Monoclonal antibodies to carcinoembryonic antigen: ionic strength as a factor in the selection of antibodies for immunoscintigraphy. *Cancer Res.*, **43**, 3857–64

136. Colcher, D., Horan Hand, P., Nuti, M. and Schlom, J. (1983). Differential binding to human mammary and nonmammary tumors of monoclonal antibodies reactive with carcinoembryonic antigen. *Cancer Invest.*, **1**, 127–38

137. Kupchik, H. Z., Zurawski, V. R., Nurrel, J. G. R., Zamcheck, N. and Black, P. H. (1981). Monoclonal antibodies to carcinoembryonic antigen produced by somatic cell fusion. *Cancer Res.*, **41**, 3306–10

138. Lindgren, J., Bang, B., Hurme, M. and Makela, O. (1982). Monoclonal antibodies to carcinoembryonic antigen (CEA): characterization and use in a radioimmunoassay for CEA. *Acta Pathol. Microbiol. Immunobiol. Scand.*, **C90**, 159–62

139. Wagner, C., Yang, Y. H. J., Crawford, F. G. and Shively, J. E. (1983). Monoclonal antibodies for carcinoembryonic antigen and related antigens as a model system: a systemic approach for the determinations of epitope specificities of monoclonal antibodies. *J. Immunol.*, **130**, 2308–14

140. Wagner, C., Clark, B. R., Rickard, K. J. and Shively, J. E. (1983). Monoclonal antibodies for carcinoembryonic antigen and related antigens as a model system: determination of affinities and specificities of monoclonal antibodies by using biotin-labeled antibodies and avidin as precipitating agent in a solution phase radioimmunoassay. *J. Immunol.*, **130**, 2302–7

141. Mitchell, K. F. (1980). A carcinoembryonic antigen (CEA) specific monoclonal hybridoma antibody that reacts only with high-molecular-weight CEA. *Cancer Immunol. Immunother.*, **109**, 1–5

142. Primus, F. J., Newell, K. D., Blue, A. and Goldenberg, D. M. (1983). Immunological heterogeneity of carcinoembryonic antigen: antigenic determinants on carcinoembryonic antigen distinguished by monoclonal antibodies. *Cancer Res.*, **43**, 686–92

143. Rogers, G. T., Rawlins, G. A. and Bagshawe, K. D. (1981). Somatic-cell hybrids producing antibodies against CEA. *Br. J. Cancer*, **43**, 1–4
144. Schmidt, J. and Staehelin, T. (1981). Distinction and characterization by monoclonal antibodies of epitopes on four proteins of clinical interest. *Res. Monogr. Immunol.*, **3**, 201–8
145. Hedin, A., Carlsson, L., Berglund, A. and Hammarstrom, S. (1983). A monoclonal antibody–enzyme immunoassay for serum carcinoembryonic antigen with increased specificity for carcinomas. *Proc. Natl. Acad. Sci. USA*, **80**, 3470–4
146. Imai, K., Moriya, Y., Fujita, H., Tsujisaki, M., Kawaharada, M. and Yachi, A. (1984). Immunologic characterization and molecular profile of carcinoembryonic antigen detected by monoclonal antibodies. *J. Immunol.*, **132**, 2992–7
147. Chism, S. E., Warner, N. L., Wells, J. V. *et al.* (1976). Evidence for common and distinct determinants of colon CEA, CCA-III and molecules with CEA activity isolated from breast and ovarian cancer. *Cancer Res.*, **36**, 3486
148. Hansen, J. H., Snyder, L. J., Miller, E. *et al.* (1974). CEA assay: a laboratory adjunct in the diagnosis and management of cancer. *Hum. Pathol.*, **5**, 139
149. Kam, W., Tsao, D., Itzkowitz, S. H. and Kim, Y. S. (1985). Production, characterization, and clinical utility of carcinoembryonic antigen. In *Advances in Biotechnological Processes*. Vol. 4, pp. 151–81. (Alan R. Liss)
150. Terry, W. D., Henkart, P. A., Coligan, J. E. and Todd, C. W. (1972). Structural studies of the major glycoprotein in preparations with carcinoembryonic antigen activity. *J. Exp. Med.*, **136**, 200
151. Shively, J. E., Kessler, M. J. and Todd, C. W. (1978). Amino-terminal sequences of the major tryptic peptides obtained from carcino-embryonic antigen by digestion with trypsin in the presence of Triton X-100. *Cancer Res.*, **38**, 2199
152. Nanjo, C., Shuster, J. and Gold, P. (1974). Intermolecular heterogeneity of the carcinoembryonic antigen. *Cancer Res.*, **34**, 2114
153. Shively, J. E. and Beatty, J. D. (1985). CEA-related antigens: molecular biology and clinical significance. *CRC Crit. Rev. Oncol. Hematol.*, **2**, 355–99
154. Zimmermann, W., Friedrich, R., Grunert, F., Luckenbachk, G. A., Thompson, J. and von Kleist, S. (1983). Characterization of messenger RNA specific for carcinoembryonic antigen. *Ann. NY Acad. Sci.*, **417**, 21–30
155. Yamamoto, Y., Yasumura, K., Murakoshi, M., Abe, H., Furukawa, S., Osamura, R. Y. and Watanabe, K. (1985). Application of immuno-electron microscopy to the cytologic study of benign and malignant mammary lesions with special reference to the carcinoembryonic antigen localization patterns. *Acta Cytologica*, **29**, 257–61
156. Loprinzi, C. L., Tormey, D. C., Rasmussen, P., Falkson, G., Davis, T. E., Falkson, H. C. and Chang, A. Y. (1986). Prospective evaluation of carcinoembryonic antigen levels and alternating chemotherapeutic regimens in metastatic breast cancer. *J. Clin. Oncol.*, **4**, 46–56
157. Beard, D. and Haskell, C. M. (1986). Carcinoembryonic antigen in breast cancer. *Am. J. Med.*, **80**, 241–5
158. Fletcher, R. H. (1986). Carcinoembryonic antigen. *Ann. Int. Med.*, **104**, 66–73
159. Loprinzi, C., Tormey, D., Rasmussen, P., Falkson, G., Davis, T. E., Falkson, H. C. and Chang, A. V. (1986). Prospective evaluation of carcinoembryonic antigen levels and alternating chemotherapeutic regimens in metastatic breast cancer. *J. Clin. Oncol.*, **4**, 46–56
160. Mach, J. P., Buchenner, F., Forni, M., Ritschard, J., Berche, C., Lumbroso, J., Schreyer, D., Girardet, C., Accolla, R. S. and Carrel, S. (1981). Use of radiolabeled monoclonal anti-CEA antibodies for the detection of human carcinomas by external photoscanning and tomoscintigraphy. *Immunol. Today*, **2**, 239–49
161. Rowland, G. F., Corvalan, J. R. F., Axton, C. A., Gore, V. A., Marsden, C. H., Smith, W. and Simmonds, R. G. (1984). Suppresssion of growth of a human colo-rectal tumour in nude mice by vindesine-monoclonal anti-CEA conjugates. *Prot. Biol. Fluids*, **31**, 783
162. Levine, L., Griffin, T., Haynes, L. and Sedor, C. (1982). Selective cytotoxicity for a colorectal carcinoma cell line by a monoclonal anti-carcinoembryonic antigen antibody coupled to the A chain of ricin. *J. Biol. Resp. Mod.*, **1**, 149–62
163. Hilkens, J., Buijs, F., Hilgers, J., Hageman, Ph., Sonnenberg, A., Koldovsky, U.,

Karande, K., Van Hoeven, R., Feltkamp, C. and Van de Rijn, J. (1982). Monoclonal antibodies against human milkfat globule membranes detecting differentiation antigens of the mammary gland. *Prot. Biol. Fluids*, **29**, 813–16

164. Hilkens, J., Hilgers, J., Buijs, F., Hageman, Ph., Schol, D., Van Doornewaard, G. and Van Den Tweel, J. (1984). Monoclonal antibodies against human milkfat globule membranes useful in carcinoma research. *Prot. Biol. Fluids*, **31**, 1013–16

165. Hageman, Ph., Van Den Tweel, J., Hilgers, J., Hilkens, J., Peterse, H., Delemarre, J., Van Den Valk, M., Van Doornewaard, G., Atsma, D. and Schol, D. (1984). Sweat glands and salivary glands as model system for the characterization of monoclonal antibodies against differentiation antigens of the human mammary gland. *Prot. Biol. Fluids*, **31**, 1009–12

166. Gooi, H., Jones, N., Hounsell, E., Scudder, P., Hilkens, J., Hilgers, J. and Feizi, T. (1985). Novel antigenic specificity involving the blood group antigen, Lea, in combination with onco-developmental antigen, SSEA-1, recognized by two monoclonal antibodies to human milk-fat globule membranes. *Biochem. Biophys. Res. Commun.*, **131**, 543–50

167. Feller, W., Kantor, J., Hilkens, J. and Hilgers, J. (1985). Monoclonal antibody defined antigens in plasma of breast cancer patients. *Proc. Am. Assoc. Cancer Res.*, **26**, 149

168. Rasmussen, B., Pedersen, B., Thorpe, S., Hilkens, J., Hilgers, J. and Rose, C. (1985). Prognostic value of surface antigens in primary human breast carcinomas, detected by monoclonal antibodies. *Cancer Res.*, **45**, 1424–7

169. Ceriani, R., Sasaki, M., Sussman, H., Wara, W. and Blank, E. (1982). Circulating human mammary epithelial antigens in breast cancer. *Proc. Natl. Acad. Sci. USA*, **79**, 5420–4

170. Burchell, J., Bartek, J. and Taylor-Papdimitriou, J. (1985). Production and characterization of monoclonal antibodies to human casein. A monoclonal antibody that cross-reacts with casein and alpha-lactalbumin. *Hybridoma*, **4**, 341–50

171. Soule, H., Linder, E. and Edgington, T. (1983). Membrane 126-kilodalton phosphoglyco-protein associated with human carcinomas identified by a hybridoma antibody to mammary carcinoma cells. *Proc. Natl. Acad. Sci. USA*, **80**, 1332–6

172. Khaw, B., Strauss, H., Cahill, S., Soule, H., Edgington, T. and Cooney, J. (1984). Sequential imaging of indium-111-labeled monoclonal antibody in human mammary tumors hosted in nude mice. *J. Nucl. Med.*, **25**, 592–603

173. Hand, P., Nuti, M., Colcher, D. and Schlom, J. (1983). Definition of antigenic heterogeneity and modulation among human mammary carcinoma cell populations using monoclonal antibodies to tumor-associated antigens. *Cancer Res.*, **43**, 728–35

174. Hayes, D., Zalutsky, M., Kaplan, W., Noska, M., Thor, A., Colcher, D., Schlom, J. and Kufe, D. (1986). Pharmacokinetics of radiolabeled monoclonal antibody B6.2 in patients with metastatic breast cancer. *Cancer Res.*, In press

175. Buchegger, F., Schreyer, M., Carrel, S. and Mach, J.-P. (1984). Monoclonal antibodies identify a CEA crossreacting antigen of 95 kd (NCA-95) distinct in antigenicity and tissue distribution from the previously described NCA of 55 kd. *Int. J. Cancer*, **33**, 643–9

176. Kufe, D., Nadler, L., Sargent, L., Shapiro, H., Hand, P., Austin, F., Colcher, D. and Schlom, J. (1983). Cell surface-binding properties of monoclonal antibodies reactive with human mammary carcinoma cells. *Cancer Res.*, **43**, 851–7

177. Colcher, D., Zalutsky, M., Kaplan, W., Kufe, D., Austin, F. and Schlom, J. (1983). Radiolocalization of human mammary tumors in athymic mice by a monoclonal antibody. *Cancer Res.*, **43**, 736–42

178. Dillman, R., Beauregard, J., Sobol, R., Royston, I., Bartholomew, R., Hagan, P. and Halpern, S. (1984). Lack of radioimmunodetection and complications associated with monoclonal anticarcinoembryonic antigen antibody cross-reactivity with an antigen on circulating cells. *Cancer Res.*, **44**, 2213–18

179. Dairkee, S., Greenwalt, D., Smith, H., Harkanon, S., Scannon, P. and Hackett, A. (1985). A tumor-associated anti-mammary monoclonal antibody. *Proc. Am. Assoc. Cancer Res.*, **26**, 292

180. Pirker, R., Fitzgerald, D., Hamilton, J., Ozols, R., Laird, W., Frankel, A., Willingham, M. and Pastan, L. (1985). Characterization of immunotoxins active against ovarian cancer cell lines. *J. Clin. Invest.*, **76**, 1261–7

181. Menard, S., Tagliabue, E., Canevari, S., Fossati, G. and Colnaghi, M. (1983). Generation of monoclonal antibodies reacting with normal and cancer cells of human breast. *Cancer Res.*, **43**, 1295–1300

182. Canevari, S., Fossati, G., Balsari, A., Sonnino, S. and Colnaghi, M. (1983). Immunochemical analysis of the determinant recognized by a monoclonal antibody (MBr1) which specifically binds to human mammary epithelial cells. *Cancer Res.*, **43**, 1301–5

183. Bremer, E., Levery, S., Sonnino, S., Ghidoni, R., Canevari, S., Kannagi, R. and Hakomori, S.-I. (1984). Characterization of a glycosphingolipid antigen defined by the monoclonal antibody MBr1 expressed in normal and neoplastic epithelial cells of human mammary gland. *J. Biol. Chem.*, **259**, 14773–7

184. Mariani-Constantini, R., Colnaghi, M., Leoni, F., Menard, S., Cerasoli, S. and Rilke, F. (1984). Immunohistochemical reactivity of a monoclonal antibody prepared against human breast carcinoma. *Virchows. Arch.*, **402**, 389–404

185. Edwards, D., Grzyb, K., Dressler, L., Mansel, R., Zava, D. and McGuire, W. (1986). Monoclonal antibody identification and characterization of a Mr 43 000 membrane glycoprotein associated with human breast cancer. *Cancer Res.*, In press

186. LeMaistre, C., Edwards, D., Dressler, L., Lathan, R., Mansel, R. and McGuire, W. (1985). Studies with monoclonal antibodies to breast tumors. In Ceriani, R. (ed.) *Monoclonal Antibodies and Breast Cancer.* pp. 80–5. (Boston: Martinus Nijhoff)

187. Stacker, S., Thompson, C., Riglar, C. and McKenzie, I. (1985). A new breast carcinoma antigen defined by a monoclonal antibody. *J. Natl. Cancer Inst.*, **75**, 801–11

188. Stacker, S., Lowe, M., McKatee, K., Thompson, C., Lichtenstein, M., Leyden, M., Salehi, N., Andrews, J. and McKenzie, I. (1985). Detection of breast cancer using the monoclonal antibodies 3E-1.2. In Ceriani, R. (ed.) *Monoclonal Antibodies and Breast Cancer.* pp. 233–47. (Boston: Martinus Nijhoff)

189. White, C., Dulbecco, R., Allen, R., Bowman, M. and Armstrong, B. (1985). Two monoclonal antibodies selective for human mammary carcinoma. *Cancer Res.*, **45**, 1337–43

190. Teramoto, Y., Mariani, R., Wunderlich, D. and Schlom, J. (1982). The immunohisto-chemical reactivity of a human monoclonal antibody with tissue sections of human mammary tumors. *Cancer*, **50**, 241–9

191. Burnett, K., Mashuho, Y., Hernandez, R., Maeda, T., King, M. and Martinis, J. (1986). Human monoclonal antibodies to breast tumor cells. In Chatterjee, S. (ed.) *Monoclonal Antibodies.* pp. 47–61. (Littleton, Mass.: PSG Publishing)

192. Mandeville, R., Lecomte, J., Sombo, F., Chausseau, J. and Giroux, J. (1986). Production, purification and biochemical characterization of monoclonal antibodies reacting with human breast carcinoma cells. In Chatterjee, S. (ed.) *Monoclonal Antibodies.* pp. 63–71. (Littleton, Mass.: PSG Publishing)

193. Imam, A., Drushella, M., Taylor, C. and Tokes, Z. (1985). Generation and immunohisto-logical characterization of human monoclonal antibodies to mammary carcinoma cells. *Cancer Res.*, **45**, 263–71

194. Kaul, S., Bastert, G., Drahovsky, D. and Wacker, A. (1984). Monoclonal antibodies to human mammary carcinoma cells. *Prot. Biol. Fluids*, **32**, 1017–20

195. Kaul, S., Bastert, G., Drahovsky, D. and Wacker, A. (1984). Human and murine monoclonal antibodies against human mammary carcinoma cells. *Prot. Biol. Fluids*, **32**, 831–4

196. Old, L. J. (1981). Cancer immunology: the search for specificity. G. H. A. Clowes Memorial Lecture. *Cancer Res.*, **41**, 361–75

197. Baldwin, R. W. (1981). Specific and non-specific cellular interactions modulating host resistance to tumors. In Saunders, J. P., Daniels, J. C., Serrou, B., Rosenfeld, C. and Denny, C. B. (eds.) *Fundamental Mechanisms in Human Cancer Immunology.* pp. 167–80. (New York: Elsevier/North Holland)

198. Prehn, R. T. (1972). The immune reaction as a stimulator of tumor growth. *Science*, **176**, 170–1

199. Gonwa, T. A., Peterlin, B. M. and Stobo, J. D. (1983). Human Ir genes: structure and function. *Adv. Immunol.*, **34**, 71–96

200. Zinkernagel, R. M. and Doherty, P. C. (1979). MHC-restricted cytotoxic T cells: studies on the biological role of polymorphic major transplantation antigens determining T-cell restriction-specificity, function, and responsiveness. *Adv. Immunol.*, **27**, 51–177

201. Teasdale, C., Hughes, L. E., Whitehead, R. H. and Newcombe, R. G. (1979). Factors

affecting pretreatment immune competence in cancer patients. I. The effects of age, sex and ill health. II. The corrected effects of malignant disease. *Cancer Immunol. Immunother.*, **6**, 89–99

202. Bolton, P. M., Mander, A. M., Davidson, J. M., James, S. L., Newcombe, R. G. and Hughes, L. E. (1975). Cellular immunity in cancer: comparison of delayed hypersensitivity skin tests in three common cancers. *Br. Med. J.*, **3**, 18–20

203. Park, S. K., Brody, J. I., Wallace, H. A. and Blakemore, W. S. (1971). Immunosuppressive effect of surgery. *Lancet*, 53–5

204. Cochran, A. J., Spilg, W. G. S., Mackie, R. M. and Thomas, C. E. (1972). Post-operative depression of tumour-directed cell-mediated immunity in patients with malignant disease. *Br. Med. J.*, **4**, 67–70

205. Han, T. (1972). Immunosuppressive effect of surgery in patients with breast cancer. *Clin. Res.*, **26**, 566

206. Rotstein, S., Blomgren, H., Petrini, B., Wasserman, J. and Barel, E. (1985). Long term effects on the immune system following local radiation therapy for breast cancer. I. Cellular composition of the peripheral blood lymphocyte population. *Int. J. Radiat. Oncol. Biol. Phys.*, **11**, 921–5

207. Shukla, H. S., Whitehead, R. H. and Hughes, L. E. (1980). A comparison of the mechanism of T-cell depression following radiotherapy or surgery for stage III breast cancer. *Clin Oncol.*, **6**, 39–47

208. Mackay, I. R., Goodyear, M. D., Riglar, C., Penschow, J., Wittingham, S., Russell, I. S., Kitchen, P. R. B. and Collins, J. P. (1984). Effect on immunologic and other indices of adjuvant cytotoxic chemotherapy including melphalan in breast cancer. *Cancer*, **52**, 2619–27

209. Strender, L. E., Blomgren, H., Petrini, B., Wasserman, J., Forsgren, M., Norbert, R., Baral, E. and Wallgren, A. (1981). Immunologic monitoring in breast cancer patients receiving postoperative adjuvant chemotherapy. *Cancer*, **48**, 1996–2002

210. Weinberg, M. A., Brenner, B. and Margolese, R. G. (1983). Immune responsiveness and the effects of adjuvant chemotherapy. In Margolese, R. G. (ed.) *Breast Cancer.* pp. 223–48. (New York: Churchill Livingstone)

211. Krown, S. E., Pinsky, C. M., Wanebo, H. J., Braun, D. W. Jr., Wong, P. P. and Oettgen, H. F. (1980). Immunologic reactivity and prognosis in breast cancer. *Cancer*, **46**, 1746–52

212. Shukla, H. S., Hughes, L. E., Whitehead, R. H. and Newcombe, R. G. (1986). Long-term (5–11 years) follow-up of general immune competence in breast cancer. I. Pre-treatment levels with reference to micrometastasis. *Cancer Immunol. Immunother.*, **21**, 1–5

213. Pinsky, C. M. (1979). Skin tests. In Hermerman, R. B. and McIntire, K. R. (eds.) *Immunodiagnosis of Cancer.* Vol. 2, pp. 722–38. (New York: Marcel Dekker)

214. Goust, J. M., Roof, B. S., Fudenberg, H. H. and O'Brien, P. H. (1979). T-cell markers in breast cancer patients at diagnosis. *Clin. Immunol. Immunopathol.*, **12**, 396–403

215. Stein, J. A., Adler, A., Ben-Efraim, S. and Maor, M. (1976). Immunocompetence, immuno-suppression, and human breast cancer. I. An analysis of their relationship by known parameters of cell-mediated immunity in well-defined clinical stages of disease. *Cancer*, **38**, 1171–87

216. Adler, A., Stein, J. A. and Ben-Efraim, S. (1980) Immunocompetence, immuno-suppression, and human breast cancer. II. Further evidence of initial immune impairment by integrated assessment effect of nodal involvement (N) and of primary tumor size (T). *Cancer*, **45**, 2061–73

217. Wanebo, H. J., Thaler, H. T., Hansen, J. A., Rosen, P. P., Robbins, G. F., Urban, J. A., Oettgen, H. F. and Good, R. A. (1978). Immunologic reactivity in patients with primary operable breast cancer. *Cancer*, **41**, 84–94

218. Ludwig, C. U., Hartmann, D., Landmann, R., Wesp, M., Rosenfelder, G., Stucki, D., Buser, M. and Obrecht, J. P. (1985). Unaltered immunocompetence in patients with nondisseminated breast cancer at the time of diagnosis. *Cancer*, **55**, 1673–8

219. Whitehead, R. H., Teasdale, C., Thatcher, J., Roberts, G. P. and Hughes, L. E. (1976). T and B lymphocytes in breast cancer stage relationship and abrogation of T-lymphocyte depression by enzyme treatment *in vitro*. *Lancet*, 330–3

220. Morton, D. L. and Goodnight, J. (1980). Cancer immunology and immunotherapy. In Haskell, C. M. (ed.) *Cancer Treatment.* pp. 124–53. (Philadelphia: Saunders)

221. Cunningham, T. J., Daut, D., Wolfgang, P. E., Mellyn, M., Maciolek, S., Sponzo, R. W.

and Horton, J. (1976). A correlation of DNCB-induced delayed cutaneous hypersensitivity reactions and the course of disease in patients with recurrent breast cancer. *Cancer*, **37**, 1696–1700

222. Hortobagyi, G. N., Smith, T. L., Swenerton, K. D., Legha, S. S., Buzdar, A. U., Blumenschein, G. R., Gutterman, J. U. and Hersh, E. M. (1981). Prognostic value of prechemotherapy skin tests in patients with metastatic breast carcinoma. *Cancer*, **47**, 1369–76

223. Mandeville, R., Lamoureux, G., Legault-Poisson, S. and Poisson, R. (1982). Biological markers and breast cancer. A multiparametric study. II. Depressed immune competence. *Cancer*, **50**, 1280–8

224. Adler, A., Stein, J. A. and Ben-Efraim, S. (1980). Immunocompetence, immuno-suppression, and human breast cancer. III. Prognostic significance of initial level of immunocompetence in early and advanced disease. *Cancer,* **45**, 2074–83

225. Lee, Y. N. (1984). Delayed cutaneous hypersensitivity, lymphocyte count, and blood tests in patients with breast carcinoma. *J. Surg. Oncol.*, **27**, 135–40

226. Papatestas, A. E. and Kark, A. E. (1974). Peripheral lymphocyte counts in breast carcinoma. An index of immune competence. *Cancer*, **34**, 2014–17

227. Owenby, H. E., Roi, L. D., Isenberg, R. R., Brennan, M. J. and the Breast Cancer Prognostic Study Associates (1983). Peripheral lymphocyte and eosinophil counts as indicators of prognosis in primary breast cancer. *Cancer*, **52**, 126–30

228. Rotstein, S., Blomgren, H., Petrini, B., Wasserman, J., Nilsson, B. and Baral, E. (1985). Blood lymphocyte counts with subset analysis in operable breast cancer. *Cancer*, **56**, 1413–19

229. Owenby, D. R., Owenby, H. E., Bailey, J., Frederick, J., Tilley, B., Brooks, S. C., Russo, J., Heppner, G., Brennan, M. and the Breast Cancer Prognostic Study Associates (1985). Presurgical serum immunoglobulin concentrations and the prognosis of operable breast cancer in women. *J. Natl. Cancer Inst.*, **75**, 655–63

230. Karavodin, L. M. and Golub, S. H. (1983). Immunocompetence in cancer patients. In Herberman, R. B. (ed.) *Basic and Clinical Tumor Immunology*. pp. 215–56. (Boston: Martinus Nijhoff)

231. MacCarty, W. C. (1922). Factors which influence longevity in cancer. A study of 293 cases. *Ann. Surg.*, **76**, 9–12

232. Moore, D. S. Jr. and Foote, F. W. Jr. (1949). The relatively favorable prognosis of medullary carcinoma of the breast. *Cancer*, **2**, 635–41

233. Black, M. M. and Speer, F. D. (1958). Sinus histiocytosis of lymph nodes in cancer. *Surg. Gyn. Obstet.*, **106**, 163–75

234. Culter, S. J., Black, M. M., Mork, T., Harvel, S. and Freeman, C. (1969). Further observations of prognostic factors in cancer of the female breast. *Cancer*, **24**, 653–67

235. Hamlin, I. M. E. (1968). Possible host resistance in carcinoma of the breast: a histological study. *Br. J. Cancer*, **22**, 383–401

236. Berg, J. W. (1959). Inflammation and prognosis of breast cancer. A search for host resistance. *Cancer*, **12**, 714–20

237. Elston, C. W., Gresham, G. A., Rao, G. S., Zebro, T., Haybittle, J. L., Houghton, J. and Kearney, G. (1982). The cancer research campaign (King's/Cambridge) trial for early breast cancer: clinicopathological aspects. *Br. J. Cancer*, **45**, 655–69

238. Bhan, A. K. and DesMarais, C. L. (1983). Immunohistologic characterization of major histocompatibility antigens and inflammatory cellular infiltrate in human breast cancer. *J. Natl. Cancer Inst.*, **71**, 507–16

239. Hurlimann, J. and Saraga, P. (1985). Mononuclear cells infiltrating human mammary carcinomas: immunohistochemical analysis with monoclonal antibodies. *Int. J. Cancer*, **35**, 753–62

240. Whitwell, H. L., Hughes, H. P. A., Moore, M. and Ahmed, A. (1984). Expression of major histocompatibility antigens and leukocyte infiltration in benign and malignant human breast disease. *Br. J. Cancer*, **49**, 161–72

241. Lwin, K. Y., Zuccarini, D., Sloane, J. P. and Beverley, P. C. L. (1985). An immuno-histological study of leukocyte localization in benign and malignant breast tissue. *Int. J. Cancer*, **36**, 433–8

242. Gottlinger, H. G., Rieber, P., Gokel, J. M., Lohe, K. J. and Riethmuller, G. (1985). Infiltrating mononuclear cells in human breast carcinoma: predominance of T4$^+$

284. Cannon, G. B., Barsky, S. H., Alford, T. C., Jerome, L. F., Tinley, V., McCoy, J. L. and Dean, J. H. (1982). Cell-mediated immunity to mouse mammary tumor virus antigens by patients with hyperplastic benign breast disease. *J. Natl. Cancer Inst.*, **68**, 935–43

285. Burger, D. R., Vanderbark, A. A., Finke, P., Malley, A., Frikke, M., Black, J., Acott, K., Begley, D. and Vetto, R. M. (1977). Assessment of reactivity to tumor extracts by leukocyte adherence inhibition and dermal testing. *J. Natl. Cancer Inst.*, **59**, 317–23

286. Kotlar, H. K. and Sanner, T. (1981). Humoral antitumor immune responses in patients with breast cancer measured with the leukocyte adherence inhibition technique. *J. Natl. Cancer Inst.*, **66**, 265–71

287. Powell, A. E., Sloss, A. M. and Smith, R. N. (1978). Leukocyte-adherence inhibition: a specific assay of cell-mediated immunity dependent on lymphokine-mediated collaboration between T lymphocytes. *J. Immunol.*, **120**, 1957–66

288. Koppi, T. A., Maluish, A. E. and Halliday, W. J. (1979). The cellular mechanism of leukocyte adherence inhibition. *J. Immunol.*, **123**, 2255–60

289. Halliday, W. J., Koppi, T. A., Khan, J. M. and Davis, N. C. (1980). Leukocyte adherence inhibition: tumor specificity of cellular and serum-blocking reactions in human melanoma, breast cancer, and colorectal cancer. *J. Natl. Cancer Inst.*, **65**, 327–35

290. Thomsen, D. M. P. (1983). Immunology of breast cancer. Part II. In Margoles, R. G. (ed.) *Breast Cancer.* pp. 263–87. (New York: Churchill Livingstone)

291. Marti, J. H., Grosser, N. and Thomson, D. M. P. (1976). Tube leukocyte adherence inhibition assay for the detection of antitumour immunity. II. Monocyte reacts with tumour antigen via cytophilic anti-tumour antibody. *Int. J. Cancer*, **18**, 48–57

292. MacFarlane, J. K., Thomson, D. M. P., Phelan, K., Shenouda, G. and Scanzano, R. (1982). Predictive value of tube leukocyte adherence inhibition (LAI) assay for breast, colorectal, stomach and pancreatic cancer. *Cancer*, **49**, 1185–93

293. Shenouda, G., Thomson, D. M. P. and MacFarlane, J. K. (1984). Requirement for autologous cancer extracts and lipoxygenation of arachidonic acid for human T-cell responses in leukocyte adherence inhibition and transmembrane potential change assays. *Cancer Res.*, **44**, 1238–45

294. Shenouda, G. and Thomson, D. M. P. (1984). Blocking of the response by human T-lymphocytes to extracts of autologous cancer by monoclonal antibody to class-I major histocompatibility complex gene products in the leukocyte adherence inhibition assay. *Cancer Res.*, **44**, 2762–8

295. Hellstrom, I., Hellstrom, K. E., Sjogren, H. D. and Warner, G. A. (1971). Demonstration of cell-mediated immunity to human neoplasms of various histological types. *Int. J. Cancer*, **7**, 1–16

296. Fossati, G., Canevari, S., Porta, G. D., Balzarini, G. P. and Veronesi, U. (1972). Cellular immunity to human breast carcinoma. *J. Cancer*, **10**, 391–6

297. Hellstrom, I., Sjogren, H. D., Warner, G. A. and Hellstrom, K. E. (1971). Blocking of cell-mediated tumor immunity by sera from patients with growing neoplasms. *Int. J. Cancer*, **7**, 226–37

298. Heppner, G., Henry, E., Stolbach, L., Cummings, F., McDonough, E. and Calabresi, P. (1975). Problems in the clinical use of the microcytotoxicity assay for measuring cell-mediated immunity to tumor cells. *Cancer Res.*, **35**, 1931–7

299. Canevari, S., Fossati, G. and Della Porta, G. (1976). Cellular immune reaction to human malignant melanoma and breast carcinoma cells. *J. Natl. Cancer Inst.*, **56**, 705–9

300. Vose, B. M. (1980). Natural killers in human cancer: activity of tumor-infiltrating and draining node lymphocytes. In Herberman, R. B. (ed.) *Natural Cell-mediated Immunity Against Tumors.* pp. 1081–97. (New York: Academic Press)

301. Bernards, R., Schrier, P. I., Houweling, A., Bos, J. L., van der Eb, A. J., Zijlstra, M. and Melief, C. J. M. (1983). Tumorigenicity of cells transformed by adenovirus type 12 by evasion of T cell immunity. *Nature (London)*, **305**, 776–9

302. Carlow, D. A., Herbel, R. S., Feltis, J. T. and Elliott, B. E. (1985). Enhanced expression of class I major histocompatibility complex gene (D^k) products on immunogenic variants of a spontaneous murine carcinoma. *J. Natl. Cancer Inst.*, **75**, 291–301

303. Vose, B. M. and Moore, M. (1980). Natural cytotoxicity in humans: susceptibility of freshly isolated tumor cells to lysis. *J. Natl. Cancer Inst.*, **65**, 257–63

304. Vose, B. M. and White, W. (1983). Tumour-reactive lymphocytes stimulated in mixed lymphocyte and tumour culture. Clonal analysis of effector cells in cytotoxic and prolifer-

ative assays. *Cancer Immunol. Immunother.*, **15**, 227–36

305. Wiseman, C. L., Bowen, J. M., Davis, J. W., Hersh, E. M., Brown, B. W. and Blumenschein, G. R. (1980). Human lymphocyte blastogenesis responses to mouse mammary tumor virus. *J. Natl. Cancer Inst.*, **64**, 425–30

306. Lopez, D. M., Parks, W. P., Silverman, M. A. and Distaslo, J. A. (1981). Lymphoproliferative responses to mouse mammary tumor virus in lymphocyte subsets of breast cancer patients. *J. Natl. Cancer Inst.*, **67**, 353–8

307. Cannon, G. B., Dean, J. H., Herberman, R. B., Keels, M. and Alford, C. (1981). Lymphoproliferative responses to autologous tumor abstracts as prognostic indicators in patients with resected breast cancer. *Cancer*, **27**, 131–8

308. Howard, D. R. (1983). T-antigen does not induce cell mediated immunity in patients with breast cancer. *Cancer*, **51**, 2053–6

309. Weksler, M. E., Moody, C. E. Jr. and Kozak, R. W. (1981). The autologous mixed-lymphocyte reaction. *Adv. Immunol.*, **31**, 271–312

310. Vose, B. M. and Bonnard, G. D. (1982). Specific cytotoxicity against autologous tumour and proliferative responses of human lymphocytes grown in interleukin 2. *Int. J. Cancer*, **29**, 33–9

311. Grimm, L. A., Vose, B. M., Chu, E. W., Wilson, D. J., Lotze, M. T., Rayner, A. A. and Rosenberg, S. A. (1984). The human mixed lymphocyte–tumor cell interaction test. I. Positive autologous lymphocyte proliferative responses can be stimulated by tumor cells as well as by cells from normal tissues. *Cancer Immunol. Immunother.*, **17**, 83–9

312. Gillis, S. and Smith K. A. (1977). Long-term culture of tumor-specific cytotoxic T-cells. *Nature (London)*, **268**, 154–6

313. Grimm, E. A., Mazumder, A., Zhang, H. Z. and Rosenberg, S. A. (1982). Lymphokine-activated killer phenomenon. *J. Exp. Med.*, **155**, 1823–41

314. Yssel, H., Spitz, H. and DeVries, J. (1984). A cloned human T cell line cytotoxic for autologous and allogeneic B lymphoma cells. *J. Exp. Med.*, **160**, 239–54

315. Mukherji, B. and McAlister, T. J. (1983). Clonal analysis of cytotoxic T cell response against human melanoma. *J. Exp. Med.*, **158**, 240–5

316. DeVries, J. E. and Spitz, H. (1984). Cloned human cytotoxic T lymphocyte (CTL) lines reactive with autologous melanoma cells. I. *In vitro* generation, isolation and analysis to phenotype and specificity. *J. Immunol.*, **132**, 510–19

317. Vose, B. M. (1982). Quantitation of proliferative and cytotoxic precursor cells directed against human tumours: limiting dilution analysis in peripheral blood and at the tumour site. *Int. J. Cancer*, **30**, 135–42

318. Herberman, R. B. (1981). Cells suppressing cell-mediated immune responses of cancer patients. In Serrou, B. and Rosenfeld, C. (eds.) *Human Cancer Immunology*. Vol. 2, pp. 179–211. (Amsterdam: Elsevier/North Holland Biomedical Press)

319. North, R. J. (1985). Down-regulation of the antitumor immune response. *Adv. Cancer Res.*, **45**, 1–43

320. Blomgren, H., Baral, E., Petrini, B. and Wasserman, J. (1976). Impaired lymphocyte responses to PPD-tuberculin in advanced breast carcinoma. Increased reactivity after depletion of phagocytic or adherent cells. *Clin. Oncol.*, **2**, 379–92

321. Han, T., Nemoto, T., Ledesma, E. J. and Brunoll, S. (1983). Enhancement of T lymphocyte proliferative response to mitogens by indomethacin in breast and colorectal cancer patients. *Int. J. Immunopharmacol.*, **5**, 11–15

322. Cameron, D. J. and O'Brien, P. (1982). Relationship of the suppression of macrophage mediated tumor cytotoxicity in conjunction with secretion of prostaglandin from the macrophages of breast cancer patients. *Int. J. Immunopharmacol.*, **4**, 445–50

323. Jerrells, T. R., Dean, J. H., Richardson, G. L., McCoy, J. L. and Herberman, R. B. (1978). Role of suppressor cells in depression of *in vitro* lymphoproliferative responses of lung cancer and breast cancer patients. *J. Natl. Cancer Inst.*, **61**, 1001–9

324. Moroz, C. and Kupfer, B. (1981). Suppressor cell activity of ferritin-bearing lymphocytes in patients with breast cancer. *Israel. J. Med. Sci.*, **17**, 879–81

325. Vose, B. M. and Moore, M. (1979). Suppressor cell activity of lymphocytes infiltrating human lung and breast tumours. *Int. J. Cancer*, **24**, 579–85

326. Bast, R. C. Jr., Zbar, B., Borsos, T. and Rapp, J. H. (1974). BCG and cancer. *N. Engl. J. Med.*, **290**, 1413–20; 1458–69

327. Smith, G. V., Morse, P. A., Deraps, G. D., Raju, S. and Hardy, J. D. (1973).

Immunotherapy of patients with cancer. *Surgery*, **74**, 59–68

328. Klein, E., Holtermann, O., Milgrom, H., Case, R. W., Klein, D., Rosner, D. and Djerassi, I. (1976). Immunotherapy for accessible tumors utilizing delayed hypersensitivity reactions and separated components of the immune system. *Med. Clin. N. Am.*, **60**, 389–418

329. Pardridge, D. H., Sparks, F. C., Wile, A. G. and Morton, D. L. (1977). Intratumor injection of BCG for chest wall recurrence of breast carcinoma. *ASCO Abstracts*, **18**, 326

330. Garas, J., Besbeas, S., Papamatheakis, J., Gropas, G., Maragoudakis, S., Katsexis, A., Kiparissiadis, P., Konstadakos, P. and Georgaka, A. (1975). Attempt with immunotherapy to control metastatic skin nodules from breast cancer by B.C.G. *Panminerva Med.*, **17**, 193–5

331. Rosenberg, E. and Powell, R. (1973). Active tumor immunotherapy with BCG. *South. Med. J.*, **66**, 1359–63

332. Goldman, L. E. (1975). Immunotherapy of solid tumors. I. Preliminary studies with nitrogen mustard for nonspecific immunopotentiation in human cancer. *J. Surg. Res.*, **18**, 513–21

333. Stjernsward, J. and Levin, A. (1971). Delayed hypersensitivity-induced regression of human neoplasms. *Cancer*, **28**, 628–40

334. Gutterman, J. U., Mavligit, G. M., Burgess, M. A., Cardenas, J. O., Blumenschein, G. R., Gottlieb, J. A., McBride, Ch. M., McCredie, K. B., Bodey, G. P., Rodriguez, V., Freireich, E. J. and Hersh, E. M. (1976). Immunotherapy of breast cancer, malignant melanoma, and acute leukemia with BCG: prolongation of disease free interval and survival. *Cancer Immunol. Immunother.*, **1**, 99–107

335. Hortobagyi, G. N., Gutterman, J. U., Blumenschein, G. R., Tashima, C. K., Burgess, M. A., Einhorn, L., Buzdar, A. U., Richman, S. P. and Hersh, E. M. (1979). Combination chemoimmunotherapy of metastatic breast cancer with 5-fluorouracil, adriamycin, cyclophosphamide, and BCG. *Cancer*, **43**, 1225–33

336. Hortobagyi, G. N., Blumenschein, G. R., Tashima, C. K., Buzdar, A. U., Burgess, M. A., Livingston, R. B., Valdivieso, M., Gutterman, J. U., Hersh, E. M. and Bodey, G. P. (1979). Ftorafur, adriamycin, cyclophosphamide and BCG in the treatment of metastatic breast cancer. *Cancer*, **44**, 398–405

337. Blumenschein, G. R., Hortobagyi, G. N., Richman, S. P., Gutterman, J. U., Tashima, C. K., Buzdar, A.U., Burgess, M. A., Livingston, R. B. and Hersh, E. M. (1980). Alternating noncross-resistant combination chemotherapy and active nonspecific immunotherapy with BCG or MER-BCG for advanced breast carcinoma. *Cancer*, **45**, 742–9

338. Muss, H. B., Richards, F. II, Cooper, M. R., White, D. R., Jackson, D. V., Stuart, J. J., Howard, V., Shore, A., Rhyne, A. L. and Spurr, C. L. (1981). Chemotherapy vs chemoimmunotherapy with methanol extraction residue of Bacillus Calmette-Guerin (MER) in advanced breast cancer: a randomized trial by the Piedmont Oncology Association. *Cancer*, **47**, 2295–301

339. Israel, L., Edelstein, R., Depierre, A. and Dimitrov, N. (1975). Brief communications: daily intravenous infusions of *Corynebacterium parvum* in twenty patients with disseminated cancer: a preliminary report of clinical and biologic findings. *J. Natl. Cancer Inst.*, **55**, 29–33

340. Israel, L. and Edelstein, R. (1976). Nonspecific immunostimulation with *Corynebacterium parvum* in human cancer. In *Immunologic Aspects of Neoplasia, 26th Symposium.* pp. 485–505. (Baltimore, Maryland: Williams and Wilkins)

341. Pinsky, C., DeJager, R., Wittes, R., Wong, P., Kaufman, R., Mike, V., Hansen, J., Oettgen, H. and Krakoff, I. (1977). *Corynebacterium parvum* as adjuvant to combination chemotherapy in patients with advanced breast cancer. In Crispen, R. G. (ed.) *Neoplasm Immunity: Solid Tumor Therapy.* pp. 145–51. (Philadelphia: Franklin Institute Press)

342. Roszkowski, K., Nozdryn-Piotnicki, B., Roszkowski, W., Ko, H. L., Pulverer, G. and Jeljaszewicz, J. (1983). Immunochemotherapy of breast cancer with *Propionibacterium granulosum. Cancer Immunol. Immunother*, **15**, 23–6

343. Pluzanska, A., Stempczynska, J., Szmigielski, S., Luczak, M., Jeljaszewicz, J. and Pulverer, G. (1985). Local immunotherapy with *Propionibacterium granulosum* KP-45 in advanced breast cancer. *Anticancer Res.*, **5**, 521–6

344. DeJager, R., Pinsky, C., Kaufman, R., Ochoa, M., Oettgen, H. and Krakoff, I. (1976). Chemotherapy of advanced breast cancer with a combination of cyclophosphamide,

adriamycin, methotrexate and 5-fluorouracil (CAMF) with and without *C. parvum.* *ASCO Abstracts,* **17**, 296

345. Mercurio, T., Harvey, H., White, D. and Lipton, A. (1978). A comparison of 5-fluorouracil, adriamycin, cytoxan (FAC) chemotherapy with chemoimmunotherapy using *C. parvum* ± BCG in advanced breast cancer. *ASCO Abstracts,* **19**, 349

346. Cummings, F. J., Gelman, R. and Horton, J. (1985). Comparison of CAF versus CMFP in metastatic breast cancer: analysis of prognostic factors. *J. Clin. Oncol.,* **3**, 932–40

347. Fisher, B., Rubin, H., Sartiano, G., Ennis, L. and Wolmark, N. (1976). Observations following *Corynebacterium parvum* administration to patients with advanced malignancy. *Cancer,* **38**, 119–30

348. Band, P. R., Jao-King, C., Urtasun, R. and Haraphongse, M. (1975). A phase I study of intravenous *Corynebacterium parvum* in solid tumors. *AACR Abstracts,* **16**, 9

349. Buzdar, A. U., Blumenschein, G. R., Smith, T. L., Powell, K. C., Hortobagyi, G. N., Yap, H. Y., Schell, F. C., Barnes, B. C., Ames, F. C., Martin, R. G. and Hersh, E. M. (1984). Adjuvant chemotherapy with fluorouracil, doxorubicin, and cyclophosphamide, with and without Bacillus Calmette-Guerin and with or without irradiation in operable breast cancer. A prospective randomized trial. *Cancer,* **53**, 384–9

350. Cohen, E., Scanlon, E. F., Caprini, J. A., Cunningham, M. P., Oviedo, M. A., Robinson, B. and Knox, K. L. (1982). Follow-up adjuvant chemotherapy and chemoimmunotherapy for stage II and III carcinoma of the breast. *Cancer,* **49**, 1754–61

351. Plagne, R., Misset, J. L., Belpomme, D., Guerrin, J., Le Mevel, B., Metz, R., Chollet, P., Delgado, M., Fargeot, P., Fumoreau, P., Jeanne, C., Ferriere, P., Schneider, M., de Vassal, F., Jasmin, C., Schwarzenberg, L., Hayat, M., Machover, D., Ribaud, P., Dorval, T. and Mathe, G. (1982). BCG adjuvant immunotherapy after adjuvant chemotherapy for operable breast cancer. A 'group inter-france' randomized trial. *AACR Abstracts,* **23**, 157

352. Hubay, C. A., Pearson, O. H., Manni, A., Gordon, N. H. and McGuire, W. L. (1985). III. Antiestrogens in combination with chemotherapy in early breast cancer. Adjuvant endocrine therapy, cytotoxic chemotherapy and immunotherapy in stage II breast cancer: 6-year result. *J. Steroid Biochem.,* **23**, 1147–50

353. Tormey, D. C., Weinberg, V. E., Holland, J. F., Weiss, R. B., Glidewell, O. J., Perloff, M., Falkson, G., Falkson, H. C., Henry, P. H., Leone, L. A., Rafla, S., Ginsberg, S. J., Silver, R. T., Blom, J., Carey, R. W., Schein, P. S. and Lesnick, G. J. (1983). A randomized trial of five and three drug chemotherapy and chemoimmunotherapy in women with operable node positive breast cancer. *J. Clin. Oncol.,* **1**, 138–45

354. Lacour, J., Lacour, F., Spira, A., Michelson, M., Petit, J.-Y., Delage, G., Sarrazin, D., Contesso, G. and Viguier, J. (1980). Adjuvant treatment with polyadenylic-polyuridylic acid (polya, polyu) in operable breast cancer. *Lancet,* 161–4

355. Lacour, J., Lacour, F., Spira, A., Michelson, M., Petit, J.-V., Delage, G., Sarrazin, D., Contesso, G. and Viguier, J. (1984). Adjuvant treatment with polyadenylic-polyuridylic acid in operable breast cancer: updated results of a randomised trial. *Br. Med. J.,* **288**, 589–92

356. Hovanessian, A. G., Youn, J. K., Buffet-Janvresse, C., Riviere, Y., Michelson, M., Lacour, J. and Lacour, F. (1985). Enhancement of natural killer cell activity and 2-5A synthetase in operable breast cancer patients treated with polyadenylic; polyuridylic acid. *Cancer,* **55**, 357–62

357. Verhaegen, H., De Cree, J., De Cock, W. and Verbruggen, F. (1975). Levamisole and the immune reponse. *N. Engl. J. Med.,* **289**, 1148

358. Rojas, A. F., Mickiewicz, E., Feierstein, J. N., Glait, H. and Olivari, A. J. (1976). Levamisole in advanced human breast cancer. *Lancet,* 211–16

359. Henson, J. C., Mattheim, W. H., Engelsman, E. *et al.* (1983). Assessment of immunotherapy with levamisole combined with postoperative chemotherapy of N⁺ primary breast cancer. *Proc. 3rd EORTC Breast Cancer Working Conference,* Amsterdam (abstract)

360. Schreml, W., Lang, M., Betzler, M., Schlag, P., Lohrmann, H.-P., Heimpel, H. and Herfarth, C. (1983). Adjuvant chemo(immuno-)-therapy of primary breast cancer with adriamycin-cyclophosphamide (and levamisole) – six year evaluation. *Eur. J. Cancer Clin. Oncol.,* **19**, 607–13

361. Kay, R. G., Mason, B. H., Stephens, E. J., Arthur, J. F., Hitchcock, G. C., Trindall, P. L.,

Rodgers, R. and Mullins, P. (1983). Levamisole in primary breast cancer. A controlled study in conjunction with 1-phenylalanine mustard. *Cancer*, **51**, 1992–7

362. Grohn, P., Heinonen, E., Klefstrom, P. and Tarkkanen, J. (1984). Adjuvant postoperative radiotherapy, chemotherapy, and immunotherapy in stage III breast cancer. *Cancer*, **54**, 670–4

363. Klefstrom, P. (1980). Combination of levamisole immunotherapy and polychemotherapy in advanced breast cancer. *Cancer Treat. Rep.*, **64**, 65–72

364. Hakes, T. B., Currie, V. E., Kaufman, R. J., Kinne, D., Oettgen, H. and Pinsky, C. (1982). CMF ± levamisole (L) breast adjuvant chemotherapy: 5 year analysis. *Proc. Am. Soc. Clin. Oncol.*, **1**, 319

365. Singh, K. K. and Sinha, C. M. (1982). The encouraging role of chemo-immunotherapy in the management of recurrent breast cancer. *Int. J. Cancer*, **19**, 153–8

366. Hortobagyi, G. N., Yap, H. Y., Blumenschein, G. R., Gutterman, J. U., Buzdar, A. U., Tashima, C. K. and Hersh, E. M. (1978). Response of disseminated breast cancer to combined modality treatment with chemotherapy and levamisole with or without Bacillus Calmette-Guerin. *Cancer Treat. Rep.*, **62**, 1685–92

367. Cunningham, T. J., Olson, K. B., Laffin, R., Horton, J. and Sullivan, J. (1969). Treatment of advanced cancer with active immunization. *Cancer*, **24**, 932–7

368. Anderson, J. M., Kelly, F., Gettinby, G. and Woods, S. E. (1977). Prolonged survival after immunotherapy (irradiated cancer autografts) for mammary cancers, assessed by a measure of therapeutic deficiency. *Cancer*, **40**, 30–5

369. McCune, C. S., Patterson, W. B. and Henshaw, E. C. (1979). Active specific immunotherapy with tumor cells and *Corynebacterium parvum*. A phase I study. *Cancer*, **43**, 1619–23

370. Humphrey, L. J. (1974). Approaches to immunotherapy in cancer. In *Host Defence in Breast Cancer*. p. 191. (Chicago: Year Book Medical Publishers)

371. Humphrey, L., Taschler-Collins, S. and Volenec, F. (1984). Treatment of primary breast cancer with immunotherapy. Comparison with adjuvant chemotherapy and radiation therapy. *Am. J. Surg.*, **148**, 649–52

372. Borden, E. C. and Balkwill, F. R. (1984). Preclinical and clinical studies of interferons and interferon inducers in breast cancer. *Cancer*, **53**, 783–9

373. Gutterman, J. U., Blumenschein, G. R., Alexanian, R., Yap, H. Y., Buzdar, A. U., Cabanillas, F., Hortobagyi, G. N., Hersh, E. M., Rasmussen, S. L., Harmon, M., Kramer, M. and Pestka, S. (1980). Leukocyte interferon-induced tumor regression in human metastatic breast cancer, multiple myeloma, and malignant lymphoma. *Ann. Int. Med.*, **93**, 399–406

374. Borden, E. C., Holland, J. F., Dao, T. L., Gutterman, J. U., Wiener, L., Chang, Y. C. and Patel, J. (1982). Leukocyte-derived interferon (alpha) in human breast carcinoma. *Ann. Int. Med.*, **97**, 1–6

375. Sarna, G. P. and Figlin, R. A. (1985). Phase II trial of a-lymphoblastoid interferon given weekly as treatment of advanced breast cancer. *Cancer Treat. Rep.*, **69**, 547–9

376. Sherwin, S. A., Mayer, D., Ochs, J. J., Abrams, P. G., Knost, J. A., Foon, K. A., Fein, S. and Oldham, R. K. (1983). Recombinant leukocyte A interferon in advanced breast cancer. *Ann. Int. Med.*, **98**, 598–602

377. Muss, H. B., Kempf, R. A., Martino, S., Rudnick, S. A., Greiner, J., Cooper, M. R., Decker, D., Grunberg, S. M., Jackson, D. V., Richards, F. II, Samal, B., Singhakowinta, A., Spurr, C. L., Stuart, J. J., White, D. R., Caponera, M. and Mitchell, M. S. (1984). A phase II study of recombinant a interferon in patients with recurrent or metastatic breast cancer. *J. Clin. Oncol.*, **2**, 1012–16

378. Sherwin, S. A., Knost, J. A., Fein, S. *et al.* (1982). A multiple-dose phase I trial of recombinant leukocyte A interferon in cancer patients. *J. Am. Med. Assoc.*, **248**, 2461–6

379. Silver, H. K. B., Connors, J., Salinas, F. *et al.* (1983). Treatment response in a prospectively randomized study of high vs low dose treatment with lymphoblastoid interferon (IFN). *Proc. ASCO*, **2**, 51

380. Smedley, H., Katrak, M., Sikora, K. *et al.* (1983). Recombinant human interferon in advanced breast cancer. *Br. J. Cancer*, **47**, 566–7

381. Goodwin, B. J., Brenckman, W., Moore, J. *et al.* (1984). Phase II trial of human lymphoblastoid interferon (Wellferon) in metastatic breast carcinoma. *Proc ASCO*, **3**, 60

382. Sarna, G., Figlin, R. and McCarthy, S. (1983). Phase I study of Wellferon[R] (human

lymphoblastoid a-interferon) as cancer therapy: clinical results. *J. Biol. Resp. Mod.*, **2**, 187–95

383. Herberman, R. B. and Thurman, G. B. (1983). Approaches to the immunological monitoring of cancer patients treated with natural or recombinant interferons. *J. Biol. Resp. Mod.*, **2**, 548–62

384. Oettgen, H. F., Old, L. J., Farrow, J. H., Valentine, F. T., Lawrence, H. S. and Thomas, L. (1974). Effects of dialyzable transfer factor in patients with breast cancer. *Proc. Natl. Acad. Sci. USA*, **71**, 2319–23

385. Sparks, F. C., Wile, A. G., Ramming, K. P., Silver, H. K. B., Wolk, R. W. and Morton, D. L. (1976). Immunology and adjuvant chemoimmunotherapy of breast cancer. *Arch. Surg.*, **111**, 1057–62

386. Adler, A., Stein, J. A., Kedar, E., Naor, D. and Weiss, D. W. (1984). Intralesional injection of interleukin-2-expanded autologous lymphocytes in melanoma and breast cancer patients: a pilot study. *J. Biol. Resp. Mod.*, **3**, 491–500

387. Bansal, S. C., Bansal, B. R., Thomas, H. L., Siegel, P. D., Rhoads, J. E., Cooper, D. R., Terman, D. S. and Mark, R. (1978). *Ex vivo* removal of serum IgG in a patient with colon carcinoma. Some biochemical, immunological and histological observations. *Cancer*, **42**, 1

388. Terman, D. S. (1985). Protein A and staphylococcal products in neoplastic disease. *CEC Crit. Rev. Hematol. Oncol.*, **4**, 103–24

389. Kinet, J. P., Bensinger, W. I., Balland, N., Saint-Remy, M., Frankenne, F., Hennen, G. and Mahieu, Ph. (1986). *Ex vivo* perfusion of plasma over protein A columns in human mammary adenocarcinoma. Role of the Fc-binding capacity of protein A in the side effects and the tumoricidal response. *Eur. J. Clin. Invest.*, **16**, 50–5

390. Bertram, J. H., Grunberg, S. M., Shulman, I., Apuzzo, M. L. J., Boquiren, D., Kunkel, L., Hengst, J. C. D., Nelson, J., Waugh, W. J., Plotkin, D. and Mitchell, M. S. (1985). Staphylococcal protein A column: correlation of mitogenicity of perfused plasma with clinical response. *Cancer Res.*, **45**, 4486–94

391. Fer, M. F., Beman, J. A., Stevenson, H. C., Maluish, A., Moratz, C., Delawter, T., Foon, K., Herberman, R. B., Oldham, R. K., Terman, D. S., Young, J. B. and Daskal, Y. (1984). A trial of autologous plasma perfusion over protein A in patients with breast cancer. *J. Biol. Resp. Mod.*, **3**, 352–8

392. Young, J. B., Ayus, J. C., Miller, L. K., Divine, G. W., Frommer, J. P., Miller, R. R. and Terman, D. S. (1983). Cardiopulmonary toxicity in patients with breast carcinoma during plasma perfusion over immobilized protein A. *Am. J. Med.*, **75**, 278–88

393. Messerschmidt, G., Bowles, C., Alsaker, R., McCormack, K., Corbitt, R. H., Mosley, K. R. and Deisseroth, R. B. (1983). Prognostic indicators of tumor response to *Staphylococcus aureus* cowan strain I plasma perfusion. *J. Natl. Cancer Inst.*, **71**, 535–8

394. Sukumar, S., Zbar, B., Terata, N. and Langone, J. J. (1984). Plasma therapy of primary rat mammary carcinoma: antitumor activity of tumor-bearer plasma adsorbed against inactivated CNBr sepharose or protein A-sepharose. *J. Biol. Resp. Mod.*, **3**, 303–15

395. Ray, P. K. (1985). Immunosuppressor control as a modality of cancer treatment: effect of plasma adsorption with *Staphylococcus aureus* protein A. *Contemp. Top. Immunobiol.*, **15**, 147–211

396. Daskal, Y., Mattioli, C. A. and Terman, D. S. (1984). Ultrastructural changes in breast tumors of patients following treatment with plasma perfused over immobilized protein A. *J. Biol. Resp. Mod.*, **3**, 247–54

397. Colcher, D., Zalutsky, M., Kaplan, W., Kufe, D., Austin, F. and Schlom, J. (1983). Radiolocalization of human mammary tumors in athymic mice by a monoclonal antibody. *Cancer Res.*, **43**, 736–42

398. Schlom, J., Greiner, J., Hand, P. H., Colcher, D. Inghirami, G., Weeks, M., Pestka, S., Fishter, P. B., Noguchi, P. and Kufe, D. (1984). Monoclonal antibodies to breast cancer-associated antigens as potential reagents in the management of breast cancer. *Cancer*, **54**, 2777–94

399. Krolick, K. A., Yuan, D. and Vitetta, E. S. (1981). Specific killing of a human breast carcinoma cell line by a monoclonal antibody coupled to the A-chain of ricin. *Cancer Immunol. Immunother.*, **12**, 39–41

400. Canevari, S., Oriandi, R., Ripamonti, M., Tagliabue, E., Aguanno, S., Miotti, S., Menard, S. and Colnaghi, M. I. (1985). Ricin A chain conjugated with monoclonal

Table 11.1 AIDS cases reported to Centers for Disease Control as of Dec. 1985. Outcome (USA cases)

Disease group	Adult/adolescent				Paediatric				Total			
	Cases	%	Known deaths	%	Cases	%	Known Death	%	Cases	%	Known deaths	% Dead
Both KS and PCP	870	6	552	63	4	2	4	100	874	6	556	64
KS without PCP	2856	19	1084	38	7	3	7	100	2863	19	1091	38
PCP without KS	8553	57	4525	53	123	57	87	71	8676	57	4612	53
OI without KS or PCP	2676	18	1485	55	83	38	33	40	2579	18	1518	55
Total	14955	100	7646	51	217	100	131	60	14992	100	7777	51

KS = Kaposi's sarcoma; OI = opportunistic infections; PCP = pneumocystis pneumonia

Table 11.2 AIDS cases by age at diagnosis in the United States

Age	Cases	%
Under 13	217	1
13–19	72	0
20–29	3158	21
30–39	7148	47
40–49	3160	21
Over 49	1417	9
Total	15172	100

Table 11.3 AIDS cases reported to the Centers for Disease Control as of Dec. 1985. Demographic distribution

Race/ethnicity	Adult/adolescent		Paediatric		Total	
	Cases	%	Cases	%	Cases	%
White, not Hispanic	8963	60	41	19	9004	59
Black, not Hispanic	3686	25	129	59	3815	25
Hispanic	2119	14	44	20	2163	14
Other	78	1	0	0	78	1
Unknown	109	1	3	1	112	1
Total	14955	100	217	100	15172	100

Table 11.4 All reported cases of AIDS and case-fatality rates by half-year of diagnosis, 1979–Dec. 2, 1985, United States

		Number of cases	Number of known deaths	Case–fatality rate (%)
1979	Jan.–June	3	2	67
	July–Dec.	9	8	89
1980	Jan.–June	18	15	83
	July–Dec.	29	27	93
1981	Jan.–June	87	73	84
	July–Dec.	173	147	85
1982	Jan.–June	361	277	77
	July–Dec.	633	462	73
1983	Jan.–June	1185	849	72
	July–Dec.	1531	1114	73
1984	Jan.–June	2338	1524	65
	July–Dec.	2982	1545	52
1985	Jan.–June	3726	1286	35
	July–Dec. 2	2089	444	21
Totals*		15172	7777	51

*Table totals include eight cases diagnosed prior to 1979. Of these eight cases, four are known to have died.

Table 11.5 AIDS cases reported to the Centers for Disease Control as of Dec. 2, 1985. Incidence (United States)

Risk groups	Males	(%)	Females	(%)	Total cases	(%)
Adult/adolescent						
Homosexual or bisexual men	10958	(78)	—	(—)	10958	(73)
Intravenous (i.v.) drug user	2037	(15)	520	(53)	2557	(17)
Haemophilia/coagulation disorder	111	(1)	4	(0)	115	(1)
Heterosexual contact	18	(0)	137	(14)	155	(1)
Transfusion with blood/blood products	142	(1)	95	(10)	237	(2)
None of the above/other	710	(5)	223	(23)	933	(6)
Total	13976	(100)	979	(100)	14955	(100)
Paediatric						
Haemophilia/coagulation disorder	11	(9)	0	(0)	11	5
Parent with AIDS/or at increased risk for AIDS	86	(70)	79	(83)	165	(76)
Transfusion with blood/blood products	20	(16)	9	(9)	29	(13)
None of the above/other	5	(4)	7	(7)	12	(6)
Total	122	(100)	95	(100)	217	(100)

228

Table 11.6 Risk factors for seropositivity to HLTV-III/LAV

Risk group	Factors associated with increased risk
Homosexual men	Number of partners Receptive anal intercourse Contact in high risk area
Parental drug user	Needle sharing Frequent injections
Haemophiliacs	Dose of factor 8 concentrate
Blood recipients	Number of blood transfusions Donor from risk group
Other	Heterosexual contact with risk group member Frequent heterosexual contacts Frequent prostitute contacts Needle stick exposure Parent from risk group

becoming infected[11,12]. However, this proportion may increase with longer follow-up and may approach 50% in highly selected subpopulations[13]. Most seropositive individuals, however, will remain asymptomatic for a prolonged period. Some vital statistics (Tables 11.1–5) indicate the evolution of AIDS in the United States since the Centers for Disease Control defined criteria for reporting this condition, and started accumulating data. These provide an estimate of survival as a function of disease manifestations and demographic factors. Table 11.6 outlines the risk factors associated with seropositivity.

Heterosexual transmission of AIDS is currently an issue of increasing concern. The identification of HTLV-III/LAV in semen suggests a source of heterosexual as well as homosexual transmission which appears to have been confirmed by recent reports of transmission of infection to women by artificial insemination[14]. From 10 to 70% of steady heterosexual partners of infected persons have positive HTLV-III/LAV antibodies[15,16]. Currently 1% of patients with AIDS have no identifiable risk factors apart from heterosexual contact with other persons with AIDS or with persons at increased risk. A sizeable percentage (15–20%) of men with AIDS, with no other risk factors, claim to have had frequent heterosexual contact with prostitutes[17]. In addition, recent studies indicate a significant rate of seropositivity among female prostitutes, indicating at least a carrier state for this disease[18]. However, because HTLV-III/LAV infection has been present since 1980 and heterosexual transmission accounts for less than 5% of cases with AIDS, it would seem that the prevalence of infection in heterosexuals, although increasing, may not rise dramatically[19].

Tables 11.7 and 11.8 demonstrate the incidence of AIDS in Europe where homosexuals are also the primary group at risk. Intravenous drug abusers account for 3% of all European cases. Countries not importing blood products from the United States have a lower incidence of seropositivity

Table 11.7 Reported AIDS cases and estimated rates per million population from 17 European countries

Country	Oct. 1983*	Oct. 1984	Dec. 1984	Mar. 1985	Rates†
Austria	7	–	13	13	1.7
Belgium	38	–	65	81	8.2
Czechoslovakia	0	0	0	0	0.0
Denmark	13	31	34	5	8.0
Finland	–	4	5	5	1.0
France	94	221	260	307	5.6
Federal Republic of Germany	42	110	135	162	2.6
Greece	–	2‡	6	7	0.7
Iceland	0	0	0	0	0.0
Italy	3	10	14	22	0.4
Netherlands	1	26	42	52	3.6
Norway	–	4	5	8	2.0
Poland	0	0	0	0	0.0
Spain	6	18	18	29	0.8
Sweden	4	12	16	22	2.7
Switzerland	17	33	41	51	7.9
United Kingdom	24	88	108	140	2.5
Total	249	559	762	904	2.4

*These data were reported at the First European Meeting on AIDS held in Aarhus, Denmark, October, 1983.
† Based on 1983 populations, INED, Paris.
‡ Data of July 15, 1984.

Table 11.8 AIDS cases, by patient risk group and geographic origin from 17 European countries, through March 31, 1985

Patient risk group	Nationality				
	European	Caribbean	African	Other	Total
(1) Male homosexual or bisexual	627	4	9	21	661
(2) Intravenous drug abuser	25	–	–	–	25
(3) Haemophilia patient	27	–	–	1	28
(4) Transfusion recipient (without other risk factors)	11	–	5	–	16
(5) 1- and 2-associated	10	–	–	2	12
(6) No known risk factor male	33	20	67	2	122
female	18	7	32	–	57
(7) Unknown	5	1	11	2	19
Total	756	32	124	28	940

among haemophiliacs. The proportion of HTLV-III/LAV infection transmitted by heterosexual contact, homosexual contact, intravenous drug abuse or other modes varies considerably between countries because of factors that are incompletely understood. Since the reports include a small number of patients, data required for a reliable estimate of future epidemic curve in Europe are lacking[20]. Detailed studies evaluating the incidence of HTLV-III/LAV infection in Africa are beginning to appear. The virus is endemic in Uganda, Rwanda and Zaire, and is associated with generalized aggressive atypical Kaposi's sarcoma (KS). In these countries heterosexual contact is believed to be a major route for viral transmission, with the female to male ratio being almost unity[21,22]. The delineation of the epidemiology of AIDS has not only helped improve the understanding of the disease, but has also been essential to the rational planning of therapeutic and preventive measures.

VIROLOGY

The aetiologic agents of AIDS is HTLV-III/LAV, a lymphotropic and neurotropic retrovirus, consisting of an RNA core covered by a viral envelope. The virus can be isolated from peripheral lymphocytes in up to 80% of patients with positive serum antibody[23]. In addition, the virus has been detected in semen, saliva, tears, brain, and spinal fluid[24-27].

The first stage of infection involves a specific interaction at the cell membrane between the viral envelope and a cellular receptor. In the case of lymphocytes this appears to be the T4 receptor. The virus carries within its core an enzyme that synthesizes DNA called reverse transcriptase, which allows RNA to code for double-stranded DNA. This virally directed DNA then integrates with host cell DNA. In addition to integrated DNA, unintegrated proviral DNA persists in the cytoplasm of infected cells[28]. Once infection occurs with HTLV-III/LAV, it is likely to persist for the lifetime of the cell since integrated viral genes are duplicated with the normal cellular genes. In some cases this leads to neoplastic transformation, while other cells undergo degeneration[23]. HTLV-III/LAV has several features in common with HTLV-I and HLTV-II including its genetic structure, and T-lymphocyte receptor tropism. Figure 11.1 demonstrates the genetic structure of HTLV-

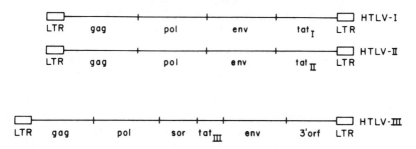

Figure 11.1 Comparison of genetic structures of HTLV-I, HTLV-II and HTLV-III/LAV

III/LAV in comparision with other retroviruses. HTLV-III/LAV contains the three basic genes common to retroviruses and necessary for replication; the gag gene coding for three viral internal structural proteins p18, p25, and p13; the pol gene for reverse transcriptase and env gene for the envelope. These genomes when integrated are flanked on each side by sequences that contain regulatory elements called long terminal repeat sequences. The long terminal repeat sequences regulate the expression of viral genes but may also regulate the expression of nearby cellular genes[29].

HTLV-III/LAV also contains a gene that encodes transcriptional activator (tat), which has been mapped to a small region in the middle of the genome. In other retroviruses the tat gene has been shown to be critical for virus replication and has been implicated in the transforming capabilities of the virus[27,29].

Although there are many similarities between HTLV-III/LAV, HTLV-I and HTLV-II, the recent demonstration of considerable sequence homology between the nucleic acid of HTLV-III/LAV and visna virus, a lentivirus infecting sheep, suggests a closer similarity to that virus than to other retroviruses. Both visna and HTLV-III/LAV are lymphocytopathic and neurotropic. In addition, they both exhibit features of antigenic drift[30].

Diagnosis of HTLV-III/LAV infection

The ability to detect serum antibodies, viral products or virus has been one of the major technical advances in this disease. The antibody response to antigenic determinants found on HTLV-III/LAV virion can be measured in a number of ways[31,32]. The simplest is the ELISA test which measures antibody to all viral proteins and is highly specific and sensitive in detecting HTLV-III/LAV infection. The original report of this technique indicated an 88% positivity in AIDS patients, and a low (approximately 0.5%) positive reaction in controls not at risk for AIDS[33]. The ELISA is an indirect assay, which utilizes inactivated HTLV-III/LAV virus lysate to coat microtitre wells; plasma antibodies are subsequently quantitated by the amount of binding to viral proteins. The ELISA test is currently the most widely utilized screening test particularly among blood donors.

Whereas the ELISA test measures antibody response to several HTLV-III/LAV antigens, the Western blot technique measures antibodies to single proteins. Virion proteins are separated by electrophoresis and reacted with human sera. The antigen–antibody complex is identified by a radioactively-labelled protein with high affinity binding to such complexes[31]. This is the most sensitive antibody test for AIDS, being positive in 100% of patients. Of interest is a recent report suggesting that ELISA-positive, Western blot-negative blood may not be as infective as ELISA-positive, Western blot-positive blood[34].

Another means of documenting infection is the isolation of virus and viral products from the body fluids of AIDS and ARC patients. Cultured T-lymphocytes or cell-free supernatants are exposed to permissive cells, for example the immortalized B-cell line FCRC-15 or immortalized T-cell line HuT-78. Virus identification can then be confirmed by several techniques

Table 11.9 Immunology of AIDS

T-cell abnormalities

Total lymphopenia
Decreased T4 subset
Reversed T4/T8 ratios
Decreased blast transformation in response to mitogen stimulation
Decreased lymphokine production
Defective T-cell and NK cell-mediated cytotoxicity
Diminished T-helper cell function for B-cell immunoglobulin production

B-cell abnormalities

Elevated levels of serum immunoglobulins
Increased circulating immune complexes
Increased spontaneous profileration
Diminished antibody response to *de novo* mitogens and antigens
Decreased response to T-cell-triggered activation

Monocyte and macrophage abnormalities

Defective monocyte chemotaxis
Diminished *in vitro* killing of extracellular and intracellular parasites
Increased IL-1 secretion and prostaglandin production
Decreased response to inducers of IL-1 production

Serologic abnormalities

Elevated β-2-microglobulin
Elevated α-2-thymosin
Elevated acid labile α-interferon
Decreased serum thymulin
Soluble suppressor factor

---

including an assay for reverse transcriptase positive particles utilizing a template primer. Cells can also be assayed for HTLV-III/LAV homologous DNA using a cloned DNA probe. Cultures can be examined for typical HTLV-III/LAV particles on electron microscopy. The development of monoclonal antibody to various viral proteins including core protein allows for specific identification of HTLV-III/LAV per cell via double antibody indirect or immunofluorescence assays[35].

Currently, there is no single standardized test for the detection of HTLV-III/LAV. With the rapid evolution of therapeutic strategies utilizing antiviral agents, the need for a standardized approach towards virologic end-points has arisen, and remains as one of the highest priorities of such trials.

IMMUNOLOGY

HTLV-III/LAV preferentially infects the T4 helper subset of lymphocytes, causing intrinsic functional lymphocyte abnormalities, and disrupting the array of interactions among various components of the immune system. Table 11.9 summarizes these immunologic abnormalities[36]. It is probable that other infections which commonly afflict susceptible populations account for some of the abnormalities.

T-cell abnormalities

One of the earliest clinical observations in AIDS patients that allowed recognition of the syndrome was an absolute decrease in the total number of circulating lymphocytes. This decrease specifically affected the subset of OKT4 or Leu 3$^+$/helper inducer cells, resulting in an inversion of the T4/T8 helper/suppressor ratio. This reversed T4/T8 ratio is not specific for AIDS and is seen in other conditions including systemic viral infections and malignancy[37,38].

A number of functional defects have been noted in both T4 and T8 lymphocytes, including decreased blast transformation in response to mitogen stimulation, decreased lymphokine production, defective T-cell-mediated cytotoxicity[39-44], and failure to respond appropriately to specific antigens such as tetanus toxoid[43]. Further investigation of T4 cells has led to the identification of a T4 subset bearing a surface marker defined by the TQ1 monoclonal antibody, which seems to be selectively depleted, whereas TQ1$^-$ cells are present in normal quantities[45]. TQ1$^+$ cells are believed to be involved in facilitating antigen-specific immune responses.

Lymphokine production, particularly interleukin-2 (IL-2), is diminished in patients with AIDS. *In vitro* studies have demonstrated decreased IL-2 production in response to suboptimal concentrations of phytohaemagglutinin (PHA). Interestingly, near normal levels are produced with higher PHA concentrations. In addition, it is possible that sera from AIDS patients contains specific IL-2 synthesis inhibitors[46].

IL-2 receptor expression has been reported variously as either diminished[47] or normal[43]. The production of other lymphokines from the T-cells of AIDS patients is also impaired, and γ-interferon production has been reported as either normal[48] or decreased. In one study there was virtually no γ-interferon production in response to specific microbial antigens[42].

T-cell-mediated cytotoxicity and natural killer (NK) cell activity is markedly reduced in AIDS patients when compared with healthy subjects[49,50]. Specific killing of cytomegalovirus (CMV)-infected target cells by T-cells, and lysis of K562 tumour target cells by NK cells are both defective. The abnormality is more striking for virus-specific cytotoxicity. However, in the presence of exogenous IL-2, both NK cell activity and virus-specific cyto-toxicity are dramatically enhanced[49,51]. This finding showed that antigen-specific cytotoxic T-cell precursors can be present in the circulation of patients with AIDS, and suggested that the mechanism for the deficient cytotoxicity was a maturational arrest of these precursors at a stage dependent on the effect of IL-2. These IL-2 effects were not interferon-mediated, as β-interferon had no significant effect when added to culture of AIDS patients' lymphocytes. Furthermore, addition of IL-2 did not induce production and release of α-interferon from the lymphocytes of AIDS patients in contrast to normal lymphocytes[51]. Nor did complete neutralization of interferon with monoclonal antibody negate the positive effect of IL-2 on NK cell cytotoxic activity.

B-cell abnormalities

Early clinical observations in AIDS patients revealed elevated levels of serum immunoglobulins, circulating immune complexes, and various autoimmune phenomena[48]. B-cells are polyclonally activated, and in fact approximately ten times the number of circulating lymphocytes spontaneously secreting non-specific antibody are found in AIDS patients compared with controls[43]. However, these lymphocytes do not proliferate or produce immunoglobulin when triggered with B-cell-specific mitogens. The defect in mitogen-stimulated antibody production was shown to involve intrinsic B-cell dysfunction perhaps related to direct B-cell infection, separate from abnormalities of T-helper cells[36,43]. Polyclonal hypergammaglobulinaemia is common in these patients and a deficiency in any specific immunoglobulin suggests a different diagnosis.

Other abnormalities in circulating proteins have been measured in serum of AIDS patients. The significance of these findings is not entirely clear at this time. β-2 microglobulin, α-1-thymosin and acid-labile α-interferon levels are reportedly elevated. Decreased serum thymulin has also been reported[52-54].

Monocyte and macrophage abnormalities

The monocyte, like the lymphocyte, may be primarily infected by the virus HTLV-III/LAV, or its function may be impaired secondarily as a result of virus-induced defects in the T4 lymphocyte subset[36]. Both extracellular killing (e.g. *Giardia lamblia*) and intracellular killing (e.g. toxoplasmosis) of parasites is defective in patients with AIDS. These defects are not overcome with IL-2; however, intracellular killing may be enhanced by the addition of α-interferon[55].

Furthermore, monocytes show increased spontaneous release of IL-1 and prostaglandin E_2, but inability to respond appropriately to the usual inducers of interleukin secretion[55]. Therefore, like B-cells, monocytes may be in a preactivated state which precludes appropriate response to specific antigens.

Soluble suppressor factor

In addition to the depletion of T4 cells induced by HTLV-III/LAV infection, a soluble protein has been isolated from the serum of AIDS patients, which is capable of inhibiting T-cell-dependent immune functions[56]. This protein is thought to be secreted by infected T4 cells. When added to cultures of normal lymphocytes and pokeweed mitogen, soluble suppressor factor inhibited proliferation and immunoglobulin synthesis. This protein closely resembles, in its amino acid structure, a portion of the envelope of HTLV-I (a retrovirus related to HTLV-III/LAV) and to p15E, an envelope protein of feline leukaemia virus (FeLV)[56]. p15E has been shown to impair the immune responses of living experimental animals. Cats injected with the substance developed cancer after exposure to feline sarcoma virus, and *in vitro* p15E has caused some of the functional lymphocyte abnormalities recognized in HTLV-III/LAV infection. The soluble suppressor factor may actually be a portion of the HTLV-III/LAV protein envelope. Another possibility is that it

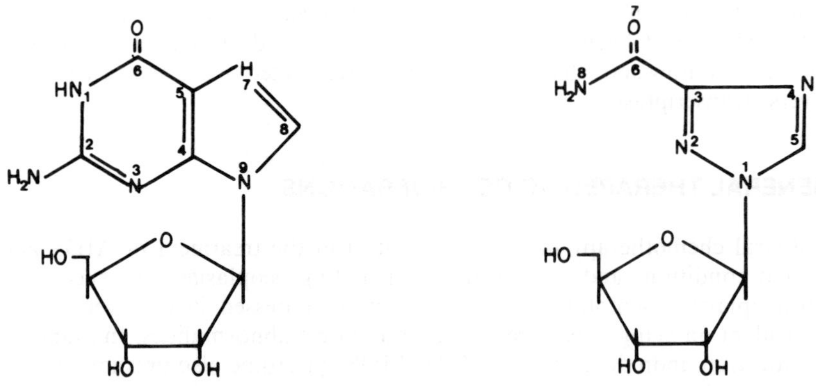

GUANOSINE **RIBAVIRIN**

Figure 11.2 Structures of guanosine and ribavirin

effect is dependent on the concentration of virus used to infect cells, the characteristics of the host cell line and the specific virus strain[60]. Recently concentrations of $50\mu g/ml$ of ribavirin have been shown *in vitro* to inhibit the replication of HTLV-III/LAV and the release of reverse transcriptase[61].

Ribavirin can be administered orally or intravenously, inhaled as an aerosol or applied topically to the skin. After oral and intravenous administration of 1000 mg/day serum plasma concentrations reached the *in vitro* mean inhibitory concentration values for herpes viruses and influenza viruses[62]. Serum half-life of the drug is approximately 9 h (range 6.5–11.0) and is about twice as long as that of other antiviral drugs such as adenosine arabinoside (Ara-a) and acyclovir[62,63]. Small-particle aerosol administration delivered adequate drug levels to infants with influenza and respiratory syncytial virus infections[64,65]. No significant toxicity has been seen in oral regimens of 600 mg/day for 28 successive days. Higher doses and longer periods of treatment may lead to toxicity – most notably decreases in haemoglobin content and haematocrit[66].

Ribavirin is selectively concentrated in red cells, and the monophosphate metabolite of the drug may then result in a competitive deficiency of ATP and interfere with the cell's metabolism or membrane components resulting in early red cell death[67]. The anaemia is rarely clinically significant, is dose-related and reversed when treatment is discontinued[68,69].

Extensive clinical testing in randomized double blind trials has shown efficacy of ribavirin in treating respiratory syncytial virus infections and lassa fever[70-74].

To date experience with ribavirin in retrovirus infection has been limited. *In vitro* concentrations of $50-100\mu mol/L$ interfere with the replication of HTLV-III/LAV in cultured T-cells[61]. In phase I trials of ribavirin mean plasma drug concentration of $3.1\mu mol/L$ was achieved after an oral dose of 1000 mg/day[66]. Following intravenous administration of 1000 mg/day and 500 mg/day for 4 days, mean plasma ribavirin levels were $94\mu mol/L$ and

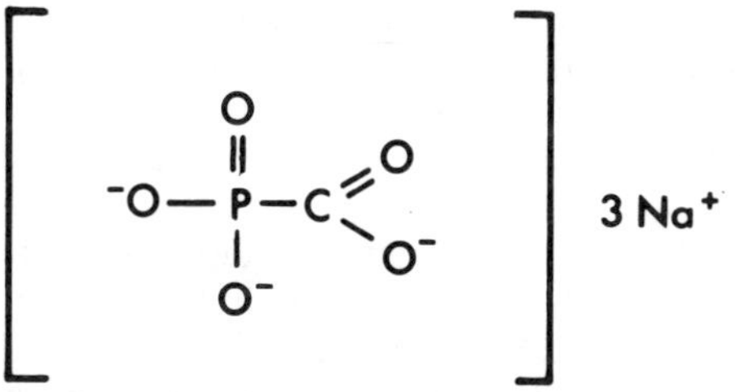

Figure 11.3 Structure of foscarnet

$68\,\mu$mol/L, respectively. These levels are in excess of the *in vitro minimal* inhibitory concentrations for the herpes virus family[60].

Toxicity in these studies included moderately severe anaemia and mild central nervous system toxicity consisting of headache, insomnia, irritability and poor concentration. Ribavirin treatment of AIDS patients has not yet been undertaken in a controlled setting.

Phosphonoformate (foscarnet)

Foscarnet, a pyrophosphate analogue (Figure 11.3), has been shown to non-competitively inhibit several viral enzymes including the DNA and RNA polymerases[75]. Reverse transcriptases from HTLV-III/LAV and other viruses are inhibited *in vitro* by foscarnet in doses ranging from 0.7 to $100\,\mu$mol[76]. Growth of HTLV-III/LAV-infected cells was suppressed by 98% with doses of $132\,\mu$mol, and was completely inhibited at $680\,\mu$mol. Growth rates of uninfected cells were not affected at the lower dose and only minimally inhibited at the higher dose.

Additional experiments[77] revealed that timing of initiation and duration of treatment was important. Either postponing addition of drug to cultures or withdrawing it prematurely incompletely inhibited RT activity and viral replication.

In cultures of T-cells from patients with ARC, foscarnet reversed the viral-induced impairment of clonal lymphocyte expansion, measured by a significant rise in T-cell colony numbers[78]. In another experiment using lymphocytes derived from patients with AIDS, seven out of 12 T-cell cultures exposed to foscarnet showed increased colony numbers, a positive trend which did not reach statistical significance[79]. Foscarnet did not stimulate normal peripheral blood leukocytes in the presence of PHA or IL-2. The mechanism of action of foscarnet in this regard is not well defined, but does not seem to be related to mitogenesis stimulated by PHA or to direct antiviral effect. One postulate is that foscarnet permits T-cell growth by activating colony precursors while preventing viral production, while another suggestion is that it may inhibit the production of soluble suppressive factors which impair immune response. The latter hypothesis was supported by the results of mixed lymphocyte experiments in which foscarnet reversed the suppression of colony formation of healthy control cells induced by lymphocytes from AIDS patients[78].

Foscarnet can only be administered intravenously in humans. Preliminary results from patients treated for CMV infections revealed plasma and CSF concentrations ranging from 40 to 75 μg/ml and 8 to 30 μg/ml respectively[80]. The drug is excreted in the urine. Its plasma half-life is between 1 and 4 h, and the drug remains in bone for very long time periods – up to 400 days.

No acute toxicity was seen in the studies of foscarnet in treatment of CMV infections in man. Evidence from animal studies suggests that the drug is relatively non-toxic. Problems related to long-term intravenous infusion include local phlebitis and volume overload. There was a suggestion of nephrotoxicity in patients who had been treated for longer than 2 weeks.

Based on its *in vitro* activity against reverse transcriptase, ability to inhibit growth of HTLV-III/LAV, and the relative lack of toxicity, foscarnet may offer some promise in the treatment of AIDS.

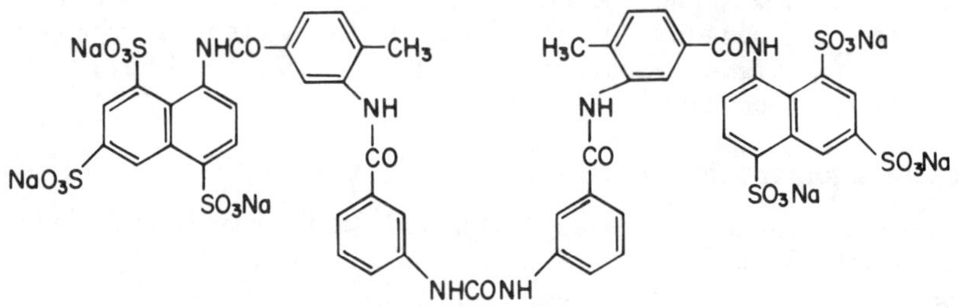

Figure 11.4 Structure of suramin

Suramin

Suramin is a hexasodium salt derivative of naphthalenetrisulphonic acid (Figure 11.4)[81]. Originally introduced in 1920 as a cure for African sleeping sickness, the drug has been extensively used in the treatment of trypanosomiasis and onchocerciasis. Its specific mechanism of action against these parasitic diseases is not known, but may be related to inhibition of various enzymes including hyaluronidase, ATPase, hexokinase and DNA polymerase[82]. Suramin has also recently been shown to competitively inhibit viral reverse transcriptase *in vitro*. At concentrations of 50 μg/ml suramin blocks the infectivity of HTLV-III/LAV in cultures of normal T4 lymphocytes and H9 cells. Higher drug levels, between 100 and 1000 μg/ml, clearly protected against the cytopathic viral effect while not inhibiting normal T-cell growth[83].

Suramin is given by slow intravenous administration as the drug is poorly absorbed by the oral route. When given by subcutaneous or intramuscular injection it causes intense local irritation.

Following intravenous injection suramin combines with plasma proteins, and may persist in the blood for up to 6 months[82]. The drug is cleared by the kidneys at a slow rate, with a half-life of about 40 days. Variable drug accumulation occurs which may account for some therapeutic failures in the diseases for which the drug is indicated.

Acute toxicity encountered in suramin treatment includes nausea, vomiting, abdominal pain and urticarial eruptions. Very rarely, in 0.02–0.05% of cases, neuromuscular irritability and cardiovascular collapse associated with coma may occur. Late reactions (usually within 24 h) include fever, photophobia, lacrimation, palpebral oedema, abdominal distension and constipation. Cutaneous hyperaesthesias of the soles and palms may begin within the first 24 h after injection and may persist for a week or longer. The affected skin may desquamate. Renal damage is the most common delayed reaction noted several days after injection. Both the proximal tubules and the glomeruli can be affected and a self-limited, mild proteinuria is extremely common and generally not an indication for stopping therapy[82].

Preliminary reports of suramin therapy in patients with ARC and AIDS have been recently published. In one study, ten patients received a total dose of 6.2 g over 5 weeks. All patients were HTLV-III/LAV antibody seropositive but positive viral cultures and reverse transcriptase activity were documented in only four cases. Viral replication was diminished in all four of these patients during the course of treatment and was actually undetectable in three. However, 1 week following discontinuation of treatment, viral growth resumed in all cases. Viral cultures in three patients who had been culture-negative at the start of therapy remained negative at the conclusion of treatment. There was no significant improvement in either the patients' clinical status or immunological parameters including total WBC, total lymphocytes, T4/T8 ratio or delayed hypersensitivity skin tests to a routine panel of antigens[84].

A second study was conducted in Rwanda; five patients with a clinical diagnosis of ARC were treated with 20 mg/kg of suramin intravenously every 5 days for 35 days. HTLV-III/LAV antibody status was not documented, nor were viral cultures or reverse transcriptase activity measured. Quantification of T-cell subsets and delayed hypersensitivity skin tests were followed as parameters of immunologic competence. Objective clinical improvement was detected after the first dose – indicated by disappearance of lymphadenopathy arthralgias and diarrhoea. Further improvement in opportunistic infections was also claimed in one patient with pulmonary tuberculosis, and another with undocumented, presumptive pneumocystis pneumonia and nephrotic syndrome. Restoration of immune competence was claimed, in that three previously anergic patients mounted delayed hypersensitivity skin reactions to PPD and PHA after treatment, and T4/T8 lymphocyte ratios rose in four treated patients. In this non-randomized uncontrolled test of suramin in ARC, a positive antiviral effect was suggested[85].

A third group at the Goethe University in West Germany treated eight patients with ARC or AIDS. A total dose of 6.2 g was administered over 6 weeks by a maintenance dose of 1 g every 2–3 weeks, in order to maintain a serum suramin level of 100 μg/ml[86]. These investigators found no clinical or immunological improvement over a 7-month follow-up, and indeed two patients actually deteriorated in a manner typical of ARC. Recent clinical data suggested that a trough serum concentration of less than 100 μg/ml allowed viral reactivation. Current trials are directed towards long-term maintenance treatment in order to maintain therapeutic drug levels. In addition, Kaposi's sarcoma and lymphoma in an AIDS patient showed an objective response to suramin[87]. Trials must also be extended to neoplasias in these patients.

Antimoniotungstate (HPA-23)

HPA-23, a mineral condensed polyanion of ammonium 5-tungsto-2-anti-moniate, is a competitive inhibitor of murine and human reverse transcriptase[88,89]. The drug is active *in vivo* against a wide variety of DNA and RNA viruses and has been used in humans in the treatment of scrapie[90]. It is active against retroviruses *in vitro*[91].

To date there has been limited clinical experience with this drug. A single published report from Paris presents the results of intravenous infusion of HPA-23 in four AIDS patients. Although no detailed pharmacokinetics were performed, in one patient the serum half-life was less than 20 min. Patients received two courses of 200 mg/day for 15 days each. All four patients completed treatment. Viral replication and reverse transcriptase activity were measured prior to, during, and after treatment. HPA-23 was shown to inhibit both enzyme activity and viral reproduction – anti-HTLV-III/LAV anti-bodies persisted throughout treatment, and viral activity increased when treatment was discontinued. HPA-23 had no significant effect on either total T4 lymphocyte counts or on the T4/T8 ratio.

The primary toxicity of the drug was significant thrombocytopenia, to platelet counts of less than 50 000. This was a reversible side-effect, with platelets rising to pretreatment levels 21–45 days after discontinuation of the drug. Mild elevations of hepatic transaminases were also noted. There was no renal toxicity[92].

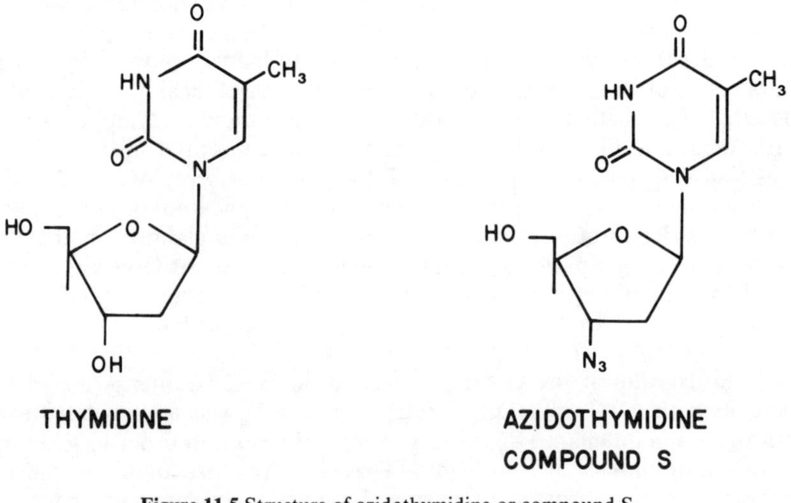

THYMIDINE

AZIDOTHYMIDINE

COMPOUND S

Figure 11.5 Structure of azidothymidine or compound S

Other antivirals

Several other new antiviral compounds have been identified, although little preclinical or clinical data has been published[93].

Compound S, or azidothymidine, is a thymidine analogue (Figure 11.5) which is converted by a cellular kinase enzyme to a competitive inhibitor of reverse transcriptase. *In vitro*, at concentrations of 5–10 μmol/L it has been shown to inhibit HTLV-III/LAV replication without affecting normal uninfected cells. Adequate serum drug levels can be obtained following oral administration, and the drug crosses the blood–brain barrier achieving concentrations of 20–25% those seen in the circulation[94-96]. Phase I studies have recently begun.

Ansamycin is a derivative of rifamycin – a drug active against human mycobacteria. Ansamycin is believed to inhibit reverse transcriptase. It has shown inhibitory effect on the replication and infectivity of HTLV-III/LAV *in vitro*. The drug has been used extensively in the treatment of *Mycobacterium avium-intracellulare*, a common opportunistic infection in AIDS patients, but has not been studied specifically as a treatment against retroviral infection[97].

Based on different mechanisms of action, combinations of antiviral drugs may be synergistic, as *in vitro* studies with interferon and reverse transcriptase inhibitors may indicate. Interferon inhibits replication of several animal retroviruses both *in vivo* and *in vitro*[98,99]. A suppressive effect *in vivo* has been shown for recombinant α-interferon-A against HTLV-III/LAV. Some inhibition was seen at doses as low as 4 units/ml and rose in a direct dose–response relationship. Doses between 256 and 1024 units/ml achieved complete inhibition of viral replication[100]. The addition of foscarnet to low non-inhibitory doses of interferon resulted in a synergistic increase in antiviral activity[100]. In addition, early *in vitro* data suggest possible synergy between compound S and suramin. In any of these attempts clearing of disease manifestations is only the first objective; the viral reservoirs in the CNS and elsewhere must also be considered as an important therapeutic aspect.

IMMUNE MODULATION

Even with the advent of adequate antiviral therapy, strategies need to be developed to correct the underlying immune defect. Immune modulating agents have recently gained wide use in patients with malignancy and congenital immunodeficiencies, and provide a treatment approach to patients with AIDS. To date results have not been promising. Immunologic endpoints have been difficult to define, and the clinical significance, in terms of survival and tumour response, of the immunologic endpoints of such trials are difficult to interpret. While some changes in immune function, such as improved NK activity or increased sensitivity to skin antigens, can be induced with immune modifiers, these usually do not correlate with clinical benefit. Immune modifiers so far used fall in three categories:

(1) Biologic, utilizing factors normally produced by the body's own immune system (most commonly lymphokines),
(2) Pharmacologic, which include drugs developed in the laboratory capable of modifying immunity, and
(3) Adoptive, which imply passive transfer of immunity.

Table 11.11 Immune modifiers

Group	Drug	Number of patients	Results
Biologic modifiers	TP5	32	↑ MLR, mitogen-induced IL-2 production, no change T4/T8
	Thymopentin	10	no response
	Thymostimulin	15	ongoing
	IL-2	12	no change NK or mitogen response
	IL-2	5	no change NK or mitogen response
	Imreg-1	33 AIDS/ ARC	↑ PHA, PWM response, IL-2 production
Pharmacologic modifiers	Isoprinosine	12 AIDS 24 ARC	no significant change
	Isoprinosine	6 AIDS 4 ARC	↑ mitogen response only
	Azimexon	16 ARC 12 AIDS	↑ lymphocyte count, T4/T8 + skin tests in ARC only
	CL246738	20 AIDS	ongoing
Adoptive modification	Thymic transplant	14 AIDS	↑ lymphocyte counts transient
	Bone marrow transplant	2	no improvement in immunity
	Bone marrow transplant	1	↑ OKT4, NK activitity

All these strategies are designed to eventually induce lymphocyte proliferation and 'activation' (Table 11.11)[101].

Biologic modifiers include thymic hormones, Imreg-1, interferons and interleukins.

Thymic hormones are currently being evaluated in Phase I/II studies. Paradoxically some have found high levels of thymic hormone activity (α-1 thymosin) in patients with AIDS[102], perhaps due to loss of feed-back inhibition related to T-cell depletion. On the other hand some have found low levels of thymosine[103]. Thymic hormones induce the differentiation of thymic-dependent T-cell precursors[104]. Small studies with Thymosin fraction 5 (TP5), a mixture of 30 different peptides, and thymopentin, a five amino acid synthetic peptide, have been reported. In a series of 32 homosexuals and haemophiliacs with abnormal T4/T8 ratios treated with TP5, 60% of patients had improvement in lymphocyte proliferative responses and increased IL-2 production. T4/T8 ratios were not normalized[105]. A small group of ten patients with AIDS and KS treated with thymopentin, however, did not exhibit any clinical or immunological improvement[106]. Currently, studies are ongoing with thymostimulin (TP1), a mixture of bovine thymus peptides, both in patients with AIDS and ARC.

Imreg-1 is a low molecular weight immunomodulator isolated from normal human leukocytes. The exact mechanism of action is uncertain, however. *In vitro* it can enhance production of IL-2 and migratory inhibitory factor (MIF) by T4 cells. Imreg-1 has been administered to 33 AIDS/ARC patients with improvement in immune parameters in 64% of subjects, as measured by PHA and PWM-induced proliferative responses, as well as PHA-induced IL-2 production. Peak effects were seen 1–2 weeks after treatment and declined to baseline by 3–4 weeks[107].

Interferons have also been used extensively, mainly in treatment of Kaposi's sarcoma. Response rates are variable as outlined below. Several studies have concurrently measured various immunological parameters in treated patients, and although some immune improvement was seen, this did not correlate with clinical responses[101,108].

Interleukin-2 (IL-2) is a glycoprotein produced by T-cells under conditions of antigenic or mitogenic stimulation which can induce proliferation and activation of T-cells. It is receiving wide attention in the treatment of malignancy. Recombinant technology has made large quantities of IL-2 available for testing. Several small studies have been reported in patients with AIDS and others are ongoing. 17 reported patients so far treated with IL-2 did not demonstrate any increases in NK activity or mitogen response. Treatment is associated with significant systemic side-effects[109–111].

Pharmacologic immune modifiers consist of a variety of drugs, including isoprinosine, Azimexon, ciamexone, and CL 246738. Isoprinosine, an inosine derivative, has been reported to restore *in vitro* impaired T-helper cell function from patients with ARC. Clinical trials, however, have not reflected this. In a recent study, 12 patients with AIDS and 24 with ARC were treated with isoprinosine. No immune reconstitution was seen in any patient as measured by lymphocyte numbers and blastogenic response to mitogens[112]. In another study of four ARC and six AIDS patients some increased mitogenic response was seen in ARC patients only[113]. Current interest with the drug focusses on the recent report of antiviral activity at low doses by inhibition of reverse transcriptase[114]. Azimexon, a 2-cyan-aziridinyl compound, has been reported to cause improvement in symptomatology in 16 ARC patients, but had no effects on 12 AIDS patients treated. In treated ARC patients, absolute lymphocyte counts, PHA mitogenic response and mean number of positive skin tests were all increased to statistically significant levels. Drug-related haemolytic anaemia, however, limited its long-term use[115]. Ciamexone, a derivative of Azimexon, has comparable immune modulating properties *in vitro*, but is less toxic and is now entering clinical studies. Assays of cell-free supernatants from cultures of normal lymphocytes preincubated with Azimexon and then PHA, suggest that the immune augmentation is associated with increased IL-2 production[116].

CL 246738 is an acridine derivative which intercalates in leukocyte DNA and subsequently lymphokine release. A Phase I study is ongoing in AIDS patients[117].

Adoptive immune therapeutic approaches, such as thymic transplantation utilizing thymic tissue from infants undergoing cardiac surgery, have been employed in a small number of patients. Thymic tissue is cultured for 3 weeks to provide lymphocyte-free epithelial cells. These cells are then injected either intraperitoneally or intrahepatically; some transient improvements were seen in 14 patients with AIDS treated in this way as measured by absolute increases in lymphocyte numbers[118]. Bone marrow transplantation is also being investigated, either alone[119,120] or more recently with antiviral drug pretreatment[121]. In the small number of patients treated so far no long-term benefit is seen.

In summary, results of immune modulating studies so far reported have been minor and transient, not surprising in view of the fact that patients so far treated had persistent HTLV-III/LAV infection. Clearly efforts to improve immune function will not be effective in the presence of active virus. Further studies will employ a combination of antivirals and immune stimulants.

AIDS VACCINE

Other prospects for controlling the AIDS epidemic involve prevention and prophylaxis. One obvious tactic is the development of a vaccine against HTLV-III/LAV. In the past, antiviral vaccines have used live attenuated virus, or killed virus (either whole or split). New cloning techniques, ability to synthesize polypeptides *in vitro* and potential for gene insertion in virus vectors, provide opportunities for large scale production of a highly immunogenic vaccine. Recent work has shown the presence of neutralizing antibodies to HTLV-III/LAV envelope antigens in patients who are positive on both ELISA and Western-blot analyses[122,123].

P41 is the antigen most likely related to non-protective antibody production. In order to be effective vaccine components, viral antigens should be highly conserved as well as immunogenic. Because of the antigenic drift postulated in HTLV-III/LAV, there appears to be a variability in about 20% of the envelope proteins when African, American and Asian virus isolates are compared[124,125]. This antigenic heterogeneity presents a potential obstacle to vaccine development. Attempts to avoid the problem of envelope protein variability have led some investigators to concentrate on carbohydrate moieties of the glycoproteins[126], and others to pursue recombinant DNA techniques to purify known immunogenic antigens.

Once the appropriate antigens are identified, they must be purified and produced in large quantity. Mass *in vitro* culture of live active virus seems risky and inefficient. Genetic engineering methods have already led to *in vitro* production of several viral proteins[127,128]. Another technique involves passive vaccination with anti-idiotype antibodies directed against specific envelope proteins – rather than inoculation directly with viral antigens. This approach also circumvents the issue of potential injection of immunosuppressive agents, and the associated risk of disease when whole viruses or virus particle are used[126].

Before human trials can begin, animal immunization to determine safety and efficacy should be undertaken. Rhesus monkeys can be infected with HTLV-III/LAV; but their response to infection is highly variable and not predictable. The chimpanzee is probably the best animal model for testing vaccines, but unfortunately the chimpanzee is a protected, rare species, does not breed in captivity, is very costly and is in short supply for medical research[129,130].

After animal trials are completed virus-negative human recipients must be tested in a preliminary fashion to determine safety and feasibility. Finally large-scale randomized placebo-controlled clinical trials with prolonged follow-up must be conducted prior to widespread adoption of the vaccine for prophylaxis.

AIDS-RELATED NEOPLASIA

Kaposi's sarcoma (KS)

The initial description of this neoplasm was first published in 1872 by Moricz Kaposi, a Hungarian physician[131]. The tumour was reported as a chronic, cutaneous pigmented haemangio sarcoma. The epidemiology was delineated by De Amicis, to highlight the unusual predisposition of Italian and Eastern European men of Jewish origin[132]. This is now known as the classical form of Kaposi's sarcoma. The disease has since been also described in an endemic form in equatorial Africa[133] referred to as African KS. Since 1981, there has been a sharp increase in the incidence of Kaposi's sarcoma in well defined risk groups in association with AIDS[134]. This form of the disease is now termed epidemic Kaposi's sarcoma (EKS) and occurs in up to 30% of patients with AIDS, predominantly among homosexual men and not intravenous i.v. drug users[135]. The majority of patients with EKS are antibody-positive[136]. Of interest is the high incidence of seropositivity in the atypical aggressive African form of the disease also implicating the virus in this variant[137]. The clinical features of patients with EKS are reminiscent of other KS patients in the setting of immunosuppression, whether due to specific underlying disorders such as lymphoreticular neoplasms[138-140] or due to iatrogenic causes such as those occurring in renal transplant patients[141-146]. This underscores the 'opportunistic' nature of EKS and its relationship to underlying immune deficiency. Epidemic Kaposi's sarcoma, in contrast to the classical variety, is often aggressive in behaviour with multiple cutaneous, mucosal and often visceral lesions at presentation[135]. Up to one-third of the patients have systemic symptoms of fever and weight loss[147]. Of note, is that despite the disseminated nature of the disease and significant morbidity, mortality in these patients is related mainly to opportunistic infection. In fact, patients with EKS who have never developed an opportunistic infection have a predicted 80% 2-year survival compared to less than 20% survival in those who have had an opportunistic infection at some time during the course of their illness[148,149]. Experience in other forms of KS has served as background for the evolution of treatment approaches. However, it remains unclear how applicable classical and African studies are to the epidemic variety, particularly on the short- and long-range effects of chemotherapy on a disease already associated with immune suppression.

The systemic nature of the disease appeared to require primarily systemic approaches, although a role for radiotherapy still exists in selected cases[150]. In an attempt to standardize responses to therapeutic trials as well as provide prognostic information, a staging system was recently proposed which takes into account the extent of disease as well as the presence or absence of systemic symptoms[147].

Multiple therapeutic trials have been reported in the treatment of EKS. Preliminary observations led to the formulation of therapeutic studies using ABV (doxorubicin, bleomycin and vinblastine), ABV + ADV (actinomycin D, DTIC and vincristine) for patients with visceral involvement and systemic symptoms[151,152], and VP16 (etoposide) only for patients with less advanced disease[153]. Results are summarized in Table 11.12. All regimens had considerable antitumour activity but the median duration of effect did not exceed 1 year. There was no reversal of immune depression. Because of the significant toxicity seen with combination chemotherapy, further trials have focussed on single or double agent therapy, with vinblastine[154], vincristine[155,156], vinblastine/bleomycin[157], and demethoxydaunorubicin[158], all with some antitumour activity (Table 11.12). Studies are ongoing with ICRF-187, an intravenous form of its insoluble enantiomer ICRF-159, and vinblastine infusions.

Table 11.12 Epidemic Kaposi's sarcoma treatment results

Regimen	Response/total (%)	Reference
VP16 (NYU)	12 CR + 19 PR/41 (76)	151
ABV (NYU)	7 CR + 19 PR/31 (84)	153
ABV (UCSF)	1 CR + 6 PR/ 9 (78)	165
ABV/ADV (NCI)	3 CR + 9 PR/14 (86)	152
Vinblastine/bleomycin (NYU)	0 CR + 24 PR/31 (62)	156
Vinblastine (UCSF)	1 CR + 9 PR/38 (27)	154
Vincristine	0 CR + 4 PR/ 5 (80)	155
	0 CR + 11 PR/18 (61)	156
Demethoxydaunorubicin (DMDR) (NYU)	0 CR + 2 PR/15 (13)	158
Bleomycin (NYU)	0 CR + 7 PR/ 9 (78)	157
Dapsone	1/1, 0/9	166, 167
Isotretinoin	0/6	168
IFN LrA (MSK)	3 CR + 2 PR/13 (38)	159
IFN rA2 (UCSF)	1 CR + 7 PR/20 (40)	160
IFN Lyb1 (NCI)	0 CR + 2 PR/10 (20)	161
IFN Lyb1 (MDA)	4 CR + 4 PR/12 (66)	162
IFNr Gamma (NYU)	0 CR + 1 PR/18 (5)	169
VP16 +IFN A2 (sequential) (NYU)	0 CR + 1 PR/12 (8)	164
VP16 + IFN A2 (concurrent) (NYU)	0 CR + 1 PR/14 (7)	164
ICRF 159 (UCSF)	0 CR + 1 PR/23 (4)	170
ICRF 187 (NYU)	Ongoing	

CR = complete remission; PR = partial remission.

Another line of investigation has been the evaluation of interferons, potentially attractive because of *in vitro* antiviral, antineoplastic and immune modulating properties. Results of clinical studies are also summarized in Table 11.12. These show a wide range of response rates, perhaps influenced by stage of disease and immune status of the patient. In addition, effects on immune function have been inconsistent and toxicity can be significant[159-163]. Combinations of cytotoxic chemotherapy with etoposide and interferon have not been encouraging[164]. A relationship between responsiveness and lesser bulk of disease has been noted by several authors both for chemotherapy and interferons.

Current interest focusses on the use of the antiviral drugs, even though the relationship of EKS to the virus is uncertain; the objective is reversal of the immune suppression which may lead to tumour response. Of note, however, is that no patients treated with antiviral agents have shown immune reconstitution to date, and studies of these agents, some of which included patients with Kaposi's sarcoma lesions, have not reported responses. It may be that combinations of antivirals, immune modulators and chemotherapy may be needed in the treatment of Kaposi's sarcoma.

Lymphoma

Since the beginning of the AIDS epidemic, there has been an emerging awareness of increased incidence of malignancies, other than Kaposi's sarcoma (KS), complicating this disease.

Ziegler *et al.* drew attention to the occurrence of Burkitt's-like lymphomas in homosexual men at risk for AIDS[171]. In a subsequent multi-institutional study of 90 homosexual men with lymphomas, all but 15 had some features of pre-AIDS or AIDS prior to diagnosis. Generalized lymphadenopathy was present in 33 patients (37%), opportunistic infections, KS, or both occurred in 42 (47%). In contrast to lymphomas arising in the general population, 62% were of high grade, 29% intermediate and 7% low grade. All except two had extranodal lymphomas, most commonly involving bone marrow, central nervous system, bowel and mucocutaneous sites. Phenotypically all were of B-cell origin[172]. The implication of HTLV-III/LAV in the aetiology of AIDS, and the availability of antibody testing, has enabled further definition of these lymphomas. Levine *et al.*[173] recently reported on 27 homosexual men with lymphoma; 22 (81%) were of high grade and five (19%) of low grade disease. HTLV-III/LAV antibody was present in 13 (87%) of 15 with high grade lymphoma and in two (40%) of five with low grade disease. In contrast only one (9%) of 11 control heterosexuals with high grade lymphoma and 17 (55%) of 31 asymptomatic homosexual men were HTLV-III/LAV antibody-positive. 85% of patients presented with extranodal disease. Ioachim *et al.*[174] reported on 21 cases of lymphoma in men at high risk for AIDS, again emphasizing the B-cell origin, high grade nature and extranodal origin of these tumours. Of interest was the inclusion of three patients with Hodgkin's disease, all of whom had reversed T4/T8 ratios; in the one patient tested, HTLV-III/LAV antibody was positive[174]. Other investigators have also noted an increased incidence of Hodgkin's lymphoma in patients with AIDS[152,175] indicating a possible association with HTLV-III/LAV infection.

In all reported series the HTLV-III/LAV associated lymphomas have been aggressive in behaviour. Response rates with various combination chemotherapy and/or radiation range from 30 to 50%. Relapse rates are high with median survival ranging from 5 to 8 months[172,173]. Mortality and morbidity is correlated with other manifestations of HTLV-III/LAV infection, in patients with prior features of AIDS (KS, OI or both), or (LAS) mortality and morbidity with 91% and 79% respectively. In patients with no other features of AIDS, mortality and morbidity was 42%[172].

In face of the clear association between lymphomas and HTLV-III/LAV infection, the Centers for Disease Control have recently amended the case definition of AIDS to include patients with non-Hodgkin's lymphoma of high grade (pathologic type diffuse, undifferentiated) and of B-cell or unknown immunologic phenotype in the setting of positive serology or viral culture for HTLV-III/LAV[176].

Several hypotheses have been advanced to explain the association of immune deficiency and neoplasia. The original 'immune surveillance' postulate of Burnet, attributed to cell-mediated immunity the role of constantly destroying the emergence of neoplasms by early recognition of neoplastic cells as alien[177]. Organ transplantation has highlighted the association of certain malignancies with subsequent iatrogenic immune suppression. The incidence of non-Hodgkin's lymphomas rises dramatically in the setting of immune suppression, constituting 26% of all tumours arising in renal transplant recipients and 71% in cardiac transplants[178].

The link between lymphomas and immune depression has also focussed on a possible viral aetiology of these tumours, in particular Epstein–Barr virus (EBV). As previously suggested by Klein[179], Burkitt's-like lymphoma may develop from EBV infection that induces polyclonal B-cell division and defective differentiation. This could result in the emergence of a single clone, with cytogenetic changes that activates a C-oncogene. This hypothesis is strengthened by the report of two homosexual patients with Burkitt's-like lymphoma: both had genome translocations, one at t (8,14) and the other at t (8,22), both had high EBV titres[180]. Of interest is that the c myc oncogene has been localized at breakpoint for the t (8,14) translocation[181].

Histopathologic studies in lymph nodes in patients with LAS show that the risk of developing malignancy correlated with the pattern of follicular involution with small hypocellular germ centres and paracentral hyperplasia[182]. This pattern is similar to that seen with viral lymphadenitis[183,184], further supporting the viral hypothesis.

Other malignancies

There has been a definite increase in the incidence of squamous cell carcinoma of the oral cavity[185] and anorectum[186,187] since 1980–81 in homosexual males. The incidence of these tumours may relate to recurrent local trauma or activation of viruses such as papilloma virus. Further information as to the incidence, treatment, and outcome of these malignancies is lacking. A recent report of two homosexual males with embryonal cell carcinoma of the testis occurring in the setting of generalized lymphadenopathy and reversed T4/T8 ratios, may further extend the spectrum of cancer complicating AIDS[188].

HTLV-III/LAV infection is clearly associated with an increased incidence of malignancy among risk groups. Whether this relates to the immune deficiency induced by the virus, or activation of other endogenous or exogenous viruses, is still unclear but is likely to be a combination of both factors and is the subject of intense investigation. The malignancies associated with AIDS are high grade in histology and aggressive in behaviour. There is no standard therapeutic approach. Chemotherapeutic approaches have been as disappointing in this setting as in the treatment of neoplasias arising in other immunodeficient states. Future attempts at treatment may incorporate antivirals and immune modulators in addition to the more conventional approaches. The possible occurrence of preneoplastic syndromes has also been observed. Lymphoid interstitial pneumonia, in patients with positive HTLV-III/LAV antibody and abormal T4/T8 ratios, responsive to treatment with steroids and cyclophosphamide, may represent such a syndrome[189]. In addition, clinical manifestations of B-cell hyperplasia, characterized by massive splenomegaly, pancytopenia and fever, many precede the onset of lymphoma in some patients with HTLV-III/LAV infection[190].

OPPORTUNISTIC INFECTION

As well as trials employing antiviral and immunomodulating agents in the treatment of AIDS, several new drugs are being tested in the treatment of some of the infection's complications (Table 11.13).

Table 11.13 New drugs being tested in the treatment of opportunistic infection

Infection	Drug	Results
CMV	DHPG	14/18 improved
Cryptosporidiosis	DFMO	1 complete response/9
M. avium	γ-IFN	ongoing
PCP	sulphas maintenance vs. no maintenance	
	DFMO second line	ongoing

Two agents are currently being evaluated in cytomegalovirus infection. Phosphonoformate has received attention in Europe; in the United States dihydrophenylguanine (DHPG), an acyclic guanine analogue, is currently in early Phase II studies. Results of these studies have been promising; however, they are not placebo-controlled, positive culture sites do not correlate with sites of symptoms, and viral culture negativity may not correlate with clinical response. DHPG is well tolerated, but cessation of treatment leads to relapse in the majority of patients, showing that maintenance therapy is indicated[191].

Difluoromethyl ornithine (DFMO), an ornithine analogue that inhibits enzymatic transformation of ornithine to putrescine, is currently being evaluated in the treatment of cryptosporidiosis, a protozoal infection causing chronic diarrhoea in AIDS. In a recent report one of nine patients treated with DFMO achieved a long lasting complete response, as measured by disappearance of the organism from stool and resolution of clinical symptoms[192].

The recognition that up to 40% of patients will develop a second episode of pneumocystis pneumonia has prompted evaluation of maintenance treatment. Controlled, double-blind studies are in progress comparing the efficacy of Bactrim and Fansidar vs. placebo[193]. Second line therapy with DFMO after Bactrim failure is also being investigated[194].

γ-IFN is currently being evaluated in *Mycobacterium avium* disease resistant to clofazamine and ansamycin. *In vitro* studies suggest that activation of NK cells by interferon renders them resistant to infection.

CONCLUSION

Over the past year we have moved rapidly into therapeutic studies with specific antiviral agents. It is now clear that presently employed clinical and immunologic endpoints may not be relevant to antiviral studies. Rather, a virologic endpoint is of prime importance. Several questions need to be answered for meaningful data to be obtained. Firstly, there is a need for a standard technique to evaluate HTLV-III/LAV presence in various body fluids. Secondly, there has been an emerging awareness that AIDS represents the worst end of the spectrum of HTLV-III/LAV infection; future clinical studies should perhaps address milder forms of infection (ARC, LAS). To this purpose, an accurate, predictive, uniform staging classification needs to be developed. One such classification has recently been proposed and requires further testing and elucidation[195]. Thirdly, because of the persistence of retroviral infections, chronic administration of antivirals needs to be considered. Particular attention must therefore be paid to chronic toxicity assessment, as well as ease of administration of drug. In view of lack of data regarding the natural history of HTLV-III/LAV viraemia and shedding, antiviral studies should be placebo-controlled, in order to discriminate between drug effect and the natural course of infection.

Immune modulators are ineffective by themselves in the treatment of AIDS, and should be given in combination with active antiviral agents. Immunologic endpoints need to be specifically developed for such studies, and if possible correlated with clinical responses. Again, patients with milder forms of the disease may have a better chance of response. Anti-HTLV-III/LAV vaccines, while still in the development phases, potentially provide the best preventive approach to AIDS. Studies are continuing in the treatment of the complications of AIDS – the malignancies and opportunistic infections. While addressing important specific questions, it is clear that correction of the underlying immune disorder is critical in the treatment of AIDS.

References

1. Centers for Disease Control (1981). Pheumocystis pneumonia. Los Angeles, *MMWR*, **30**, 250–2
2. Centers for Disease Control (1981). Kaposi's sarcoma and pneumocystis pneumonia among homosexual men. New York City and California. *MMWR*, **30**, 305–8
3. Selik, R. M., Haverkos, H. W. and Curran, J. W. (1984). Acquired immune deficiency syndrome (AIDS) trends in the United States 1978–1982. *Am. J. Med.*, **76**, 493–500
4. Auerbach, D. M., Darrow, W. W., Jaffe, H. W. and Curran, J. W. (1984). Cluster of cases of the acquired immunodeficiency syndrome. Patients linked by sexual contact. *Am. J. Med.*, **76**, 487–92
5. Curran, J. W., Lawrence, D. N., Jaffe, H. *et al.* (1984). Acquired immune deficiency syndrome (AIDS) associated with transfusion. *N. Engl. J. Med.*, **310**, 69–75
6. Barre-Sinousi, F., Chermann, J. C., Rey, F. *et al.* (1983). Isolation of a T lymphotropic retrovirus from a patient at risk for acquired immune deficiency syndromes (AIDS). *Science*, **220**, 868–70
7. Popovic, M., Sarngadharan, M. G., Read, E. and Gallo, R. C. (1984). Detection, isolation, and continuous production of cytopathic retrovirus (HTLV III) from patients with AIDS and pre AIDS. *Science*, **224**, 497–500
8. Sarngadharan, M. G., Popovic, M., Bruch, L., Schuphach, J. and Gallo, R. C. (1984). Antibodies reactive with human T lymphotropic retrovirus (HTLV-III) in the serum of patients with AIDS. *Science*, **224**, 506–8
9. Miller, B., Stansfield, S. K., Zack, M. M. *et al.* (1984). The syndrome of unexplained generalized lymphadenopathy in young men in New York City, is it related to the acquired immune deficiency syndrome? *J. Am. Med. Assoc.*, **251**, 242–6
10. Centers for Disease Control (1982). Persistent, generalized lymphadenopathy among homosexual males. *MMWR*, **31**, 249
11. Mataur-Wagh, U., Enlow, R., Spigland, I. *et al.* (1984). Longitudinal study of persistent generalized lymphadenopathy in homosexual men: relation to acquired immuno-deficiency syndrome. *Lancet*, **1**, 1033
12. Jaffe, H. W., Darrow, W. W., Echenberg, D. F. *et al.* (1985). The acquired immuno-deficiency syndrome in a cohort of homosexual men: a six year follow up study. *Ann. Intern. Med.*, **103**, 210–14
13. Klein, R. S., Harris, C. A., Small, C. B. *et al.* (1984). Oral candidiasis in high risk patients as the initial manifestation of the acquired immunodeficiency syndrome. *N. Engl. J. Med.*, **311**, 358
14. Stewart, G. J. *et al.* (1985). Transmission of human T cell lymphotropic virus type III (HTLV III) by artificial insemination by donor. *Lancet*, **2**, 581–3
15. Harris, C. A., Cabradilla, C., Robert-Guroff, M. *et al.* (1985). Immunodeficiency and HTLV-III/LAV serology in heterosexual partners of AIDS patients. In *The International Conference on the Acquired Immunodeficiency Sydrome.* p. 22 Abstract.
16. Kreiss, J. K., Kitchen, L. W., Prince, H. E., Kasper, C. K. and Essex, M. (1985). Antibody to human T-lymphotropic virus type III in wives of hemophiliacs. Evidence for hetero-sexual transmission. *Ann. Intern. Med.*, **102**, 623–6
17. Centers for Disease Control (1984). Update: acquired immunodeficiency syndrome (AIDS). United States. *MMWR*, **33**, 681–4
18. Van de Perre, P. *et al.* (1985). Female prostitutes: a risk group for infection with human T cell lymphotropic virus type III. *Lancet*, **2**, 524–6
19. Curran, J. W. (1985). The epidemiology and prevention of the acquired immuno-deficiency syndrome. *Ann. Intern. Med.*, **103**, 657–62
20. McEvoy, M. *et al.* (1985). Some problems in the prediction of future numbers of cases of the acquired immunodeficiency syndrome in the U.K. *Lancet*, **2**, 541–2
21. Clumeck, N., Sonnet, J., Taelman, H. *et al.* (1984). Acquired immunodeficiency in African patients. *N. Engl. J. Med.*, **310**, 492.
22. Van De Perre, P., Munyambuga, D., Zissis, G. *et al.* (1985). Antibody to HTLV III in blood donors in Central Africa. *Lancet*, **1**, 336–7
23. Gallo, R. C. and Wong-Staal, F. (1985). A human T-lymphotropic retrovirus (HTLV III) as the cause of the acquired immunodeficiency syndrome. *Ann. Intern. Med.*, **103**, 679–89

24. Lafleur, F. L., Friedman-Kien, A. E., Hennessey, N. P. *et al.* (1986). Prevalence of HTLV-III infection in peripheral blood (PB), seminal mononuclear cells (SMC) and cell-free semen (CFS) of AIDS-related complex (ARC) and AIDS-associated Kaposi's sarcoma (KS) patients (pts): preliminary analysis. Submitted to *International Conference on Acquired Immunodeficiency Syndrome (AIDS)*

25. Groopman, J. E., Salahuddin, S. Z., Sarngadharan, M.G. *et al.* (1984). HTLV-III/LAV in saliva of people wth AIDS related complex and healthy homosexual men at risk for AIDS. *Science*, **226**, 447-9

26. Fujikowa, L. S., *et al.* (1985). Isolation of human T lymphotropic type virus III from tears of a patient with the acquired immune deficiency syndrome. *Lancet*, **2**, 529

27. Levy, J. A. *et al.* (1985). Isolation of AIDS. Associated retroviruses from cerebrospinal fluid and brain of patients with neurological symptoms. *Lancet*, **2**, 586-8

28. Shaw, G. M., Hahn, B. H., Arya, S. K., Groorman, J. E., Cauo, R. C. and Wong-Staal, F. (1984). Molecular characterization of human T-cell leukemia lymphotropic virus type III, in the acquired immune deficiency syndrome. *Science*, **226**, 1165-71

29. Montagnier, L. (1985). Lymphadenopathy associated virus: from molecular biology to pathogenicity. *Ann. Intern. Med.*, **103**, 689-693

30. Gonda, M. A., Wong-Staal, F., Gallo, R. C. *et al.* (1985). Sequence homology and morphologic similarity of HTLV III and visna virus a pathogenic lentivirus. *Science*, **227**, 173-7

31. Schupbach, J., Popovic, M., Gilden, R. V. *et al.* (1984). Serological analysis of a subgroup of human T lymphotropic retrovirus HTLV-III associated with AIDS. *Science*, **224**, 503

32. Petricciani, J. C. (1985). Licensed tests for antibody to human T lymphotropic virus type III. *Ann. Intern. Med.*, **103**, 726-9

33. Fischinger, P. and Bolognesi, (1985). Prospects for diagnostic tests, intervention and vaccine development in AIDS. In De vita, V., Hellman, S. and Rosenberg, S. (eds.) *AIDS Etiology, Diagnosis, Treatment and Prevention.* pp. 55-88. (Philadelphia: Lippincott)

34. Esteban, J. I., Shih, W.-K. J. and Tai Chang Chih (1985). Importance of western blot analysis in predicting infectivity of anti HTLV-III/LAV positive blood. *Lancet*, **2**, 1083-6

35. Poiesz, B., Personal communication

36. Bowen, D. L., Lane, H. C. and Fauci, A. S. (1985). Immunopathogenesis of the acquired immune deficiency syndrome. *Ann. Intern. Med.*, **103**, 704-9

37. Stahl, R. E., Friedman-Kien, A. E., Dubin, R., Marmor, M. and Zolla-Pazner, S. (1982). Immunologic abnormalities in homosexual men: relationship to Kaposi's sarcoma. *Am. J. Med.*, **73**, 171-8

38. Rogers, M. F., Morens, D. M., Stewart, J. A. *et al.* (1983). National case-control study of Kaposi's sarcoma and *Pneumocystis carinii* pneumonia in homosexual men. 2. Laboratory results. *Ann. Intern. Med.*, **99**, 151-8

39. Ciobanu, N., Welk, K., Kruger, G. *et al.* (1983). Defective T cell response to PHA and mitogenic monoclonal anitbodies in male homosexuals with AIDS and its *in vitro* correction by IL-2. *J. Clin. Immunol.*, **3**, 332-40

40. Gupta S. and Safai, B. (1983). Deficient autologous mixed lymphocyte reaction in Kaposi's sarcoma associated with deficiency of Leu 3$^+$ responder T cells. *J. Clin. Invest.*, **71**, 296-300

41. Schroff, R. W., Gottlieb, M. S., Prince, H. E. *et al.* (1983). Immunological studies of homosexual men with immunodeficiency and Kaposi's sarcoma. *Clin. Immunol. Immunopathol.*, **27**, 300-14

42. Murray, H. W., Rubin, M., Masur, H. and Roberts, R. B. (1984). Impaired production of lymphokines and immune (gamma) interferon in AIDS. *N. Engl. J. Med.*, **310**, 883-9

43. Lane, H. C., Depper, J. M., Greene, W. C. *et al.* (1985). Qualitative analysis of immune function in patients with AIDS: evidence for a selective defect in soluble antigen recognition. *N. Engl. J. Med.*, **313**, 79-84

44. Quinnan, G. V., Siegel, J. P., Epstein, J. S. *et al.* (1985). Mechanisms of T-cell functional deficiency in AIDS. *Ann. Intern. Med.*, **103**, 710-14

45. Nicholson, J. K., McDougal, J. S., Spira, T. J. *et al.* (1984). Immunoregulatory subsets of the T helper and T suppressor cell population in homosexual men with chronic unexplained lymphadenopathy. *J. Clin. Invest.*, **73**, 191-201

46. Siegel, J. P., Djeu, J. Y., Stocks, N. I., Massur, H. *et al.* (1985). Sera from patients with AIDS inhibit production of IL-2 by normal lymphocytes. *J. Clin. Invest.*, **75**, 1957-64

47. Prince, H. E., Kermani-Arab, V. and Fahey, J. L. (1984). Depressed IL-2 receptor expression in AIDS and lymphadenopathy syndromes. *J. Immunol.*, **133**, 1313–17

48. Rook, A. H., Masur, H., Lane, C. H., Frederick, W. *et al.* (1983). IL-2 enhances the depressed NK and CMV specific cytotoxic activities of lymphocytes from patients with AIDS. *J. Clin. Invest.*, **72**, 398–403

49. Rook, A. H., Manishewitz, J. F., Frederick, W. *et al.* (1985). Deficient, HLA restricted, CMV-specific cytotoxic T-cells and NK cells in patients with AIDS. *J. Infect. Dis.*, **152**, 627–30

50. Rook, A. H., Hook, J. J., Quinnan, G. V., Lane, H. C. *et al.* (1985). IL-2 enhances the NK cell activity of AIDS patients through a gamma-interferon independent mechanism. *J. Immunol.*, **134**, 1503–7

51. Lane, H. C., Masur, H., Edgar, L. C. *et al.* (1983). Abnormalities of B-cell activation and immunoregulation in patients with AIDS. *N. Engl. J. Med.*, **309**, 453–9

52. Bhalla, R. B., Safai, B., Mertelsmann, R. and Schwartz, M. K. (1983). Abnormally high concentrations of beta-2-microglobulin in AIDS patients. *Clin. Chem.*, **29**, 1560

53. Hersh, E. M., Reuben, J. M., Rios, A. *et al.* (1983). Elevated serum thymosin alpha, levels associated with immune dysregulation in male homosexuals with a history of infectious diseases or Kaposi's sarcoma. *N. Engl. J. Med.*, **308**, 45–6

54. DeStefano, E., Friedman, R. N., Friedman-Kien, A. E. *et al.* (1982). Acid-labile human leukocyte interferon in homosexual men with Kaposi's sarcoma and lymphadenopathy. *J. Infect. Dis.*, **146**, 451–9

55. Smith, P. D., Ohura, K., Masur, H. *et al.* (1984). Monocyte function in AIDS: defective chemotaxis. *J. Clin. Invest.*, **74**, 2121–8

56. Laurence, J. (1985). The immune system in AIDS. *Scientific American*, **December**, 84–93

57. Stephen, E. L., *et al.* (1980). Ribavirin pharmacology. In *Ribavirin: A Broad Spectrum Antiviral Agent.* pp. 169–83. Smith, R. A. and Kirkpatrick, W. (eds.) (New York: Academic Press, Harcourt Brace Jovanovich Publishers)

58. Crumpacker, C. S. (1984). Overview of ribavirin treatment of infection caused by RNA viruses. In Smith, R. A., Knight, V. and Smith, J. A. D. (eds.) *Clinical Applications of Ribavirin.* pp. 33–9. (New York: Academic Press, Harcourt Brace Jovanovich Publishers)

59. Huggins, J. W. *et al.* (1984). Efficacy of ribavirin against virulent RNA virus infections. In Smith, R. A., Knight, V. and Smith, J. A. D. (eds.) *Clinical Applications of Ribavirin.* pp. 49–65. (New York: Academic Press, Harcourt Brace Jovanovich Publishers)

60. Sidwell, R. W. (1984). *In vitro* and *in vivo* inhibition of DNA viruses by ribavirin. In Smith, R. A., Knight, V. and Smith, J. A. D. (eds.) *Clinical Applications of Ribavirin.* pp. 19–33. (New York: Academic Press, Harcourt Brace Jovanovich Publishers)

61. McCormick, J. B., Getchell, J. P., Mitchell, S. W. and Hicks, D. R. (1984). Ribavirin suppresses replication of LAV in cultures of human adult T lymphocytes. *Lancet*, **2**, 1367–9

62. Conner, J. D. *et al.* (1984). Ribavirin pharmacokinetics in children and adults during therapeutic trials. In Smith, R. A., Knight, V. and Smith, J. A. D. (eds.) *Clinical Applications of Ribavirin.* pp. 107–25. (New York: Academic Press, Harcourt Brace Jovanovich Publishers)

63. Catlin, D. H. (1980). ^{14}C ribavirin: distribution and pharmacokinetic studies in rats, baboons and man. In Smith, R. A. and Kirkpatrick, W. (eds.) *Ribavirin: A Broad Spectrum Antiviral Agent.* pp. 215–30. (New York: Academic Press, Harcourt Brace Jovanovich Publishers)

64. Gilbert, B. E. *et al.* (1984). Ribavirin small particle aerosol treatment of influenza in college students 1981–1983. In Smith, R. A., Knight, V. and Smith, J. A. D. (eds.) *Clinical Applications of Ribavirin.* pp. 125–45. (New York: Academic Press, Harcourt Brace Jovanovich Publishers)

65. Schiff, G. M. *et al.* (1984). Small particle aerosol of ribavirin in therapy of influenza – Cincinnati study. In Smith, R. A., Knight, V. and Smith, J. A. D. (eds.) *Clinical Applications of Ribavirin.* pp. 165–73. (New York: Academic Press, Harcourt Brace Jovanovich Publishers)

66. Canonico, P. G., Kende, M. and Huggins, J. W. (1984). The toxicity and pharmacology of ribavirin in experimental animals. In Smith, R. A., Knight, V. and Smith, J. A. D. (eds.) *Clinical Applications of Ribavirin.* pp. 65–79. (New York: Academic Press, Harcourt Brace Jovanovich Publishers)

67. Shulman, N. R. (1984). Assessment of hematologic effects of ribavirin in humans. In Smith, R. A., Knight, V. and Smith, J. A. D. (eds.) *Clinical Applications of Ribavirin.* pp. 79–93. (New York: Academic Press, Harcourt Brace Jovanovich Publishers)

68. Smith, R. A. and Kirkpatrick, W. (eds.) (1980). *Ribavirin: A Broad Spectrum Antiviral Agent.* (New York: Academic Press, Harcourt Brace Jovanovich Publishers)

69. Hall, C. B. *et al.* (1983). Aerosolized ribavirin treatment of infants with respiratory syncytial virus infection. A randomized double blind study. *N. Engl. J. Med.*, **308**, 1443–7

70. Hall, C. B. *et al.* (1984). Ribavirin in the treatment of respiratory syncytial viral infections. In Smith, R. A., Knight, V. and Smith, J. A. D. (eds.) *Clinical Applications of Ribavirin.* pp. 165–73. (New York: Academic Press, Harcourt Brace Jovanovich Publishers)

71. Hall, C. B. *et al.* (1985). Ribavirin treatment of respiratory syncytial viral infection in infants with underlying cardiopulmonary disease. *J. Am. Med. Assoc.*, **254**, 3047–52

72. Taber, L. H., Gilbert, B. E. and Wilson, S. Z. (1984). Ribavirin aerosol treatment of respiratory syncytial virus bronchiolitis in infants, 1981–1983. In Smith, R. A., Knight, V. and Smith, J. A. D. (eds.) *Clinical Applications of Ribavirin.* pp. 155–65. (New York: Academic Press, Harcourt Brace Jovanovich Publishers)

73. McCormick, J. B., King, I. J. and Webb, P. A. (1986). Lassa fever: effective therapy with ribavirin. *N. Engl. J. Med.*, **314**, 20–7

74. McCormick, J. B. *et al.* (1984). Chemotherapy of acute lassa fever with ribavirin. In Smith, R. A., Knight, V. and Smith, J. A. D. (eds.) *Clinical Applications of Ribavirin.* pp. 187–92. (New York: Academic Press, Harcourt Brace Jovanovich Publishers)

75. Stridh, S., Helgstrand, E., Lannero, B. *et al.* (1979). The effect of pyrophosphate analogues on influenza virus RNA polymerase and influenza virus multiplication. *Arch. Virol.*, **61**, 245–50

76. Oberg, B. (1983). Antiviral effects of phosphonoformate. *Pharmacol. Ther.*, **19**, 387–415

77. Sandstrom, E. G., Kaplan, J., Byington, R. E. and Hirsch, M. (1985). Inhibition of human T-cell lymphotropic virus type III *in vitro* by phosphonoformate. *Lancet*, **1**, 1480–2

78. Beldekas, J. C., Levy, E. M., Black, P., Von Krogh, G. and Sandstrom, E. (1985). *In vitro* effect of foscarnet on expansion of T-cells from people with LAS and AIDS. *Lancet*, **2**, 1128–9

79. Beldekas, J. C. (1986). In press

80. Friedman-Kien, A. Personal communication

81. DeClercq, E. (1979). Suramin: a potent inhibitor of the reverse transcriptase of RNA tumor viruses. *Cancer Lett.*, **8**, 9–22

82. Hawking, F. (1978). Suramin, with special reference to onchocerciasis. *Adv. Pharmacol Chemother.*, **15**, 289–322

83. Mitsuya, H. *et al.* (1984). Suramin protection of T cells *in vitro* against infectivity and cytopathic effect of HTLV III. *Science*, **226**, 172–4

84. Broder, S. *et al.* (1985). Effects of suramin on HTLV III/LAV infection presenting as Kaposi's sarcoma on AIDS-related complex: clinical pharmacology and suppression of virus replication *in vivo*. *Lancet*, **2**, 627–30

85. Rouvroy, D. *et al.* (1985). Short-term results with suramin for AIDS-related conditions. *Lancet*, **1**, 878

86. Busch, W. *et al.* (1985). Suramin treatment for AIDS. *Lancet*, **2**, 1247

87. Levine, A. Personal communication

88. Jasmin, C., Chermann, J. C., Herve, G., Theze, A., Souchay, P., Boy-Lousteau, C., Raybaud, N., Sinoussi, F. and Raynau, M. (1974). *In vivo* inhibition of murine leukemia and sarcoma viruses by the heteropolyanion 5-tungsto-2-antimoniate. *J. Natl. Cancer Inst.*, **53**, 469–74

89. Chermann, J. C., Sinoussi, F. C. and Jasmin, C. (1975). Inhibition of RNA dependent DNA polymerase of murine oncornaviruses by ammonium-5-tungsto-2-antimoniate. *Biochem. Biophys. Res. Commun.*, **65**, 1229–36

90. Kimberlin, R. H. and Walker, C. A. (1983). The antiviral compound HPA-23 can prevent scrapie when administered at the time of infection. *Arch. Virol.*, **78**, 9–18

91. Dormont, D., Spire, B., Barre-Sinoussi, F., Montaigner, L. and Chermann, J. C. (1985). Inhibition of RNA-dependent DNA polymerases of AIDS and SAIDS retroviruses by HPA-23 (ammonium-21-tungsto-9-antimoniate). *Ann. Inst. Pasteur/Virol.*, **136E**, 75–83

92. Rozenbaum, W. *et al.* (1985). Antimoniotungstate (HPA 23) treatment of three patients with AIDS and one with prodrone. *Lancet*, **1**, 450–1
93. Hirsch, M. S., and Kaplan, J. C. (1985). Prospects of therapy for infections with human T lymphotropic virus Type III. *Ann. Intern. Med.*, **103**, 750–5
94. Furman, P. A., St. Clair, M., Weinhold, K., Fyfe, J. A., Nusinoff-Lehrman, S. and Barry, D. W. (1985). Selective inhibition of HTLV-III by BWA509U (abstract no. 44). In *Program and Abstracts of the 25th Interscience Conference on Antimicrobial Agents and Chemotherapy*, Minneapolis, American Society for Microbiology
95. Hardy, W. D., Zuckerman, E. E., Nusinoff-Lehrman, S. and Barry, D. W. (1985). Antiviral effects of BWA509U against a naturally occurring feline acquired immune deficiency syndrome (abstract no. 438). In *Program and Abstracts of the 25th Interscience Conference on Antimicrobial Agents and Chemotherapy*, Minneapolis, American Society for Microbiology
96. Mitsuya, H., Weinhold, K. J., Furman, P. A., St. Clair, M. H., Nusinoff-Lehrman, S., Gallo, R. C., Bolognesi, D., Barry, D. W. and Broder, S. (1985). 3′-azido-3′deoxy-thymidine (BWA509U): an antiviral agent that inhibits the infectivity and cytopathic effect of human T-lymphotropic virus type III/lymphadenopathy-associated virus *in vitro*. *Proc. Natl. Acad. Sci. USA.*, **82**, 7096–100
97. Anand, R., Moore, J. L., Srinivason, A. *et al.* (1985). Ansamycin inhibits replication and infectivity of HTLV III/LAV (abstract). *International Conferences on AIDS*, Philadelphia, American College of Physicians
98. Sen, C. G., Herz, R., Davatelis, V. and Pestka, S. (1984). Antiviral and protein-inducing activities of recombinant human leukocyte interferons and their hybrids. *J. Virol.*, **50**, 445–50
99. Hirsch, M. S., Ellis, D. A., Profitt, M. R. and Black, P. (1973). Effects of interferon on leukemia virus activation in graft-versus-host disease. *Nature New Biol.*, **244**, 1–6
100. Ho, D. D., Hartshorn, K. L., Rota, T. R., Andrews, C. A., Kaplan, J. C., Schooky, R. T. and Hirsch, M. S. (1985). Recombinant human interferon alpha-A suppresses HTLV-III replication *in vitro*. *Lancet*, **1**, 602–4
101. Lotze, M. (1985). Treatment of immunological disorders in AIDS. In DeVita, V., Hellman, S. and Rosenberg, S. (eds.) *AIDS Etiology, Diagnosis, Treatment and Prevention*. p. 235. (Philadelphia: Lippincott Company)
102. Hersh, Em., Reuben, J. M., Rios, A. *et al.* (1983). Elevated serum thymosin, levels associated with evidence of murine dysregulation in male homosexuals with a history of infectious disease or Kaposi's sarcoma. *N. Engl. J. Med.*, **308**, 45
103. Kreiss, J. K., Lawrence, D. N., Kasper, C. K. *et al.* (1984). Antibody to human T cell leukemia virus membrane antigens, B2 immunoglobulin levels and thymosis, levels in hemophiliacs and their spouses. *Ann. Intern. Med.*, **100**, 178
104. Low, T. K., Thurman, G. B., Meadoo, M. *et al.* (1979). The chemistry and biology of thymosin, isolation characterization and biological activities of thymosin, and polypeptide B, from calf thymus. *J. Biol. Chem.*, **24**, 981
105. Schulof, R., Simon, G., Sztein, M., Orenstein, J., Gallo, R., Goldstein, A. *et al.* (1985). Pilot study to evaluate the *in vivo* effects of thymosin fraction (TFS) in male homosexuals and hemophiliacs with impaired cellular immunity. *International Conference on AIDS*, April, 40 (abstract)
106. Friedman-Kien, A. Personal communication
107. Gottlieb, A., Farmer, J., Levine, A., Gill, P., Flaum, M. and Gottlieb, M. S. (1985). Reconstitution of T-cell function in AIDS and ARC patients by use of the endogenous, leukocyte-derived immunomodulator Imreg-1. *International Conference on AIDS*, April, 26 (abstract)
108. Volberding, P., Maran, T., Abrams, D. *et al.* (1983). Recombinant alpha interferon (IFN) therapy of Kaposi's sarcoma (KS) in the acquired immune deficiency syndrome (AIDS). *Blood*, **62** (Suppl 1), 118A
109. Lotze, M. T., Robb, R. J., Frana, L. W. *et al.* (1984). Systemic administration of inter-leukin 2 in patients with cancer and AIDS: initial results of a Phase I trial. *Proc. Am. Soc. Clin. Oncol.*, **3**, 51
110. Lane, H. C., Siegal, J., Rook, A. H. *et al.* (1986). Use of interleukin-2 in patients with the acquired immune deficiency syndrome. *J. Biol. Resp. Mod.*, In press

111. Lotze, M. T., Robb, R. J., Frana, L. W. *et al.* (1984). Toxicity, half life and immune effects of purified jurrat derived interleukin 2 (IL-2) in patients with cancer and AIDS. In Gottlieb, M. S. and Groopman, J. E. (eds.) *Acquired Immune Deficiency Syndrome.* p. 409. (New York: Alan R. Liss)

112. Mansell, P., Reuben, J., Odem, M., Rios, A. and Hersh, E. (1985). The use of isoprinosine in an attempt to improve immune function in AIDS and AIDS related complex. *International Conference on AIDS*, April, 42 (abstract)

113. Reddy, M. M., Man Var, O. *et al.* (1984). In-vivo immunomodulation by isoprinosine in patients with the acquired immunodeficiency syndrome and related complexes. *Ann. Intern. Med.,* **101**, 206

114. Pompidou, A., Zagury, D., Gall, R. *et al.* (1985). *In vitro* inhibition of LAV/HTLV III infected lymphocytes by dithiocarb and inosine pranobes. *Lancet*, **2**, 1423

115. Patt, Y., Mansell, P., Reuben, J., Mazumder, A., Li, S. and Hersh, E. (1985). Amelioration of symptomatology and partial *in vivo* immunorestoration with azimexon. *International Conference on AIDS*, April, 42 (abstract)

116. Mertin, J., Bicker, U. and Pahlke, W. (1985). Immunomodulation by ciamexone. *International Conference on AIDS*, April, 42 (abstract)

117. Green, M. Unpublished data

118. Dupuy, J. M., Pekovic, D. D., Goldman, H., Tsoukas, C., Gilmore, N., Thibodeau, Y., Pelletier, L., Joly, M. and Duperval, R. (1985). Thymus transplantation in AIDS and recurrence of HTLV III infection. *International Conference on AIDS*, April, 41 (abstract)

119. Hassett, J. M., Jaroulis, C. G., Greenberg, M. L. *et al.* (1985). Bone marrow transplantation in AIDS. *N. Engl. J. Med.,* **309**, 665

120. Lane, H. C., Masur, H., Longo, D. L. *et al.* (1984). Partial immune reconstitution in a patient with the acquired immune deficiency syndrome. *N. Engl. J. Med.,* **311**, 1099

121. NIH workshop (1985). Unpublished data

122. Robert-Guroff, M., Brown, M. and Gallo, R. C. (1985). HTLV-III neutralizing antibodies in patients in AIDS and ARC. *Nature (London)*, **316**, 72–4

123. Weiss, R. A., Clapham, P. R., Cheingsong-Popov, R. *et al.* (1985). Neutralizing of HLTV-III by sera of AIDS and AIDS-risk patients. *Nature (London)*, **316**, 69–72

124. Essex, M., Allan, J., Kauki, P. *et al.* (1985). Antigens of human T-lymphotropic virus type III/lymphadenopathy-associated virus. *Ann. Intern. Med.,* **103**, 700–3

125. Barin, R., McLane, M. F., Allan, J. S. *et al.* (1985). Virus envelope protein by human T-cell leukemia virus type III (HTLV-III) represents major target antigen for antibodies in AIDS patients. *Science*, **228**, 1094–6

126. Francis, D. P. and Petricciani, J. C. (1985). The prospects for and pathways toward a vaccine for AIDS. *N. Engl. J. Med.,* **313**, 1586–90

127. Chang, N. T., Huang, J., Glurayeb, J. *et al.* (1985). An HTLV-III peptide produced by recombinant DNA is immunoreactive with sera from patients with AIDS. *Nature (London)*, **315**, 151–4

128. Crowl, R., Ganguly, K., Gordon, M. *et al.* (1985). HTLV-III env. gene products synthesized in *E. Coli* are recognized by antibodies present in the sera of AIDS patients. *Cell*, **41**, 979–86

129. Kanki, P. J., McLane, M. F., King, M. W. Jr. *et al.* (1985). Serologic identification and characterization of a macaque T-lymphotropic retrovirus closely related to HTLV-III. *Science*, **228**, 1199–201

130. Daniel, M. D., Letvin, N. L., King, N. W. *et al.* (1985). Isolation of T-cell tropic HTLV-III like retrovirus from macaques. *Science*, **228**, 1201–4

131. Kaposi, M. (1872). Idiopathiscles multiples pigment sarkom der Haut. *Arch. Dermatol. Suph.,* **4**, 265–72

132. De Amicis, T. (1982). Studies clinicoedanatomo patologico sir dodici nuove ossruozioni di deuno polimelanosarcoma idiopatterico. *Napoli Tipografio A Troui*

133. Kaminer, B. and Murrary, J. P. (1950). Sarcoma idiopathium multiple hemorrhagicism of Kaposi's with spread reference to its incidence in the South African Negro and two core reports. *S. Afr. J. Clin, Sir.,* **1**, 1–25

134. Slavin, G., Cameron, H. M., Forbes, C. *et al.* (1971). Kaposi's sarcoma in Uganda: a clinico-pathological study. *Int. J. Cancer,* **8**, 122–35
in AIDS. *Int. J. Cancer*, **8**, 122–35

135. DeVita, V., Hellman, S. and Rosenberg, S. (1985) Kaposi's sarcoma in AIDS. In Krigel, R. and Friedman-Kiln, A. (eds.) *AIDS, Etiology, Diagnosis, Treatment and Preventions.*

136. (Philadelphia: Lippincott) distinguishes atypical and endemic Kaposi's sarcoma in Africa. *Lancet*, **1**, 359–61

137. Fauci, A. S., Macher, M., Longo, D. L. *et al.* (1984). Acquired immune deficiency syndrome, epidemiologic, clinical, immunologic and therapeutic considerations. *Ann. Intern. Med.*, **100**, 92

138. Reynolds, W. A., Winkelmann, R. K. and Soule, E. H. (1965). Kaposi's sarcoma: a clinicopathologic study with particular reference to its relationship to the reticuloendothelial system. *Medicine (Baltimore)*, **44**, 419

139. Safai, B., Mike, V., Giraldo, G. *et al.* (1980). Association of Kaposi's sarcoma with second primary malignancies: possible etiopathogenic implications. *Cancer*, **45**, 1472–9

140. Ulbright, T. M. and Santa Cruz, D. J. (1981). Kaposi's sarcoma relationship with hematologic, lymphoid and thymic neoplasia. *Cancer*, **47**, 963–73

141. Hardy, M. A., Goldfarb, P., Levine, S. *et al.* (1976). *De novo* Kaposi's sarcoma in renal transplantation: case report and brief review. *Cancer*, **38**, 144–8

142. Penn, I. (1979). Kaposi's sarcoma in organ transplant recipients. *Transplantation*, **27**, 8–11

143. Harwood, A. R., Osoba, D., Hofstader, S1. *et al.* (1979). Kaposi's sarcoma in recipients of renal transplants. *Am. J. Med.*, **67**, 759–65

144. Harwood, A. R. (1984). Kaposi's sarcoma in renal transplant patients. In Friedman-Kien, A. E. and Laubenstein, L. J. (eds.) *AIDS: The Epidemic of Kaposi's Sarcoma and Opportunistic Infections.* pp. 41–4. (New York: Masson)

145. Stibling, J., Weitzner, S. and Smith, G. V. (1978). Kaposi's sarcoma in renal allograft recipients. *Cancer*, **42**, 442–6

146. Iversen, O. H., Wetteland, P., Jervell, A. *et al.* (1980). Kaposi's sarcoma in a renal allograft recipient under long term immunosuppressive therapy. *Scand. J. Urol. Nephrol.*, **14**, 126–8

147. Krigel, R. L., Laubenstein, L. J. and Muggia, F. M. (1983). Kaposi's sarcoma: a new staging classification. *Cancer Treat. Rep.*, **67**, 6–10

148. Krigel, R. L. (1984). Prognostic factors in Kaposi's sarcoma. In Friedman-Kien, A. E. and Laubenstein, L. J. (eds.) *AIDS: The Epidemic of Kaposi's Sarcoma and Opportunistic Infections.* pp. 69–72. (New York: Masson)

149. Krigel, R. L. (1984). Kaposi's sarcoma. In Issel, B. F., Muggia, F. M. and Carter, S. K. (eds.) *Etoposide (VP-16): Current Status and New Developments.* pp. 325–30. (Orlando, Fl: Academic)

150. Cooper, J. S., Fried, P. R. and Laubenstein, L. J. (1984). Initial observations of the effect of radiotherapy on epidemic Kaposi's sarcoma. *J. Am. Med. Assoc.*, **252**, 934–5

151. Laubenstein, L. J., Krigel, R. L., Odajnyk, C. M. *et al.* (1984). Treatment of epidemic Kaposi's sarcoma with VP-16 (etoposide) or a combination of doxorubicin, bleomycin, and vinblastine. *J. Clin. Oncol.*, **2**, 1115–20

152. Longo, D., Steis, R., Lane, C. *et al.* (1984). Malignancies in the AIDS patient; natural history, treatment strategies and preliminary results. *Ann. N. Y. Acad. Sci.*, **437**, 421–30

153. Laubenstein, L. J., Krigel, R. L., Hymes, K. B. *et al.* (1983). Treatment of epidemic Kaposi's sarcoma with VP-16-213 (etoposide) and a combination of doxorubicin, bleomycin and vinblastine (ABV). *Proc. Am. Soc. Clin. Oncol.*, **2**, 228

154. Volberding, P., Abrams, D., Ziegler, J. *et al.* (1985). Vinblastine therapy of AIDS related Kaposi's sarcoma. *International Conference on AIDS*, April, 21

155. Rieber, E., Mittelman, A., Wormser, G. P. *et al.* (1984). Vincristine and Kaposi's sarcoma in the acquired immunodeficiency syndrome. *Ann. Intern. Med.*, **101**, 876 (letter)

156. Mintzer, D. M., Real, F. X., Jovinol, L. *et al.* (1985). Treatment of Kaposi's sarcoma and thrombocytopenia with vincristine in patients with the acquired immunodeficiency syndrome. *Ann. Intern. Med.*, **102**, 200–2

157. Wernz, J., Laubenstein, L., Hymes, K., Walsh, C. and Muggia, F. (1986). Chemotherapy and assessment of response in epidemic Kaposi's sarcoma (EKS) with bleomycin (B)/velban (V). *Proc. Am. Soc. Clin. Oncol.*, **5**, 4

158. Muggia, F., Chachoua, A., Green, M. D., Wernz, J., Laubenstein, L. and Krigel, R. (1986). Oral 4-demethoxydaunorubicin (DMDR) in epidemic Kaposi's sarcoma (EKS). *Proc. Am. Soc. Clin. Oncol.*, **5**, 136

159. Krown, S. E., Real, F. X., Cunningham-Rundles, S. *et al.* (1983). Interferon in the treatment of Kaposi's sarcoma. Letter to the Editor. *N. Engl. J. Med.*, **309**, 923–4

160. Groopman, J. E., Gottlieb, M. S., Goodman, J. *et al.* (1984). Recombinant alpha-2 interferon therapy for Kaposi's sarcoma associated with the acquired immunodeficiency syndrome. *Ann. Intern. Med.*, **100**, 671–6

161. Fauci, A. S., Macher, Am., Largo, D. *et al.* (1984). NIH Conference. Acquired immunodeficiency syndrome: epidemiologic, clinical, immunologic and therapeutic considerations. *Ann. Intern. Med.*, **100**, 92–106

162. Rios, A., Mansell, P., Newall, G. *et al.* (1984). The use of lymphoblastoid interferon Hu IFN (1y) in the treatment of acquired immunodeficiency syndrome (AIDS) related Kaposi's sarcoma (KS). *Proc. Am. Soc. Clin. Oncol.*, **3**, 63

163. Odajnyk, C., Laubenstein, L., Friedman-Kien, A. E. *et al.* (1984). Therapeutic trial of gamma-interferon in patients with epidemic Kaposi's sarcoma (EKS). *Proc. Am. Soc. Clin. Oncol.*, **3**, 61

164. Lonberg, M., Odajnyk, C., Krigel, R. *et al.* (1985). Sequential and simultaneous alpha 2 interferon (IFN) and VP16 in epidemic Kaposi's sarcoma (EKS). *Proc. Am. Soc. Clin. Oncol.*, **4**, 2

165. Lewis, B., Abrams, D., Ziegler, J. *et al.* (1983). Single agent and combination chemotherapy of Kaposi's sarcoma in acquired immune deficiency syndrome. *Proc. Am. Soc. Clin. Oncol.*, **2**, 59

166. Paulsen, A., Hultberg, B., Thomsen, K. *et al.* (1984). Regression of Kaposi's sarcoma in AIDS after treatment with dapsone (letter). *Lancet*, **1**, 560

167. Hruza, G. J., Friedman-Kien, A. E., Laubenstein, L. J. *et al.* (1985). Response for AIDS associated KS. *Lancet*, **2**, 642

168. Ziegler, J. L., Volberding, P. A. and Hu, L. M. (1984). Failure of isotretinoin in Kaposi's sarcoma (letter). *Lancet*, **2**, 641

169. Green, M. Unpublished data

170. Volberding, P., Abrams, D., Kaplan, L. *et al.* (1985). Therapy of AIDS related Kaposi's sarcoma with ICRF-159. *International Conference on AIDS*, April, 21

171. Ziegler, J. T., Drew, W. L., Miner, R. C. *et al.* (1985). Outbreak of Burkitt's-like lymphoma in homosexual men. *Lancet*, **2**, 631–3

172. Ziegler, J. T., Beckstead, J. A., Volberding, P. A. *et al.* (1984). Non-Hodgkin's lymphoma in 90 homosexual men, relationship to generalized lymphadenopathy and acquired immunodeficiency syndrome (AIDS). *N. Engl. J. Med.*, **311**, 565–70

173. Levine, A., Gill, P. S., Meyer, P. R. *et al.* (1985). Retrovirus and malignant lymphoma in homosexual men. *J. Am. Med. Assoc.*, **254**, 1921–5

174. Ioachim, H. L., Cooper, M. and Hellman G. (1985). Lymphomas in men at high risk for acquired immune deficiency syndrome (AIDS): a study of 21 cases. *Cancer*, **56**, 2831–43

175. Muggia, F. M. Unpublished data

176. Centers for Disease Control (1985). Revision of case definition of acquired immune deficiency syndrome for National Reporting. United States. *MMWR*, **34**, 25–6

177. Burnet, F. M. (1970). *Immunological Surveillance.* (New York: Oxford University Press)

178. Penn, I. (1983). Lymphomas complicating transplantation patients. *Transplant. Proc.*, **15**, 2790–7

179. Klein, G. (1979). Lymphoma development in mice and humans: diversity of initiation is followed by convergent cytogenetic evolution. *Proc. Natl. Acad Sci. USA*, **76**, 2442

180. Chaganti, R. S. K., Jhanwar, S. C., Koziner, B. *et al.* (1983). Specific translocations characterize Burkitt's-like lymphoma of homosexual men with acquired immunodeficiency syndrome. *Blood*, **61**, 1269

181. Neel, B. G., Jhanwar, S. C., Chaganti, R. S. K. *et al.* (1982). Two human c-oncogenes are located on the long arm of chromosome 8. *Proc. Natl. Acad. Sci. USA*, **79**, 7842

182. Fernandez, R., Mouradian, J., Metroka, C. *et al.* (1983). The prognostic value of histopathology in persistent generalized lymphadenopathy in homosexual men. *N. Engl. J. Med.*, **308**, 186

183. Zuker Franklin, D. (1983). Looking for the cause of AIDS. *N. Engl. J. Med.*, **308**, 837

184. Ewing, E. P., Spira, T. J., Chandler, T. W. *et al.* (1983). Unusual cytoplasmic body in lymphoid cells of homosexual men with unexplained lymphadenopathy. *N. Engl. J. Med.*, **308**, 819

185. Lozada, F., Silverman, S. and Conant, M. (1982). New outbreak of oral tumors, malignancies and infectious diseases strikes young male homosexuals. *Calif. Dent. J.*, **10**, 39

186. Daling, J. R., Weiss, N. S., Klopfenstein, L. L. *et al.* (1982). Correlates of homosexual behaviour and the incidence of anal cancer. *J. Am. Med. Assoc.*, **247**, 1988

187. Peters, R. K. and Mack, J. M. (1983). Patterns of anal carcinoma by gender and marital status in Los Angeles County. *Br. J. Cancer*, **48**, 629

188. Logothetis, C. J., Newell, G. R. and Samuel, M. L. (1985). Testicular cancer in homosexual men with cellular immune deficiency: report of 2 cases. *J. Urol.*, **133**, 484-6

189. Laubenstein, L. J., Kamelhar, D. L., Garay, S. M., Greene, J. B. and Poiesz, B. (1986). Lymphoid interstitial pneumonia (LIP) in adult AIDS: treatment with cytoxan and prednisone. Submitted to *International Conference on Acquired Immunodeficiency Syndrome (AIDS)*, Paris, France, June 23-25

190. Laubenstein, L., Raphael, B., Chachoua, A., Scholes, J., Mouradian, J. and Metroka, (1986). Clinical manifestations of B-cell hyperplasia in response to HTLV-III/LAV infection. Abstracts of the *International Conference on Acquired Immunodeficiency Syndrome (AIDS)*, Paris, France, June 23-25

191. Chachoua, A., Dietrich, D. and Newall, J. (1986). Dihydrophenyl guanine (DHPG) in the treatment of CMV infection in patients with AIDS. *Proc. Am. Soc. Clin. Oncol.*, **5**, 4

192. Dietrich, D., Chachoua, A. and Faust, M. (1986). Diflourmethyl ornithine (DFMO) in the treatment of cryptospordiosis in patients with AIDS. *Am. Soc. Gastroenterol.*, **90**, 1395 (abstract)

193. Holzman, R. and Chachoua, A. (1986). Personal communication

194. Dietrich, D., Chachoua, A., Green, J. and Garay, S. (1986). Eflornithine in treatment of resistant pneumocystis pneumonia in patients with AIDS. *International Conference on AIDS*, Abstract submitted

195. Redfield, R., Wright, D. and Tramont, E. (1986). Special report: the Walter Reed (staging) classification for HTLV-III/LAV infection. *N. Engl. J. Med.*, **314**, 131-2

Index